GENERAL and ORAL
PATHOLOGY
FOR DENTAL HYGIENE PRACTICE

GENERAL and ORAL PATHOLOGY

FOR DENTAL HYGIENE PRACTICE

Sandra L. Myers, DMD
Associate Professor
University of Minnesota, School of Dentistry
Minneapolis, MN

Alice E. Curran, DMD, MS
Associate Professor
University of North Carolina at Chapel Hill,
School of Dentistry
Chapel Hill, NC

F.A. Davis Company • Philadelphia

F. A. Davis Company
1915 Arch Street
Philadelphia, PA 19103
www.fadavis.com

Printed in the United States of America

Last digit indicates print number: 10 9 8 7 6 5 4 3 2 1

Publisher: T. Quincy McDonald
Developmental Editor: Jennifer Ajello
Director of Content Development: George Lang
Art and Design Manager: Carolyn O'Brien

As new scientific information becomes available through basic and clinical research, recommended treatments and drug therapies undergo changes. The author(s) and publisher have done everything possible to make this book accurate, up to date, and in accord with accepted standards at the time of publication. The author(s), editors, and publisher are not responsible for errors or omissions or for consequences from application of the book, and make no warranty, expressed or implied, in regard to the contents of the book. Any practice described in this book should be applied by the reader in accordance with professional standards of care used in regard to the unique circumstances that may apply in each situation. The reader is advised always to check product information (package inserts) for changes and new information regarding dose and contraindications before administering any drug. Caution is especially urged when using new or infrequently ordered drugs.

Library of Congress Cataloging-in-Publication Data

Myers, Sandra L., 1949-
  General and oral pathology for dental hygiene practice / Sandra L. Myers,
Alice E. Curran.
     p. ; cm.
  Includes bibliographical references and index.
  ISBN-13: 978-0-8036-2577-8
  ISBN-10: 0-8036-2577-4
  I. Curran, Alice E. II. Title.
  [DNLM: 1. Mouth Diseases—pathology. 2. Dental Hygienists. 3. Oral
Hygiene. WU 140]
  RK60.7
  617.6'01—dc23
                                2013010392

*We dedicate this textbook
to all our students, past and present.
Without you,
our experiences as dental educators
would not have been possible.*

Contributors

Mansur Ahmad, BDS, PhD
Associate Professor
University of Minnesota
School of Dentistry
Minneapolis, MN

Walter Bowles, DDS, MS, PhD
Associate Professor
University of Minnesota
School of Dentistry
Minneapolis, MN

Catherine Champagne, PhD
Chapel Hill, NC

Raj Gopalakrishnan, BDS, PhD
Associate Professor
University of Minnesota
School of Dentistry
Minneapolis, MN

Nelson Rhodus, DMD, MPH
Professor
University of Minnesota
School of Dentistry
Minneapolis, MN

Molly Rosebush, DDS, MS
Assistant Professor, Oral and Maxillofacial
   Pathology
Diplomate, American Board of Oral and
   Maxillofacial Pathology
Louisiana State University School of Dentistry
New Orleans, LA

Chelsia Sim, BDS, MS
National Dental Centre of Singapore
Singapore

Reviewers

Kristi Taylor Davis, DDS
Assistant Professor
Department of Dental Hygiene
University of Louisiana at Monroe
Monroe, LA

Terry Dean, DMD
Associate Professor
Department of Allied Health & Dental Hygiene
Western Kentucky University
Bowling Green, KY

Lisa Hebl, BS, RDH, Med
Clinical Coordinator
Dental Hygiene Program
Associate Professor
Department of Allied Health
Kirkwood Community College
Cedar Rapids, IA

Kenneth Horowitz, DDS
Instructor, Dental Hygiene
Department of Dental Hygiene
Biological and Health Sciences Division
Foothill College
Los Altos Hills, CA

Barbara A. Jansen, DDS
Program Director
Department of Dental Hygiene
Middle Georgia Technical College
Warner Robins, GA

Patricia A. Mannie, RDH, MS
Dental Hygiene Instructor
Department of Dental Hygiene
St. Cloud Technical & Community College
St. Cloud, MN

Kristina Okolisan-Mulligan, RDH, BS, MA
Clinical Assistant Professor
Department of Diagnostic and Biomedical
  Sciences
University of Detroit
Mercy Dental School
Detroit, MI

Linda Lee Paquette, CDA, RDA, RDH, MS
Faculty
Department of Dental Programs
Santa Rosa Junior College
Santa Rose, CA

Christine L., Robb Dip. DH, BA, MEd
Assistant Professor
School of Dental Hygiene
Dalhousie University
Halifax, NS Canada

Judith E. Romano, RDH, MA
Department Chair
Department of Dental Hygiene/Dental Assisting
Hudson Valley Community College
Troy, NY

Katherine A. Woods, PhD, RDH
Professor
Department of Dental Hygiene
St. Petersburg College
Pinellas Park, FL

General and Oral Pathology for Dental Hygiene Practice is an introductory textbook written for dental hygiene students studying general and oral pathology, and as a resource for dental educators and clinicians. Our career journeys have included training and clinical practice in dental assisting, dental hygiene, dentistry, and oral and maxillofacial pathology. We have more than 76 years combined experience in dentistry, oral and maxillofacial pathology, and dental education. Throughout the years we have received numerous requests to write a pathology textbook targeting dental hygiene that contains current material contributed from experts in their respective fields. This inspired us to write such a text that is also student-oriented, instructor-friendly, and includes online supplementary materials. *General and Oral Pathology for Dental Hygiene Practice* is a direct result of our combined passion for dental hygiene education, dentistry, and oral pathology. Our goal is to use educational tools that promote critical thinking and transfer learning outcomes to clinical dental hygiene practice.

Approach

First, we understand that not everyone who teaches pathology in the dental hygiene curriculum has advanced training in general and oral pathology. Our textbook seeks to "train the trainer" by use of supplementary materials. These instructor resources not only enhance student learning but also promote instructor confidence in the material.

Second, our colleagues in dental hygiene education report that currently available texts often do not provide a sufficient depth of background knowledge important for understanding and assessing pathology. For instance, oral lesions associated with systemic conditions are described, but essential discussion of the underlying disease mechanism may be sparse or missing. Additionally, etiologies and risk factors for diseases are not consistently emphasized. To address this issue, we begin each chapter with concise foundational and basic principles of pathology related to disorders or lesions presented in the chapter. The effects of disease processes on the oral cavity and human body are emphasized as they relate to clinical practice. The text is organized into nine chapters around seven core topics in pathology: 1) reactive/inflammatory disorders, 2) infectious diseases, 3) immune-based disorders, 4) developmental disorders, 5) genetic disorders, 6) neoplasms, and 7) oral manifestations of systemic disorders.

Third, we have updated the material to incorporate the most recent changes in pathology nomenclature and classification. For example, we have included human papilloma virus-related pathologies in the chapter on infectious diseases rather than in the chapter on neoplasia, where they have traditionally been located. This emphasizes that infectious agents can induce neoplastic changes. We believe this approach enhances retention of knowledge and promotes active learning by minimizing repetition of disease topics in multiple chapter locations, which can be confusing for new learners. The result is enhanced subject integration rather than duplication within the text and other courses in the curriculum.

One of our goals in writing this text is to underscore the central and critical role pathology plays in patient care. To this end, we have consistently endeavored to point out where, how, and why particular pathological findings are important to both clinicians and patients. The specific terminology of pathology is featured and promoted to facilitate communication between all members of the health-care team. A suite of online student and instructor resources is used to present the topics in a format tailored to a new generation of learners.

Our approach uses a chapter layout that allows for easy visualization of content. This includes an outline and key learning objectives at the beginning of each chapter. Important vocabulary is highlighted within the text and included in a comprehensive glossary. Approximately 500 high-quality color images, in addition to illustrations, figures, and tables, are included.

Features

The following key features enhance the learning process, link education with clinical practice, and help students prepare for the National Board Dental Hygiene Examination:

Clinical Implications: Clinical implication boxes correlate chapter content to clinical practice so that the student gets a real-world glimpse at how general and oral pathology is relevant to the practice of dental hygiene today.

Critical Thinking Exercises: Critical thinking exercises use a case scenario and a series of thought-provoking questions that encourage the student to think through the chapter content and apply their new knowledge.

Chapter Review Questions: The chapter review questions are in National Board Dental Hygiene Examination format so students can become familiar with and be prepared to answer questions in this format.

Supplementary Materials

An accompanying companion website at http://davisplus. fadavis.com is available for both students and instructors. The ancillaries available on DavisPlus for students can be accessed using the Plus code included under the scratch-off label inside the front cover of each new text. These premium ancillaries include: practice clinical case scenarios, questions with similar format to the National Board Dental Hygiene Examination, and animations that help illustrate disease processes in a dynamic way. Teaching support for instructors includes an extensive accessible image bank, a PowerPoint presentation for every chapter in the text, and a robust electronic test bank with questions with similar format to the National Board Dental Hygiene Examination.

The importance of a learning partnership between student and instructor became clear to us over our many years of teaching. Students are motivated to learn when they understand why the material is important and see how it applies to clinical practice situations. Instructors can be more engaged in presenting material when resources are available that present subject matter in a format that is current, interesting, promotes learning, and correlates to clinical practice. We believe the outcomes of strong student-instructor partnerships include clinicians with stronger clinical skills who embrace their role in providing improved patient care. We hope our book contributes to this outcome and that all who use it will be inspired by our passion for pathology.

Sandra L. Myers
Alice E. Curran

Acknowledgments

The first edition of any textbook is a daunting task and this is certainly true for *General and Oral Pathology for Dental Hygiene Practice*. We would like to acknowledge the many individuals who have contributed to this book and guided us through our first adventure in publication. Without their help, this would not have been possible.

Our current and former editors at F. A. Davis deserve a tremendous amount of gratitude. They include: Quincy McDonald, Senior Acquisitions Editor; Jennifer Ajello, Development Editor; Liz Schaeffer, Developmental Editor/Electronic Products Coordinator; Mackenzie Lawrence, Freelance Editor/Project Manager; and Jackie Lux, Marketing/Convention Coordinator. We appreciate their expertise and their infinite patience as we navigated this new world.

We acknowledge our chapter contributors who took time from their hectic lives to help draft interesting and challenging material: Mansur Ahmad BDS, PhD; Walter Bowles DDS, MS, PhD; Catherine Champagne PhD; Raj Gopalakrishnan BDS, PhD; Nelson Rhodus DMD, MPH; Molly Rosebush DDS, MS; and Chelsia Sim BDS, MS.

An oral pathology textbook is nothing without good photographs from which students learn to recognize disease in their patients. Our colleagues who generously stepped forward to share images from their personal archives cannot be thanked enough: Abdel-Ghany Al-Saidi DDS; Carl Allen DDS, MSD; Mark Anderson DDS; Bruce F. Barker DDS; Soraya Beiraghi DDS, MSD, MS, MSD; Indraneel Bhattacharyya DDS, MSD; James Castle DDS, CAPT, DC, USN; Risa Chaisuparat DDS; Kitrina G. Cordell DDS, MS; Darren P. Cox DDS, MBA; Andre Paes Batista DeSilva DDS; Kerry Dove DMD; John E. Fantasia DDS; George Gallagher DMD, DMSc; Thalji Ghadeer DDS, MS; Susan Hadler MD; James Hughes DDS, MS; Michael A. Kahn DDS; Shanti Kaimal BDS, MDS, MS; John R. Kalmar DMD, PhD; Robert D. Kelsch DMD; Ioannis Koutlas DDS, MS; Walter Kucaba DDS, MS; John Ludlow DDS, MS; Alan Lurie DDS, PhD; Denis P. Lynch DDS, PhD; Richard Madden DDS, MS; Beth McKinney RDH, MS; Kristin K. McNamara DDS, MS; Nicole Miller DDS; Glenn Minsley DMD; Madhu Mohan DMD; Danny Mora DMD; Leslie Orzech DMD; Ricardo Padilla DDS; Ali Pourian DDS, MS; Pavithra Pugalagiri BDS, MS; Yeshwant Rawal BDS, MDS, MS; Renee Reich DDS; Jonathan Reside DDS, MS; Michael Rohrer DDS, MS; James Rokos DDS, MS; Vladimir Leon-Salazar DDS, MS; Shelly Stecker DDS, MS; Lan Su DMD, PhD; Kurt F. Summersgill DDS, PhD; Jeffrey Thomas DDS; Brian Vandersea DDS; J. Craig Whitt DDS, MS; Dag Zapatero DDS; and Theodore Zislis DDS.

We also thank the University of Minnesota School of Dentistry for allowing us access to images from the archives of the late Dr. Robert J. Gorlin. We also need to credit Northwest Dentistry for use of several photographs from an article Sandra Myers wrote.

We would like to acknowledge the reviewers whose valuable and insightful comments and suggestions greatly enhanced the final product. Their time and expertise are greatly appreciated.

Special thanks to Dr. Christine Harrington, Ohio State University; Alexandra Komichek RDH, MS, University of North Carolina; Patricia Lenton GDH, MA, University of Minnesota; and Hanae Tsujimoto RDH, MS, University of Minnesota for their contributions to our ancillaries.

Our goal with this book is to spread the passion for oral pathology to the next generation of dental hygienists. We would be remiss if we did not acknowledge our own mentors who over many years inspired us to follow our dreams and become dental assistants, dental hygienists, dentists, oral pathologists, and finally, educators. They include: Drs. Harold C. Reid, Wei-Yung Yih, LeGrand H. Woolley, Murray H. Bartley Jr., Charles C. Thompson, Norman H. Rickles, Robert J. Bruckner, Nelson Rhodus, and Robert J. Gorlin; Suzanne Box RDH, MS; Drs. Samir K. ElMofty, Douglas Damm, Dean White, Jim Drummond, Charles Waldron, Peter A. Pullon, and Ronnie Weathers.

Contents

Introduction to Oral and Maxillofacial Pathology and the Study of Disease

Overview of Oral and Maxillofacial Pathology
The Practice of Oral and Maxillofacial Pathology
Assessment of Oral Pathologic Lesions
Patient Assessment and History
Signs and Symptoms

Head, Neck, and Intraoral Examinations
Terminology Used in Describing Oral Pathologic Lesions
Supplemental Diagnostic Aides
Differential Diagnosis
Variants of Normal

Learning Outcomes

At the end of this chapter, the student will be able to:

1.1. Define and describe all key terms included in the chapter.

1.2. Explain the ways general and oral maxillofacial pathology impacts dental hygiene practice.

1.3. Describe characteristics included in physical assessment of the patient and explain why they are important.

1.4. Compare and contrast characteristics of signs and symptoms.

1.5. Explain why using descriptive terminology for pathological conditions is important in dental hygiene practice.

1.6. Demonstrate key elements of a proper head, neck, and intraoral examination.

1.7. Explain the role of supplemental diagnostic aides in establishing a diagnosis.

1.8. Recognize common variants of normal oral structure.

OVERVIEW OF ORAL AND MAXILLOFACIAL PATHOLOGY

Pathology (Greek. *pathos* "suffering" + *logia* "study") is defined as the study or science of **disease** and includes its causes, development, course, and effects. The most common diseases affecting the oral cavity are dental caries and periodontal disease. Prevention and treatment of these two diseases comprise the main focus of dental and dental hygiene practice. However, many other diseases affect the oral and maxillofacial structures. Some are unique to the oral cavity, whereas others are oral manifestations of diseases elsewhere in the body. Although diagnosis is generally not within the scope of dental hygiene practice, disease recognition is of great concern to the dental hygienist who is in an optimal position to examine the entire oral cavity, discuss signs and symptoms with patients, and provide patient education. Therefore, a basic knowledge of disease is essential for successful dental hygiene practice.

The study of oral pathology encompasses **general pathology,** the study of basic disease processes such as infection, autoimmunity, and neoplasia. The study of **systemic pathology** includes diseases that affect specific organ systems, such as cardiovascular, respiratory, gastrointestinal, or endocrine. Knowledge of both general and systemic pathology is important for the dental hygienist in treating patients with both localized and systemic pathology.

Oral and maxillofacial pathology is the study of diseases that affect the oral cavity and facial structures. Oral pathologists are dentists with advanced training in oral pathology devoted to the diagnosis of oral disease. This chapter provides an overview of oral and maxillofacial pathology. It provides important information on the recognition, assessment and documentation of disease, as well as a basic foundation for effective communication between clinicians and patients. Additionally, examples of variations of common oral findings that are considered within the range of normal but often mistaken for pathology are reviewed.

The Practice of Oral and Maxillofacial Pathology

Oral and maxillofacial pathology is the dental specialty that identifies and manages diseases affecting the oral and maxillofacial regions and investigates the causes, processes, and effects of these diseases. The practice of oral and maxillofacial pathology involves the diagnosis of disease through the use of clinical, radiographic, microscopic, and/or biochemical examinations. Oral pathologists collaborate with many other dental and medical professionals to advance oral health care needs of their patients by providing consultation and diagnostic services.

Forensic odontology is a branch of forensic medicine that deals with matching characteristics of the teeth or oral cavity with existing dental records. Forensic odontologists identify victims of accidents or contribute expertise to other tragedies with legal ramifications. Although oral pathologists may serve as forensic pathologists, one does not have to be an oral pathologist to participate on a forensic team. In fact, many dental hygienists use their superior knowledge of the oral cavity to serve on forensic teams that include physicians, dentists, crime scene investigators, funeral directors, and other experts.

Assessment of Oral Pathologic Lesions

The first step in the assessment of oral pathologic conditions is recognition of a **lesion,** a general term defined as "a pathological change in an organ or tissue that alters normal form or function." Identification and assessment of oral lesions is best performed using a methodical approach that includes a complete patient history; assessment of signs and symptoms; a complete head, neck, and intraoral exam; and use of clinical and laboratory diagnostic procedures.

Patient Assessment and History

Patient assessment is the cornerstone of dental hygiene practice. It is fundamental in the early detection of pathological conditions and systemic problems that may pose a serious threat to the patient and or dental team. Determining health status in patients is also extremely important for two reasons. First, it may lead to the identification of undiagnosed medical conditions. Second, it enables ongoing evaluation of known conditions for progression and changes that may impact dental treatment. Deferral of dental treatment may be required and the patient may need referral to an appropriate health-care provider if new conditions or changes in existing conditions are detected.

Patient assessment includes obtaining complete medical, dental, and social histories, physical evaluation of the patient, and performing head and neck and intraoral examinations. Ultimately, patient assessment determines decisions about clinical treatment and directly impacts quality of patient care.

Patient assessment begins the first moment a patient is observed in the waiting room or dental operatory. Physical evaluation and the process of updating or taking a comprehensive medical and dental history are critical before undertaking head and neck and intraoral examinations. This is important because some medical problems have oral manifestations that are easily observed, such as spontaneous gingival bleeding in hemophilia; while other medical problems, such as hypertension, have no oral manifestations, but their medications may produce visible oral side effects.

Clinical Implications

Many patients do not consider the herbal supplements and vitamins they take to be "medications." Herbal supplements may produce important side effects, and many people are allergic or otherwise sensitive to these often powerful agents. Be sure to include these items in your medical history review.

The social history includes important information on drug, alcohol, and tobacco consumption. Alcohol along with tobacco contributes to the development of pathologic lesions found in the oral cavity, including oral cancer. Questions about other habits, including type of oral health care products and use of alternative therapies, may also contribute important information for evaluation of risk factors for pathology in patients.

Diagnosis is the identification of a disease from its signs and symptoms. Although diagnosis is not within the scope of dental hygiene practice, recognition of abnormalities and their proper documentation, as well as patient education, are. To properly document abnormalities, it is important to become familiar with the terminology of pathology.

The **etiology** of a disease refers to its cause. If a disease has more than one etiology, these are referred to as **etiologic factors or agents**. Examples of etiologic factors include trauma, genetic abnormality, and infection. **Iatrogenic** etiology means the lesion occurred as a result of treatment. A **facticial** lesion is an injury that is self-induced, either internationally or unintentionally. If the cause of a disease is unknown, the term **idiopathic** is used.

Signs and Symptoms

Signs are objective findings observed by the clinician that the patient may or may not be aware of. An example is a painless white patch on the lateral border of the tongue. **Symptoms** are subjective findings perceived by the patient but not observable by the clinician. Examples are fatigue, headache, anxiety, and sensations such as tingling, itching, burning, bad taste, soreness, or numbness.

Symptomatic means the lesion is causing pain or other symptoms perceived by the patient. *Asymptomatic* means the lesion is not causing pain or symptoms. Patients are often unaware of a lesion until a clinician brings it to their attention.

Head, Neck, and Intraoral Neck Examinations

In order for a disease or lesion to be diagnosed, it must first be recognized. The patient may bring it to the attention of the clinician, or it may be discovered during routine examination. Structures in the head and neck to be examined include the muscles of the face and neck, salivary glands, lymph nodes, oral mucosa, and skin. Careful examination will reveal normal anatomical structures, variations from normal, or pathologic changes.

Head and neck examinations are accomplished through procedures known as inspection, palpation, auscultation, and percussion. **Inspection** is the critical appraisal involving examination, measurement, and comparison with normal. **Palpation** occurs when the examiner feels the size, shape, or firmness of the tissues. One or several fingers are used to feel below the surface skin for thickenings and masses not visible on the mucosal surface. **Auscultation** is the act of listening to body sounds to evaluate if a structure is normal or abnormal. This can be performed by listening with the unaided ear or with a stethoscope. Auscultation is used in evaluation of the temporomandibular joint (TMJ) to detect crepitus (grating or crackling) or popping. **Percussion** is tapping on a surface to determine the condition of the underlying structure. It can be performed with the fingers, hand, or an instrument. This is helpful in determining both the sensitivity and relative density of the structure (i.e., whether it is solid or hollow). Percussion is used in the evaluation of muscles and bones, and is also applied to the teeth to determine sensitivity.

Table 1-1 reviews the basic steps in the *extraoral* head and neck examination and illustrates the type and variety of lesions that may be discovered at each step.

Table 1-2 reviews the basic steps of the *intraoral* examination and illustrates intraoral lesions that may be discovered at each step.

Terminology Used in Describing Oral Pathologic Lesions

Significant clinical findings must be clearly described and documented in the patient record using proper descriptive terminology. Consistent descriptive terminology is essential for:

1. Accurate record-keeping
2. Comparison of lesions between visits
3. Clear communication among colleagues
4. Development of a differential diagnosis based on clinical appearance

When describing a lesion, the anatomic location, color, shape, borders, and consistency all need to be recorded. See Table 1-3 for descriptive terminology and examples of lesions that illustrate each term. For obvious reasons, consistency cannot be illustrated here.

In addition to basic descriptive terminology, the following specific terminology is generally used for some of the most commonly encountered lesions.

Vesicle: a small blister (< 5 mm) located below the epithelium that is filled with clear fluid. These

(Text continued on page 15)

Table 1.1	Steps for the Extraoral Head and Neck Examination and Examples of Lesions That May Be Encountered
Steps for Head and Neck Examination	**Significant Finding and Chapter Number**
Begin at the base of the neck just above the clavicles. Palpate up the anterior segment of the neck bilaterally to examine the anterior cervical lymph nodes, thyroid gland, and cricoid cartilage.	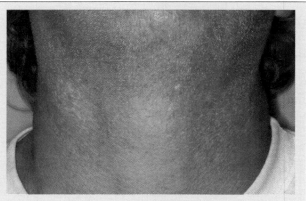 Lymphadenopathy of cervical lymph node (7)
Palpate the anterior medial aspect of the neck to just under the chin; move beneath the chin and firmly backwards along the inferior aspect of the mandible, evaluating lymph nodes and salivary glands.	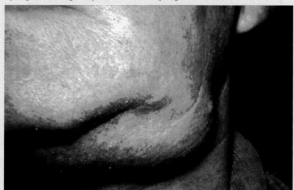 Mass in lateral neck (7)
Continue down the lateral neck along the sternocleido-mastoid muscle. Turn the patient's head to one side and then the other to examine the many lymph nodes in the posterior cervical, jugular, and supraclavicular chains.	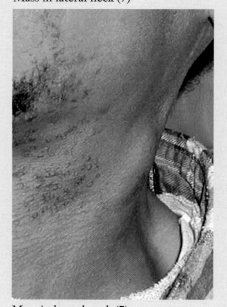 Mass in lateral neck (7)

Table 1.1	Steps for the Extraoral Head and Neck Examination and Examples of Lesions That May Be Encountered—cont'd

Steps for Head and Neck Examination	Significant Finding and Chapter Number
Bilaterally palpate the neck base, up the back of the neck and the occipital portion of the skull. Continue behind and then in front of the ears, ending at the preauricular area.	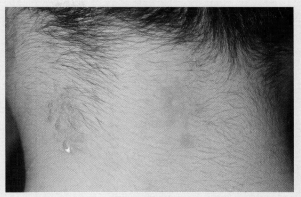 Herpes zoster (3)
Bilaterally palpate the TMJ as the mouth is slowly opened and closed.	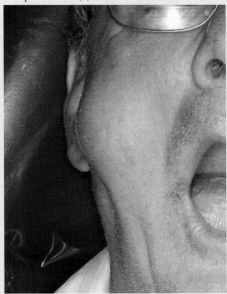 Osteoma of the TMJ (8)
Bilaterally palpate the face around the parotid salivary glands, the masseter and buccinator muscles, and the facial lymph nodes.	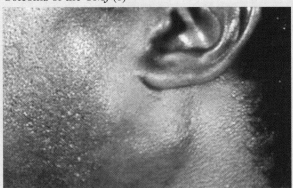 Benign salivary gland tumor (7)

Continued

Table 1.1	Steps for the Extraoral Head and Neck Examination and Examples of Lesions That May Be Encountered—cont'd
Steps for Head and Neck Examination	**Significant Finding and Chapter Number**
End on the anterior part of the mandible around the lips and chin.	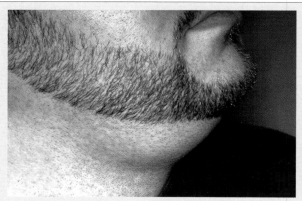 Submental swelling (2)

Table 1.2	Steps for Intraoral Examination and Lesions That May Be Encountered
Steps for Intraoral Examination	**Significant Finding and Chapter Number**
Retract upper and lower lips to expose the labial mucosa and the upper and lower vestibules. Palpate each lip.	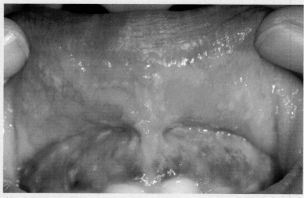 Pyostomatitis vegetans (9)
Retract left and right cheeks and the buccal mucosa. The cheeks are palpated bimanually.	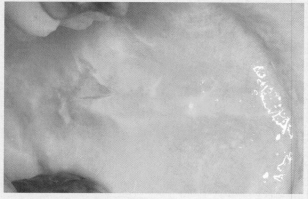 Ulceration buccal mucosa (2)

Table 1.2	Steps for Intraoral Examination and Lesions That May Be Encountered—cont'd
Steps for Intraoral Examination	**Significant Finding and Chapter Number**
Inspect and palpate hard and soft palates and uvula.	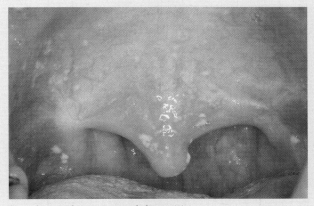 Pseudomembranous candidiasis (3)
Depress the dorsum of the tongue, while the patient says "aah," so this area can be clearly visualized.	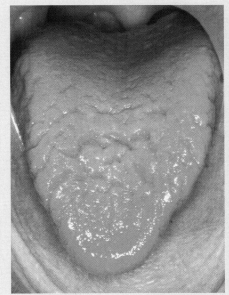 Fissured tongue (1)
Using a piece of gauze, retract the tongue so the floor of mouth and lateral borders can be visualized.	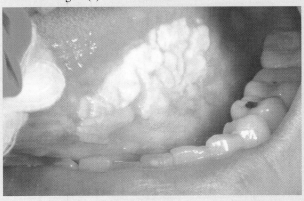 Leukoplakia (2)

Continued

Table 1.2	Steps for Intraoral Examination and Lesions That May Be Encountered—cont'd
Steps for Intraoral Examination	**Significant Finding and Chapter Number**
Inspect and palpate the lateral borders and dorsum of the tongue as far posterior as possible.	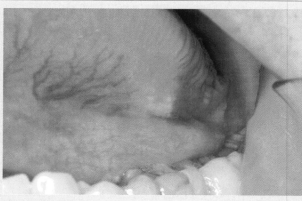 Leukoplakia (2)
Palpate the floor of the mouth bimanually. Use index finger of one hand to press the floor of the mouth down against fingers of the opposite hand, placed externally under the chin and mandible.	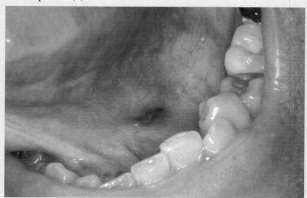 Amalgam tattoo (2)
Examine the periodontium.	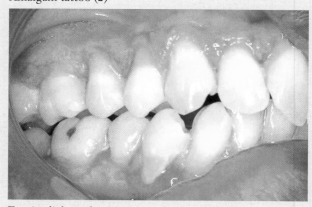 Erosive lichen planus (4)

Table 1.2	Steps for Intraoral Examination and Lesions That May Be Encountered—cont'd
Steps for Intraoral Examination	**Significant Finding and Chapter Number**
Examine the teeth.	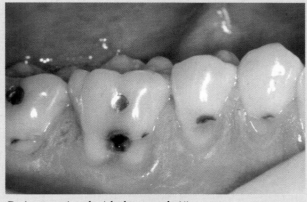 Caries associated with dry mouth (4)

Table 1.3	Descriptive Terminology: Mucosal Pathology	
Color		
Yellow	Small yellow spots on the buccal mucosa	
White	White patch in vesibule	
Red	Erythematous inflamed gingiva	
Red and white	Red patch with scattered white spots on gingiva, buccal mucosa and retromolar pad	

Continued

Table 1.3	Descriptive Terminology: Mucosal Pathology—cont'd	
Color		
Blue	Submucosal blood vessels lateral/ventral tongue	
Blue-red	Dark blue-red spots of hemorrhage on buccal mucosa	
Brown	Ill-defined patch of brown discoloration facial gingiva and mucosa	
Black	Well-defined gray-black discoloration of lingual gingiva and mucosa	
Opalescent	Diffuse white-gray change to the buccal mucosa	
Translucent	Fluid-filled swelling in the floor of mouth	

Table 1.3	**Descriptive Terminology: Mucosal Pathology—cont'd**

Shape

Exophytic: protrudes from the surface	**Types of Exophytic Lesions**	
	Pedunculated: protrudes on a stalk.	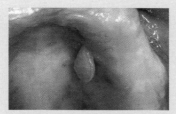
	Sessile: base is the widest part; there is no stalk.	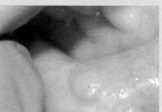
	Plaque: localized abnormal patch.	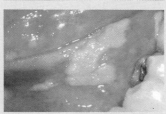
	Papule: solid lesion < 1 cm	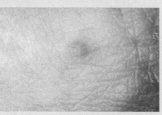
	Nodule: solid lesion ≥ 1 cm.	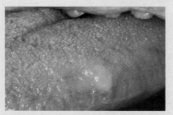
	Pustule: creamy-white, <1 cm, blister-like containing pus.	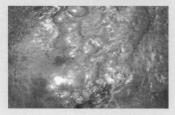

Continued

Table 1.3	Descriptive Terminology: Mucosal Pathology—cont'd

Shape

Endophytic: below level of surrounding normal tissue	**Types of Endophytic Lesions**	
	Ulcer: complete loss of epithelium with exposure of the underlying connective tissue.	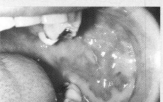
	Erosion: shallow area with denuded epithelium.	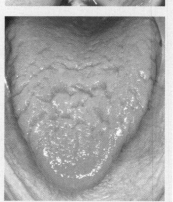
	Fissure: clefts or crack in soft tissues, often linear.	
	Sinus tract: a channel or communication between an abscess and the surface.	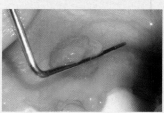
Flat	**Types of Flat Lesions**	
	Macule: <1 cm, prominent, well-defined, area of discoloration on the skin or mucosa; usually dark but can be any color.	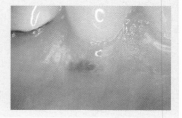

Table 1.3	Descriptive Terminology: Mucosal Pathology—cont'd

Shape

Reticular: lace-like pattern

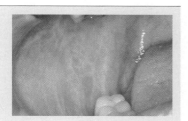

Borders

Well-Circumscribed

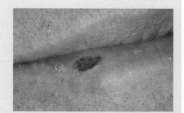

Diffuse

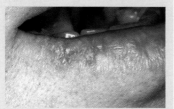

Regular

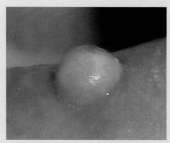

Irregular

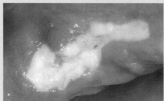

Continued

Table 1.3	Descriptive Terminology: Mucosal Pathology—cont'd

Borders

Elevated		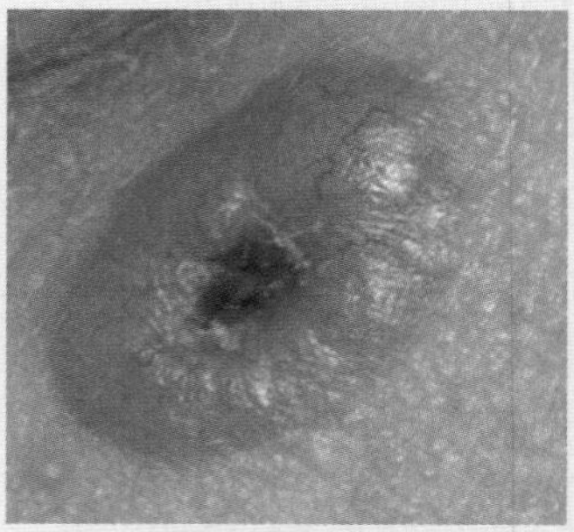
Flat		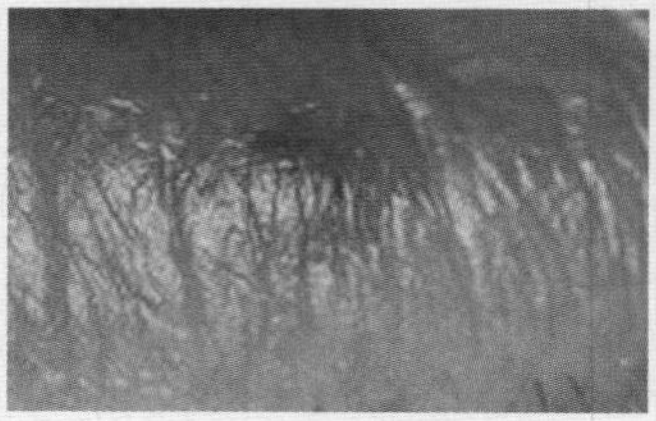

Surface Texture

Smooth		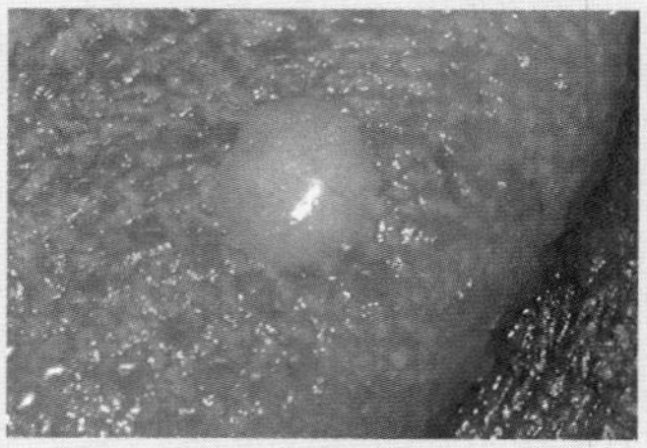
Rough	**Types of Rough Lesions** Papillary: finger-like	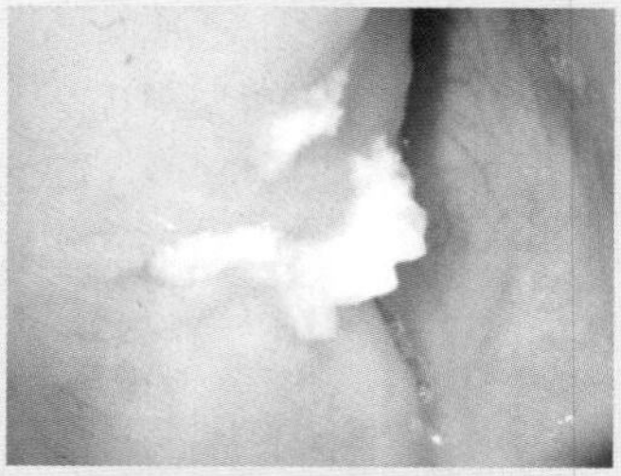
	Verrucous: fine, wart-like	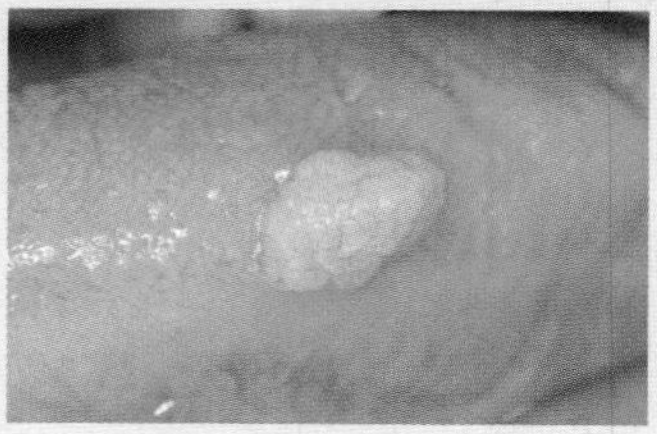

Table 1.3	Descriptive Terminology: Mucosal Pathology—cont'd

Surface Texture

Corrugated: wrinkled or folded	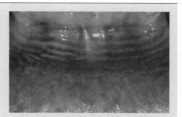
Ulcerated: epithelium is lost; surface is necrotic or absent	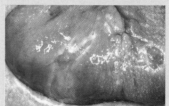
Erosive: shallow or superficial ulceration without necrosis	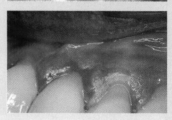

Consistency

Soft

Spongy

Compressible

Fluctuant: fluid filled

Firm

Indurated: extremely firm

Bony hard

are seen in herpes simplex and herpes zoster infections. (See Chapter 3.)

Bulla: a blister > 5 mm (*bullae* pl.). These larger fluid-filled lesions are observed in blistering conditions such as pemphigus and pemphigoid. (See Chapter 4.)

Pustule: a small (< 1 cm), creamy-white, inflamed, blister-like elevation containing pus. These are seen in acne and chickenpox. (See Chapter 3.)

Cyst: an epithelial-lined cavity below the body surface containing liquid or semi-solid material. Apical (radicular) cysts occur along the root or at the apex of nonvital teeth. (See Chapter 5.)

Macule: a small (< 1 cm), well-defined, nonelevated area of discoloration on the skin or mucosa. Freckles and oral melanotic macules on the lip are examples. (See Chapter 2.)

Papule: small (< 1 cm), solid elevations that are not fluid-filled or pus-filled. Papules may be seen in lichen planus of the skin. (See Chapter 4.)

Nodule: a solid, well-circumscribed, palpable mass ≥1 cm that arises from deeper tissues. Fibromas present as palpable nodules. (See Chapter 2.)

Tumor: by definition refers to any swelling or collection of cells appearing as a mass or lump, commonly used to refer to a **neoplasm**. Neoplasms may be benign or malignant. Lipomas and carcinomas are examples. (See Chapter 7.)

Erosion: refers to a condition in which the superficial epithelial surface of skin or mucosa is missing. It may occur as a result of trauma or disease, such as when vesicles and bullae break. (See Chapters 2 and 3.)

Ulcer: refers to an area of missing surface epithelium that extends down into the deeper tissues. Ulcers may result from trauma, infections, or neoplasms such as squamous cell carcinoma. (See Chapter 7.)

Scar: tissue defects comprised mainly of collagen, left over after a wound has healed. They are most commonly seen on the skin. (See Chapter 2.)

Plaque: describes a flat, slightly raised patch or a layer of material deposited on a tissue surface. Reticular lichen planus in the oral cavity is an example. (See Chapter 4.)

Fissure: linear clefts or cracks occurring in soft tissues. An example is fissured tongue. (See Chapter 5.)

Sinus tract: a channel from deep tissues that communicates between an area of suppuration (pus) and surface epithelium or mucosa. A sinus tract may develop between an apical abscess and the oral mucosa. (See Chapter 2.)

Supplemental Diagnostic Aides

In many instances, a definitive diagnosis cannot be determined based only on the clinical examination. Additional diagnostic procedures may be required to obtain further information. Examples include:

Imaging: including periapical, bitewing, and panoramic radiographs, cone beam (CT) scans, and magnetic resonance imaging (MRI). Table 1-4 describes terms used when interpreting radiographic images and examples of lesions that illustrate them.

Table 1.4 Descriptive Terminology: Radiographic Lesions		
Term	**Description**	**Example and Chapter Number**
Unilocular pericoronal radiolucency	Single compartment around crown of unerupted tooth.	Dentigerous cyst (5)
Unilocular apical radiolucency	Single compartment around apex of tooth.	Apical cyst or apical periodontitis (2)

Table 1.4	Descriptive Terminology: Radiographic Lesions—cont'd	
Term	**Description**	**Example and Chapter Number**
Multilocular radiolucency	Many small conjoined compartments.	Ameloblastoma (7)
Multifocal radiolucency	Many small areas not joined.	Cherubism (5)
Poorly defined radiolucency	Border fades into surrounding bone.	Osteomyelitis (2)

Continued

Table 1.4 Descriptive Terminology: Radiographic Lesions—cont'd		
Term	**Description**	**Example and Chapter Number**
Radiopacity (well-defined)	Cortical border clearly visible.	Condensing osteitis (2)
Radiopacity (poorly defined)	Cortical bone fades into surrounding tissue	Osseous dysplasia, endstage (2)
Mixed radiolucent/radiopaque	Variation in density within the lesions.	Compound odontoma (7)

Table 1.4	Descriptive Terminology: Radiographic Lesions—cont'd	
Term	**Description**	**Example and Chapter Number**
Ground glass (Frosted glass)	Hazy opacity with ill-defined borders.	Fibrous dysplasia (5)
Cotton-wool (cotton balls)	Irregular, rounded, fluffy patches of radiopaque bone.	Paget disease (2)

Biopsy is the removal of diseased or suspicious-looking tissue to diagnose or determine the extent of a disease. An **excisional biopsy** is performed when a lesion is small and can be totally removed; an **incisional biopsy** is a small sample of tissue taken from a larger lesion. The excised tissue is placed in **formalin** (Fig. 1-1), which preserves it during transportation to a pathology laboratory, where it is *processed*. Five-micron thick sections are cut using a device called a *microtome* (Fig. 1-2) and placed on a glass slide (Fig 1-3). The tissue is stained, dried, and then examined under the microscope.

Clinical Implications

Patients often fear undergoing a biopsy because they mistakenly equate it with the diagnosis of cancer. Dental hygienists are in a position to educate patients that biopsy does not automatically imply cancer, but rather is a procedure used to assure proper diagnosis for a wide spectrum of diseases.

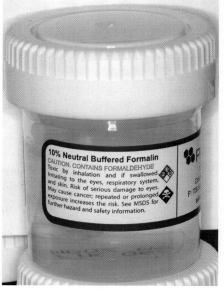

Figure 1–1   Formalin. Ten percent buffered formalin is the ideal tissue preservative.

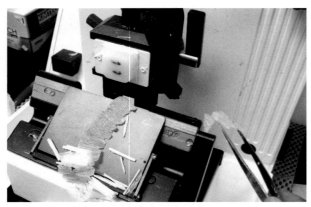

Figure 1–2   Microtome. Sharp blade to cut 5-micron thick slices of tissue that are embedded in paraffin for stability.

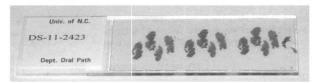

Figure 1–3   Microscopic Slide. Finished glass slide with tissue that has been stained for visibility under the microscope.

Exfoliative cytology, also called cytological smear, involves scraping surface cells from the skin or mucous membranes. The cells are applied thinly to a glass slide for preservation and staining, and then examined under the microscope. Oral cytological smears are helpful in the diagnosis of candidiasis (Chapter 3). "Brush biopsies" or "brush tests" are used to collect cells for cytological evaluation. Because the cells are disassociated from each other during the process, conclusions about the diagnosis may be limited depending on the pathologic condition evaluated.

Clinical Implications

Oral cytological smears are not invasive procedures and require no anesthesia. Therefore, in many states, performing cytological smears is within the scope of dental hygiene practice.

Laboratory tests may be required to help the pathologist reach a definitive diagnosis. These include:

1. *serological* (blood) tests, such as a complete blood count (CBC), to determine if there is a higher than normal number of inflammatory cells, which may be indicative of infection. (See Chapter 3.)
2. *urinalysis* looks for compounds filtered out by the kidneys, such as hydroxyproline in the urine, a byproduct of bone destruction in Paget disease of bone. (See Chapter 2.)
3. *microbiological cultures,* such as a bacterial culture, to determine if the microorganism is resistant to certain antibiotics. (See Chapter 3.)
4. *antibody tests* measure antibodies in the blood stream, such as SSA and SSB found in patients with Sjögren's syndrome. (See Chapter 4.)
5. DNA-PCR (polymerase chain reaction) is used to identify the DNA of disease-causing viruses, such as HIV. (See Chapter 3.)
6. ELISA (enzyme-linked immunosorbent assay) detects hormones, bacterial antigens, and antibodies. (See Chapter 4.)
7. *salivary function tests* are used to measure the quantity and consistency of saliva in patients with diseases affecting the salivary glands, such as Sjögren syndrome. (See Chapter 4.)
8. *electromyography* is used for the diagnosis of neurological and neuromuscular problems, such as temporomandibular joint (TMJ) disorders.

Differential Diagnosis

Those features that are specifically characteristic of a particular disease or lesion are referred to as **pathognomonic.** Blistering skin lesions distributed along the skin or oral mucosa served by specific nerve pathways or dermatomes are pathognomonic of herpes zoster (shingles). The appearance of a small white cauliflower-like lesion, sometimes with finger-like projections, is *pathognomonic* of oral papilloma (see Chapter 3).

For many lesions, pathognomonic features are not always present, so a strategy must be used to arrive at the final diagnosis. A **differential diagnosis** is a list of diseases that share signs and symptoms. Diseases on this list are then investigated with specific diagnostic tools to help separate and rule them in or out. The goal is to narrow the list down to a final specific or *definitive diagnosis.* See Table 1-5 for an example of a differential diagnosis.

Once a diagnosis is established by the sequence of medical, dental, and social history review, assessment of signs and symptoms, and collection of cells or tissues, the disease may be treated or managed. Options for treatment and management depend on the diagnosis. These may include medications, complete surgical excision of a remaining lesion, referral to

Table 1.5	Examples of a Differential Diagnosis

Differential Diagnosis of a White Lesion of the Buccal Mucosa That Cannot Be Wiped Off

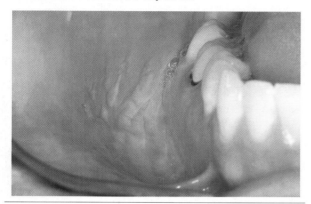

Lesion	Chapter
Leukoedema	1
Tobacco pouch keratosis	7
Lichen planus	4
White sponge nevus	5

Differential Diagnosis of a Firm Mucosal-Colored Nodule of the Lower Lip

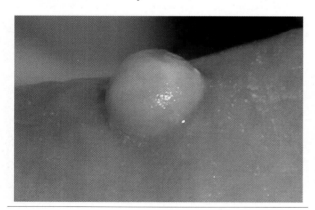

Lesion	Chapter
Irritation fibroma	2
Neuroma	7
Lipoma	7
Minor salivary gland tumor	7

other medical professionals such as a physician, or continued clinical monitoring.

Variants of Normal

Variants of normal are frequently encountered during the routine head and neck examination. With experience, they can be easily recognized and not confused with pathology. Some of these include the following:

Linea alba appears as a white line along the plane of occlusion. It may occur either unilaterally or bilaterally. Indentations from the opposing teeth may be exacerbated in cases of clenching or bruxism (Fig. 1-4) (see Chapter 2).

Leukoedema presents as a generalized translucent or opalescent covering, located over the buccal mucosa. It is most commonly observed in dark-skinned individuals. The lesion initially appears translucent white or opalescent and then disappears when the tissue is stretched (Fig. 1-5).

Physiologic pigmentation can be seen on the oral tissues of dark-skinned individuals. Melanin pigmentation can vary depending on the patient's ethnicity (Fig. 1-6).

Fordyce granules are ectopic sebaceous glands identical to those normally found in the skin. They are the "oil glands" of the skin. They appear as yellow nodules along the buccal and labial mucosa that actively secrete sebum. They are of no consequence and do not indicate any disease process (Fig. 1-7).

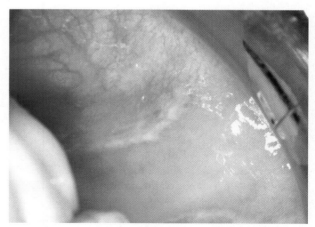

Figure 1–4 Linea alba. Thick white line along the buccal mucosa where teeth routinely occlude.

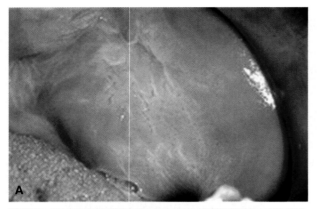

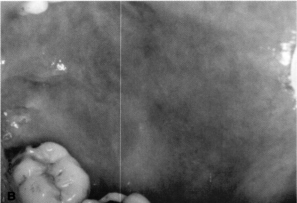

Figure 1–5 Leukoedema. Milky white translucent appearance to the buccal mucosa.

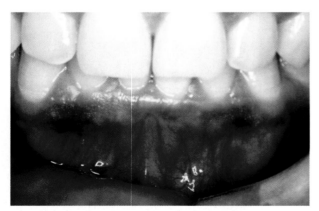

Figure 1–6 Physiologic pigmentation. Ethnic pigmentation in lower vestibule.

Hairy tongue is seen as elongated filiform papillae that produce a hair-like appearance. They can pick up yellow or brown stain and present an aesthetic problem for the patient. Smoking or ingesting certain medications, such as antibiotics, increases the risk for developing hairy tongue (Fig. 1-8).

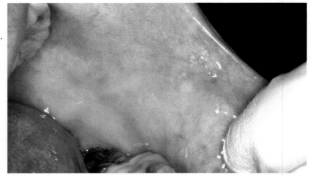

Figure 1–7 Fordyce granules. Ectopic sebaceous glands give a yellow-specked appearance to the buccal mucosa.

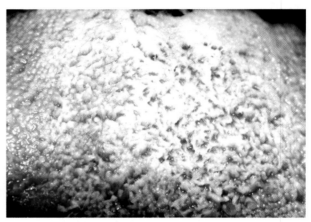

Figure 1–8 Hairy tongue. Elongated filiform papillae of the dorsal tongue.

Torus *palatinus* and *mandibularis* represent excessive growth of normal bone that occurs in the absence of other disease processes. Torus palatinus occurs along the midline and is the result of excessive bone growth at the suture line (Fig. 1-9). Torus mandibularis most often occurs bilaterally along the lingual surface of the mandible (Fig. 1-10). If the patient has more than one torus, the plural is **tori**. They are both examples of **exostoses,** bony growths that can occur anywhere along the surface of a bone. Torus palatinus and torus mandibularis are specific types of exostoses.

Foliate papillae appear as an area of vertical folds and grooves located on the extreme posterior-lateral surface of the tongue. They are occasionally mistaken for tumors or inflammatory disease. Their long axis is vertical rather than horizontal. In most people, these papillae are small and inconspicuous, but they may be prominent (Fig. 1-11).

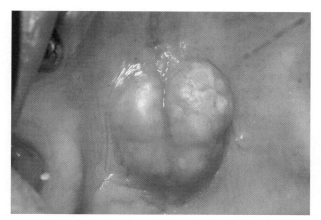

Figure 1–9   Palatal torus. Exophytic bony hard mass directly in midline of the hard palate.

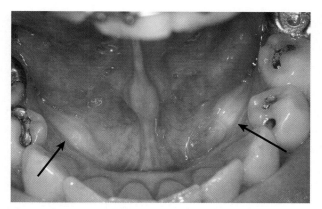

Figure 1–10   Mandibular tori. Bilateral bony hard protuberances on the lingual aspect of the mandible.

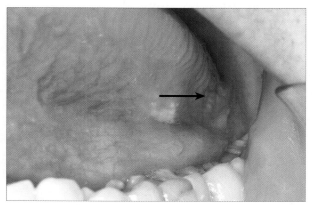

Figure 1–11   Foliate papillae. Normal soft tissue mass of lateral tongue often mistaken for disease.

Lingual tonsils are found immediately beneath the foliate papillae. They are generally inconspicuous but may but may enlarge and cause a prominence confused with a pathologic process (Fig. 1-12).

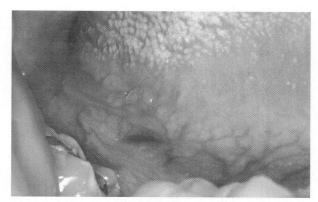

Figure 1–12   Lingual tonsils. Soft tissue mass of the lateral tongue containing tonsillar tissue.

Critical Thinking Questions

1. Describe several ways in which the dental hygienist plays an important role in the detection of systemic or oral and maxillofacial pathology.

2. Physical assessment begins the first time a patient is observed.
   - Describe some physical characteristics of disease that might be discovered initially in the dental office.
   - How is their detection important for the patient?
   - How is their detection important for dental treatment planning?

3. What are the assessment tools the dental hygienist uses in head and neck and intraoral examinations? How are these used to find pathologic lesions?

4. What are some common supplemental diagnostic procedures employed in investigating pathology? Explain when, why, and where these might be used.

5. Explain why using descriptive terminology is important. List four ways in which the use of consistent descriptive terminology is important.

Review Questions

1. **Pathology is the study of**
    A. disease processes.
    B. infectious diseases.
    C. neoplasia.
    D. All of the above

2. **A lesion is a**
    A. symptom of cancer within the tissues.
    B. defined area of pathologic tissue alteration.
    C. cytologic smear.
    D. tissue biopsy.

3. **A biopsy is**
    A. a surgical procedure.
    B. performed when the condition cannot be diagnosed with clinical procedures alone.
    C. obtained in order to determine the definitive diagnosis.
    D. All of the above

4. **Cytology**
    A. involves removal of deep tissue cells for microscopic examination.
    B. studies individual cells that are within biopsied tissue.
    C. involves removal of superficial tissue cells for microscopic examination.
    D. is contraindicated in cases of candidiasis.

5. **The first step in the assessment of oral pathology is**
    A. recognition.
    B. biopsy.
    C. cytology.
    D. laboratory testing.

6. **Patient assessment**
    A. includes obtaining medical, dental, and social histories.
    B. impacts proposed dental care.
    C. includes physical evaluation of the patient.
    D. All of the above

7. **Which one of the following statements is true?**
    A. Signs are subjective and perceived only by the patient.
    B. Signs are objective and observed by the clinician.
    C. Examples of signs are fatigue, anxiety, and sensations.
    D. Symptoms are observed by both clinicians and patients.

8. **Inspection is the critical appraisal of a patient for pathology and includes**
    A. examination.
    B. measurement.
    C. comparison with normal.
    D. All of the above

9. **Auscultation is**
    A. tapping on a surface to evaluate the underlying tissue structure.
    B. the act of listening to body sounds.
    C. used to determine hypersensitivity of teeth.
    D. performed using the fingers and/or hands.

10. **Laboratory tests to help reach a definitive diagnosis include all of the following EXCEPT:**
    A. urinalysis.
    B. microbiologic cultures.
    C. radiographs.
    D. complete blood count.

11. **An excisional biopsy of an oral lesion is performed**
    A. when a lesion is large.
    B. to cure the patient.
    C. when a lesion is small and can be totally removed.
    D. when a lesion has gone unnoticed for a prolonged period of time.

12. **Oral cytologic smears are helpful in**
    - A. diagnosing candidiasis.
    - B. evaluating allergic reactions.
    - C. identifying normal antibody titers.
    - D. identifying abnormal antibody titers.

13. **Pathognomonic features**
    - A. do not include signs.
    - B. do not include symptoms.
    - C. are virtually characteristic of a particular disease.
    - D. are only suggestive of a particular disease.

14. **A list of diseases that share signs and symptoms is known as**
    - A. a treatment plan
    - B. the differential diagnosis.
    - C. the definitive diagnosis.
    - D. abnormal variation.

15. **A distinct white line is observed bilaterally along the plane of occlusion. It most likely represents**
    - A. linea alba.
    - B. leukoedema.
    - C. fordyce granules.
    - D. physiologic pigmentation.

16. **Fordyce granules**
    - A. appear translucent white or opalescent white.
    - B. occur as a consequence of the indentations from the opposing teeth.
    - C. contain melanin pigmentation.
    - D. are ectopic sebaceous glands identical to those normally found in the skin.

17. **Elongated filiform papillae are more common in patients who**
    - A. smoke or ingest certain medications.
    - B. eat hot or spicy foods.
    - C. have leukoedema.
    - D. have linea alba.

18. **Which one of the following statements is false about tori?**
    - A. They represent excessive growths of normal bone.
    - B. They are exostoses.
    - C. They may occur in the palate or bilaterally along the lingual aspect of the mandible.
    - D. They most commonly occur in the presence of other disease processes.

19. **Which one of the following statements is false?**
    - A. Lingual tonsils are found immediately beneath the foliate papillae.
    - B. Hairy tongue indicates a serious disease process.
    - C. In the skin, fordyce granules are oil glands.
    - D. Leukoedema is most common in dark-skinned individuals.

20. **Bullae are**
    - A. small blisters or vesicles < 5 mm.
    - B. blisters > 5 mm.
    - C. solid elevations < 1 cm.
    - D. solid elevations > 1 cm.

SUGGESTED READINGS

American Academy of Oral and Maxillofacial Pathology: http://www.aaomp.org.

Bricker, S, Langlais, R, Miller, C: Oral Diagnosis, oral medicine and treatment planning, ed. 2. Lea and Febiger, Philadelphia, 2001.

Cawson, RA, Odell, EW: Cawson's Essentials of Oral Pathology and Oral Medicine, ed. 8. Churchill Livingstone, New York, 2008.

Little, JW, Falace, DA, Miller, CS, Rhodus, NL: Dental management of the medically compromised patient, ed. 7. Mosby, St. Louis, 2007.

Wilkins E: Clinical practice of the dental hygienist, ed. 13. Lippincott, Williams & Wilkins, Baltimore, 2013.

Orofacial Injury and Reactive Disorders

Learning Outcomes

At the end of this chapter, the student will be able to:

2.1. Explain the difference between reversible and irreversible cell injury.

2.2. Differentiate among the reactive processes of hyperplasia, hypertrophy, atrophy, metaplasia, dysplasia, necrosis, and ischemia.

2.3. Discuss the role of free radicals in irreversible cell injury.

2.4. Discuss the three basic types of inflammation and give an example of each.

2.5. Explain the cardinal signs of inflammation.

2.6. Explain the differences among healing by primary intention, secondary intention, and tertiary intention.

2.7. Differentiate among the clinical features of frictional keratosis, pigmented tattoos, hypermelanosis, traumatic ulcerations, burns, nicotine stomatitis, geographic tongue, hematoma, foreign body reaction, and keloid.

2.8. Differentiate among the clinical features of the proliferative repair responses pyogenic granuloma, traumatic fibroma, traumatic neuroma, and verruciform xanthoma.

2.9. Discuss the etiology and clinical identifying features of injuries to the salivary glands, gingiva, dental pulp, bones of the jaws, and the teeth.

CELL AND TISSUE RESPONSE TO INJURY

All disease originates at the cellular level. When cells are stressed or injured, they undergo a variety of adaptive changes depending on the particular stressor and the ability of the cell to respond. Basically, cells recover, adapt, or die. This chapter presents general principles of how the body responds to injury and how it restores form and function following injury. Common oral injuries and their effects on the oral cavity are presented.

Oral Pathologic Lesions Due to Injury

With the exception of caries and periodontal disease, **injury** to the oral tissues is the most common type of oral pathology seen in general dental practice. The mouth is exposed to a wide variety of objects, medications, and foods of varying textures and temperatures, any of which can inflict harm on vulnerable tissues. Types of injuries include physical (e.g., surgical trauma), chemical (e.g., exposure to caustic substances), thermal (e.g., burns), or infectious (e.g., microorganisms, discussed in detail in Chapter 3). Often the dental patient's chief complaint includes a painful area or a "lump" that may be the result of an injury and the subsequent attempt by the body to deal with injury.

There are several types of cell injuries that eventually lead to changes in form and function of tissues. Depending on the source of injury and the type of affected cell, the injury can be either reversible or irreversible (Table 2-1).

Reversible Cell Injury

Reversible cell injuries are those in which no permanent DNA damage occurs. The cells, and therefore the tissues, are able to return to normal form and/or function once an injurious agent is removed.

Hyperplasia

Hyperplasia is an increase in the size of an organ or tissue due to an increase in the number of cells. Hyperplasia can be physiologic or pathologic. **Physiologic hyperplasia** is a response to a specific stimulus in which the cells remain subject to normal regulatory control mechanisms. It may be caused by increased demand, such as that seen in a remaining kidney when one has been removed for donation (Fig. 2-1A). Physiologic hyperplasia also occurs when hormone changes result in enlargement of the breasts during pregnancy and lactation. On the other hand, **pathologic hyperplasia** can be seen in the reaction of the gingival tissues (Fig. 2-1B)

Table 2.1	Types of Cell Injury	
Reversible		**Irreversible**
Hyperplasia		Necrosis
Hypertrophy		Ischemia
Atrophy		Apoptosis
Metaplasia		Free radical damage
Dysplasia		Pathologic calcification
Intracellular pigments		Cell aging

to certain medications such as phenytoin (Dilantin), which produces an overgrowth of gingival tissue as a side effect of the drug. Gingiva is often less likely to enlarge if meticulous oral hygiene is maintained. Hyperplastic overgrowth of gingiva may be reduced surgically and medications changed to correct or control hyperplasia. This differs from neoplasia, in which the injurious agent causes gene alterations that lead to abnormal tissue enlargement. In neoplasia, growth continues despite removal of the suspected stimulus.

Hypertrophy

Hypertrophy is an increase in size of a tissue or body part due to the increase in the size of individual cells. Hypertrophy can be physiologic or pathologic. An example of **physiologic hypertrophy** is increased size of the biceps in a weight lifter due to increased work. Another example is the enlargement of the uterus during pregnancy (Fig. 2-1C). **Pathologic hypertrophy** occurs in cardiac muscle when it is overworked due to peripheral vascular disease and hypertension. Patients who grind their teeth (brux) severely or clench their jaws may show hypertrophy of the muscles of mastication due to overwork (Fig. 2-1D).

Atrophy

Atrophy refers to decrease in size of cells, organs, tissues, or body parts because of disease, hormonal alteration, injury, or lack of use. Atrophy may be physiologic or pathologic. **Physiologic atrophy** is generally not reversible. For example, once a female reaches menopause, the ovaries begin to decrease in size and atrophy. An example of reversible physiologic atrophy is muscle weakness/wasting (atrophy) that occurs when a broken arm is kept in a cast and not used (disuse atrophy) (Fig. 2-1E). An example of **pathologic atrophy** is loss of filiform papillae on the tongue following long-standing candidiasis (Fig. 2-1F). Once the fungal infection resolves

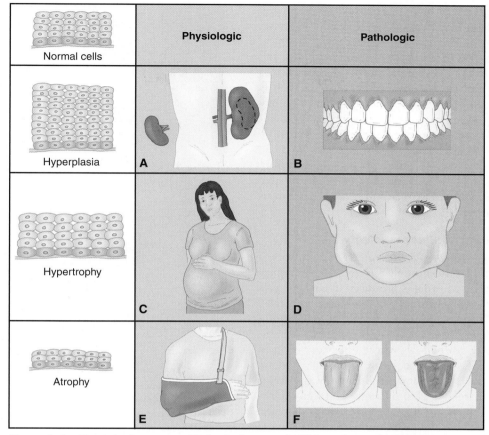

Figure 2–1   Physiologic versus pathologic changes. A. Kidney shows physiologic hyperplasia. **B.** Gingival hyperplasia is pathologic. **C.** Physiologic hypertrophy can be seen in pregnancy. **D.** Bruxism can produce muscle hypertrophy. **E.** Physiologic atrophy can occur with disuse, as in this example of a broken arm in a cast. **F.** An example of pathologic atrophy is atrophic glossitis.

(injurious agent is removed), the tongue tissue regains some or all of its former level of functioning.

Metaplasia

Metaplasia is caused by a stimulus that changes one cell type into another. An example can be seen in the epithelial lining of the respiratory tract. When the normal pseudostratified ciliated columnar epithelium of the respiratory tract comes into contact with tobacco smoke, it may transform to stratified squamous epithelium, which is thicker and more protective. But stratified squamous epithelium has no cilia or mucous to protect the respiratory tract from common irritants. Therefore, inflammatory pulmonary disorders may develop. Also, because the most common form of lung cancer is squamous cell carcinoma, the new stratified squamous epithelium presents a higher risk for developing squamous cell carcinoma of the lung. With timely elimination of an irritant, such as tobacco smoke, cells may revert to their normal state.

Another example of metaplasia occurs in the salivary glands. Normal epithelial cells of salivary gland ducts and acini undergo metaplasia from simple cuboidal epithelium to larger cells called oncocytes. The resulting nodular oncocytic metaplasia may create enlargement of the tissues and give the erroneous impression that a tumor is present. This type of metaplasia occurs most often in the parotid gland and appears to be a degenerative phenomenon related to aging.

Dysplasia

Dysplasia is defined as lack of proper maturation of a tissue. When cells are unable to mature, the tissue cannot properly develop. The classic example is the dysplasia of stratified squamous epithelium of the oral cavity. Dysplasia may be classified as mild, moderate, or severe. Mild dysplasia may be caused by mild chronic irritation that is potent enough to alter the cell's ability to develop from a normal basal cell to a mature keratinocyte. Removal of the irritant, such as a rough dental restoration or chipped tooth, may allow the cells to proceed with normal maturation. Severe dysplasia, on the other hand, may irreversibly alter cells, preventing them and the tissues involved from ever proceeding with normal maturation. Fibrous dysplasia of bone is an example, where normal bone loses its ability to mature and reverts to a fibrous state (see Chapter 6).

Endogenous Intracellular Pigments

Endogenous intracellular pigments often are indicators of cellular injury. The most widely recognized cellular pigment is **melanin**. Melanin is produced by melanocytes located in the basal layer of the epithelium (Fig. 2-2A). It functions to protect the skin and its underlying structures (Fig. 2-2B) from damage caused by ultraviolet (UV) light. Individuals whose ancestors evolved in regions close to the equator inherit a genetic propensity for excess melanin production, which helps to prevent sun-related skin damage. Naturally dark-skinned individuals are not immune to sun damage, but are resistant to it. They tend to develop melanoma of the skin at a much lower rate than fair-skinned individuals. Individuals whose ancestors evolved far from the equator have less natural melanin pigmentation and are, therefore, more susceptible to sun damage of the skin.

> ### Clinical Implications
>
> Australia, parts of which sit on the equator, has one of the highest rates of melanoma in the world. This is attributable to the fact that, in the 18th century, Australia was colonized by Northern Europeans. The ancestors of today's Australians evolved far from the equator and developed no adaptive pigmentation to pass along to their offspring. This leaves many modern-day Australians vulnerable to harmful effects of the sun, the deadliest result of which is a higher risk for melanoma (see Chapter 7).

Melanin deposition can occur as a non-specific response to injury. It can be seen in the skin following lacerations and chronic inflammatory disorders such

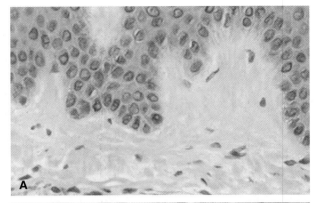
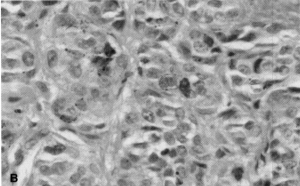

Figure 2–2   Melanin. A. Melanocytes are located in the basal layer of the epithelium. **B.** Melanin pigment in connective tissue.

as lichen planus. As the injury resolves, the melanin fades. Sometimes, however, it remains for prolonged periods of time, causing concern that a melanocytic neoplasm may be present.

Hemosiderin is a pigment derived from hemoglobin of red blood cells. It is composed of ferric oxide. A *localized* deposit of hemosiderin is seen after bruising when the red blood cells break down and the hemoglobin is released into the surrounding tissues (Fig. 2-3). Hemoglobin is then degraded into a series of pigments, the first of which is *biliverdin*, which gives the bruise a green color. The second pigment released is hemosiderin, which gives the bruise a yellow color. A *systemic* release of hemosiderin is seen when there is an overload of iron due to disease, such as hemolytic anemia. When hemosiderin is deposited into tissues and organs, it is called *hemosiderosis*. Processes by which hemosiderin is deposited into the tissues generally are reversible and cause no cellular damage. However, *hemochromatosis* is a disease of extreme iron accumulation and can lead to irreversible damage to vital organs if left untreated.

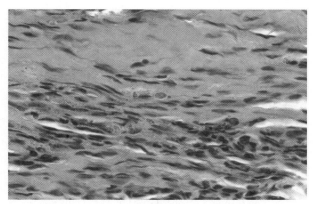

Figure 2–3   Micrograph of hemosiderin. Hemosiderin is seen after bruising. Red blood cells break down and hemoglobin is released into surrounding tissue.

Irreversible Cell Injury

Irreversible cell injury is injury that causes permanent DNA damage. The cells, and therefore the tissues, are not able to return to normal form and/or function once the injurious agent is removed.

Ischemia

Ischemia is a restriction in blood supply generally due to damaged blood vessels. The result is damage, dysfunction, or death of tissue supplied by that blood vessel, called **infarction**. For example, blockage of coronary arteries causes ischemia of the cardiac muscle, referred to as *myocardial infarction*. Blockage of cerebral arteries leads to a cerebrovascular accident (CVA), commonly called a *stroke*. Although some forms of ischemia are transient and do not result in permanent damage, ischemia typically causes permanent irreversible injury to tissues.

Necrosis

Necrosis is the death of cells and tissues that fail to adapt to changes in their environment. Pathologic necrosis occurs when normal cell functions cannot be sustained due to infection, toxins, trauma, or lack of oxygen. For example, infarction of the cardiac muscle (blockage of blood flow to the heart) causes necrosis of myocardial cells due to lack of oxygen. Once cells and tissue become necrotic, they cannot be repaired.

Several types of necrosis can develop, depending on the type of injury.

- *Coagulative necrosis* results from lack of oxygen to the cell **(hypoxia)**. As the cells die, the general cell architecture of the tissue is preserved and can be recognized microscopically. The tissue is recognizable but no viable (living) cells remain. Hypoxic damage of the kidney is a classic example of coagulative necrosis (Fig. 2-4A and B).

- *Caseous necrosis* is a form of coagulative necrosis in which the necrotic tissue takes on a "cheese-like" appearance when the area of necrotic tissue is examined clinically. The architectural features of the tissue are lost. This type of necrosis is most commonly seen in *Mycobacterium tuberculosis* infection.

- *Liquefactive necrosis* results when released enzymes digest necrotic tissues. Features of the tissue are no longer identifiable, and it is transformed into a liquid, viscous mass (Fig. 2-5). This can result from bacterial infection (abscess) or hypoxic cell death in the central nervous system (stroke). If bacteria and dead white blood cells are present, the mass may appear creamy yellow and is commonly called **pus.**

Apoptosis

Apoptosis is the process of programmed or planned cell death. This contrasts with cell death due to

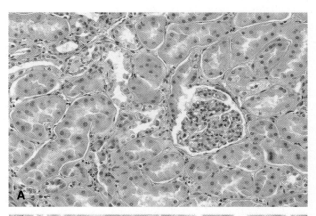

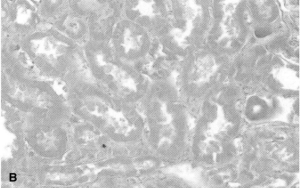

Figure 2–4   Coagulative necrosis. A. Normal kidney **B**. Kidney necrosis due to lack of oxygen; cell death with preservation of tissue form.

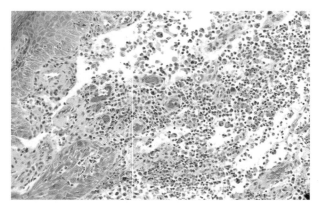

Figure 2–5   Liquefactive necrosis. Enzymatic breakdown of cells resulting in a liquid mass.

injury. Apoptosis occurs when a specific gene "turns on and turns off" during embryogenesis, allowing tissues and organs to assume their proper form. Inappropriate or excessive apoptosis causes atrophy; lack of proper apoptosis results in uncontrolled cell proliferation. Pathologic apoptosis can be seen in some tumors and inflammatory disorders.

Free Radicals

Free radicals are molecules responsible for aging, tissue damage, and a number of diseases. The molecules are unstable because they are incomplete, lacking an even number of electrons. Instead, they have a single unpaired electron in their outer shell, making them highly reactive. Free radicals seek to bond with other molecules, capturing electrons to become complete or stable. The body creates free radicals for many important functions. One example is the neutralizing or killing of bacteria and viruses. In the process they may produce collateral cell damage, causing cells to malfunction, become cancerous, or die. Free radicals may also form after exposure to chemicals, environmental toxins, radiation, or tobacco smoke, to name a few examples.

Free radicals inflict damage when they react with cell membranes or cellular DNA. Damage to cell membranes is via peroxidation of membrane lipids, a process that has been implicated in some diseases as well as in aging. **Antioxidants** are defined as molecules that inhibit or counteract oxidation. They prevent or repair damage to cells by free radicals. Problems result if the number of free radicals increases beyond the body's ability to neutralize or destroy them. The major damage is most often to DNA or cell membranes, leading to irreversible cell damage or death. Yet unanswered is whether dietary antioxidants are of significant benefit in prevention of free radical formation leading to cell damage (Fig. 2-6).

Pathologic Calcification

Pathologic calcification is defined as abnormal deposition of calcium and may be dystrophic or metastatic. *Dystrophic calcification* occurs in areas of necrosis when blood calcium is at normal levels. It indicates that the ability of cells to properly metabolize calcium has been altered or destroyed. This can be seen in arteries in advanced cases of atherosclerosis and in heart valves that have been damaged previously by rheumatic heart disease. *Metastatic calcification* occurs when blood calcium levels are elevated, a condition called *hypercalcemia*. This occurs in hyperparathyroidism, bone disease, vitamin D disorders, and renal failure. Metastatic calcification most frequently affects the gastrointestinal tract, kidneys, and lungs, causing disruptions in normal function.

Clinical Implication

Areas of dystrophic calcification can be observed in both vital and necrotic pulp tissues. Proposed causes of pulpal calcifications include irritation, injury, and reaction to the caries process. In some cases of pulp injury, calcium is deposited into the inflamed pulp. The resulting dystrophic calcifications can be seen histologically and on occasion radiographically.

Secondary dentin formation and/or dystrophic calcification may result in total obliteration of pulp chambers and canals (Fig. 2-7A and B).

Cell Aging

Cell aging is related to changes in genetic factors, diet, social conditions, and ongoing illness. Only a fixed number of divisions occur in normal cells before they die, a process called *senescence*. Senescent cells lose their ability to self-repair chromosomal damage and take up nutrients. This slowing down and loss of function manifests as the aging process.

THE INFLAMMATORY RESPONSE

Inflammation is not a disease but an attempt by the body to counteract injurious stimuli and to repair

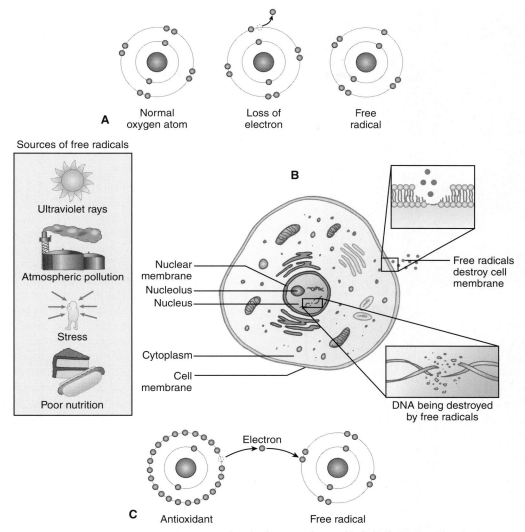

Figure 2–6   Free radicals. A. Oxygen molecules become free radicals by losing an electron. **B.** Free radicals destroy nuclear membrane and alter DNA. **C.** Free radicals are stabilized by antioxidants, which replace the missing electron.

the damage they create. It is referred to as a response because of the body's innate ability to defend itself against injury.

Inflammation and the Inflammatory Response

Inflammation is considered an essential defense mechanism necessary for health. When a tissue is involved in the inflammatory response, it is referred to as *inflamed*. The suffix *-itis* is used to indicate the specific inflammatory pathology (e.g., gingivitis or tonsillitis). Inflammation is essential in recovering

from a variety of injuries. Keep in mind that inflammation also occurs as a result of exposure to infectious microorganisms (see Chapter 3) allergens or with autoimmune diseases, and autoimmune diseases, such as rheumatoid arthritis (see Chapter 4).

The duration and extent of the inflammatory response depends on the injury. It may be local and limited, or it may become systemic and widespread if the injury is extensive. It is a dynamic process involving complex cellular and chemical reactions. Redundant systems within the body allow for variations in the inflammatory response and provide backup for deficient

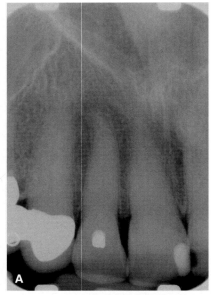

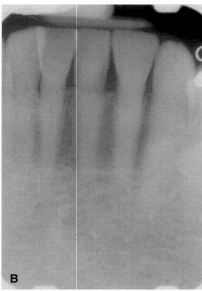

Figure 2–7   Pulp calcification. A. Pulp chamber and canals have calcified in response to injury. **B.** Calcification of pulp in lower anterior teeth.

or deactivated constituents of this response. Unfortunately, the inflammatory response can cause pain, disability, and collateral tissue damage.

Three Basic Types of Inflammation

Inflammation may be categorized as acute, chronic, or granulomatous (Table 2-2). Although there is often overlap, several clinical and microscopic features characterize each type.

Acute Inflammation

"Acute" is a general term that means abrupt onset and short duration. **Acute inflammation** occurs immediately after an injury and is characterized by exudative processes in which fluid, plasma proteins, and cells leave the bloodstream and enter the tissues. Polymorphonuclear leukocytes (PMNs, or neutrophils) are the predominant cells involved in the acute inflammatory response.

Chronic Inflammation

"Chronic" is a general term that means gradual onset over time and of longer duration. *Chronic inflammation* often follows acute inflammation, but may occur without a pre-existing acute inflammatory response. An example is deep caries affecting the dental pulp over time. Microscopically, chronic inflammation differs from acute inflammation in that lymphocytes, plasma cells, and macrophages are the predominant cells. Chronic inflammation can be described as a proliferation of cells, *neovascularization* (new blood vessel formation), and formation of new connective tissue.

Chronic inflammation may develop in two ways, depending on the nature of the inflammatory stimulus involved. It may (1) arise following an acute inflammatory response that has not resolved or (2) develop in the absence of a preceding acute response, especially in infections and autoimmune diseases, which are discussed in Chapters 3 and 4.

Granulomatous Inflammation

This is a special subtype of chronic inflammation. It occurs when cells of the chronic inflammatory response attempt to wall off substances that are perceived as foreign but that cannot be eliminated by the acute and chronic inflammatory processes alone. These walled-off zones of tissue are referred to as **granulomas** and can sometimes be detected clinically as nodules. Many pathologic nodules are referred to as granulomas; however, a nodule cannot be called a true granuloma without specific microscopic criteria. Some specific infectious microorganisms (see Chapter 3) elicit granulomatous inflammation, as do some foreign objects. Granulomas are persistent and only heal after the etiologic agent is eliminated.

Cardinal Signs and Symptoms of Inflammation

Five nonspecific common signs and symptoms characterize the inflammatory process, traditionally called the "cardinal signs of inflammation" (Table 2-3).

Table 2.2	Types of Inflammation		
	Acute	**Chronic**	**Granulomatous**
Onset	Sudden	Gradual	Gradual
Duration	Short	Long-standing	Long-standing
Predominant cell type(s)	Neutrophils, macrophages	Lymphocytes, plasma cells, macrophages	Epithelioid histiocytes, multinucleated giant cells, lymphocytes
Clinical characteristics	Pain, erythema, and edema; fever	Loss of function	Nonpainful enlargement; nodules
Outcome	Abscess; resolution; progression to chronic inflammation	Fibrosis; tissue destruction	Medical or surgical intervention

These signs are clearly observed with injury to the skin and underlying tissues.

Vascular Events

The body's initial response to physical injury, such as a paper cut or skin scrape, is vasoconstriction. Transient *pallor*, or paleness of the skin, may occur as vessels constrict, followed immediately by vasodilatation. This is clearly demonstrated in paper cuts, where bleeding is initially stopped via vasoconstriction, then followed immediately by bleeding resulting from vasodilation. Fluid movement and cell migration from blood vessels to the site of injury also results in redness and swelling. Increased blood viscosity and slower blood flow occur as fluid is lost from local blood vessels. This allows leukocytes (white blood cells) to attach to vessel walls and further increase resistance to blood flow.

Transudation and Edema

Migration of white blood cells (leukocytes) out of the blood vessels helps promote fluid and plasma protein accumulation within tissue. The process by which fluid and plasma proteins leave the blood vessels in inflammatory conditions and enter the tissues is called *exudation*. Exudates can range from serous (clear fluid with few cells) to purulent (fluid with many dead cells). *Edema* refers to an abnormally large amount of leakage of fluid from the bloodstream into the surrounding tissues, causing tissue swelling or distortion. This swelling can put pressure on nerve endings, resulting in pain. Although swelling from edema may appear harmful, it has several positive aspects, as indicated in Table 2-4.

Chemical Mediators of Inflammation

Inflammation is controlled by substances known as *chemical mediators*, each of which has a specific role at a specific stage of the inflammatory response. Three major groups of mediators include vasoactive amines, plasma proteases, and the fibrinolytic system.

Vasoactive Amines: Histamine and Serotonin

Histamine increases vascular permeability and causes the contraction of smooth muscle. *Serotonin* is a chemical messenger that can produce blood vessel narrowing and transmit signals between nerve cells.

Table 2.3	Cardinal Signs and Symptoms of Inflammation
Signs and Symptoms	**Cause**
Heat (Calor)	Increased blood flow
Redness (Rubor)	Increased blood flow
Swelling (Tumor)	Exudation
Pain (Dolor)	Fluid pressure and pain-producing agents such as kinins
Loss of function	Swelling and/or pain

Know This

Table 2.4	Beneficial Properties of Edema
Dilutes toxins in tissue	
Provides nutrients for inflammatory cells	
Contains protective antibodies	
Contains fibrinogen, which removes collagen to facilitate movement of inflammatory cells into the wound	

Plasma Proteases

Plasma proteases consist of three interrelated enzyme systems from which some chemical mediators of inflammation originate.

Kinin System

Kinins are a group of powerful blood proteins that play a central role in the inflammatory response. They can increase vascular permeability, dilate blood vessels, cause smooth muscle to contract, and trigger the pain response. *Bradykinin* and *kallidin* are two important kinins.

Fibrinolytic System

The coagulation pathway (clotting) begins when platelets adhere to injured endothelial cells and release *fibrinogen*. Thrombin converts fibrinogen to fibrin, the basis for a clot. Clot formation helps to slow or stop blood flow. The fibrinolytic system is later activated to dissolve (lyse) the clot when it is no longer needed.

Complement System

The *complement system* is composed of over 20 interactive plasma and cell membrane proteins, numbered in the order in which they were discovered. This system can be activated through antigen-antibody complexes, antibody-target complexes, or lipopolysaccharides associated with gram-negative bacteria. Once activated, the job of the complement system is to do the following:

1. Promote vascular responses
2. Recruit phagocytic white blood cells (chemotaxis)
3. Prepare targets for phagocytosis (opsonization)
4. Damage target molecules

Cessation of Inflammation

To stop inflammation, inflammatory mediators must be removed from the area, and chemotactic signals for recruitment of additional inflammatory cells must be discontinued. Removal of inflammatory cells that are already present must occur before healing is complete. This can occur through several different mechanisms, including programmed cell death (apoptosis), phagocytosis of the cells, or return of cells to the circulation via lymphatic drainage.

Cellular Interactions in the Inflammatory Process

Cells of the blood are generally classified as either red blood cells (*erythrocytes* or **RBCs**) or white blood cells (*leukocytes* or **WBCs**). The primary function of erythrocytes is to transport oxygen to and carbon dioxide away from tissues. The primary function of leukocytes is to defend the body against microorganisms and other foreign proteins.

Leukocytes are classified according to the presence or absence of cytoplasmic granules (*granular* and *agranular*) and the shape of their nucleus. A uniform ovoid nucleus is referred to as *mononuclear*; a nucleus with numerous lobes is referred to as *polymorphonuclear*. Granular leukocytes are all polymorphonuclear and are grouped according to the staining affinities of their granules: neutrophils lack staining; eosinophils stain red; basophils stain blue. The normal leukocyte count in blood varies between 5,000 and 10,000 per mm³. Values above 10,000 are referred to as *leukocytosis*, and those below 4,000 are referred to as *leukopenia*. There are three types of polymorphonuclear granulocytes based on their morphologic appearance and function (Fig. 2-8A):

1. *Neutrophils*, also called polymorphonuclear leukocytes (PMNs), comprise 50% to 70% of circulating leukocytes. Originating in the bone marrow, they are considered the first line of defense in acute inflammation. They are the first leukocytes to emerge from the blood vessels in inflammation and have a half-life of 6 to 9 hours. PMNs are identified by the

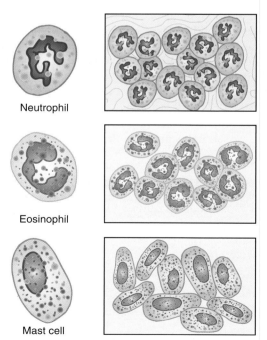

Figure 2–8   A. Polymorphonuclear granulocytes derived from basophils. Neutrophils, eosinophils, and mast cells.

presence of multi-lobed nuclei and clear cytoplasmic granules. They are guided to their targets by the process of *chemotaxis* (movement in response to a chemical stimulus), whereby they provide defense against bacterial and fungal infections. These cells contain over 20 proteolytic enzymes that destroy foreign proteins. The enzymes may cause significant collateral damage by inadvertently attacking extracellular membranes of normal host cells. In the presence of pyogenic (pus-producing) microorganisms or foreign materials resistant to phagocytosis, PMNs increase in numbers and accumulate at the site of injury. In severe inflammation, the process is overwhelmed, and pus formation predominates. Pus is composed of dead PMNs, necrotic tissue, and fluid.

2. *Eosinophils* comprise 1% to 5% of circulating leukocytes. These cells are named after their granules, which stain with eosin, a red dye. Eosinophils form the first line of defense against parasites and can survive for weeks in tissues. They have no significant role in bacterial killing. However, they do possess IgE receptors, which bind to IgE-coated parasites. See Chapter 4 for further details on the important role of eosinophils in allergic reactions.

3. *Basophils* comprise 0% to 1% of circulating leukocytes. Their granules stain blue with basic dyes, hence the name basophils. They are considered the precursor for *mast cells*, which are abundant in the peripheral tissues. They contain histamine and heparin, which are important in the allergic response. See Chapter 4 for further details on the role of basophils.

There are three types of mononuclear leukocytes (Fig. 2-8B):

1. *Monocytes* originate in bone marrow. They are phagocytes (cells capable of engulfing debris or microorganisms) that circulate in the bloodstream. Once they exit the bloodstream, they are referred to as *macrophages*. Macrophages take on different sizes and shapes depending on the tissue in which they are found. In connective tissue they are called *histiocytes*. They are the second line of defense during acute inflammation. Macrophages can live up to several months and are key players in the chronic inflammatory response as a major component of the phagocyte system. Macrophages have several functions during inflammation (Table 2-5), the most important of which is *phagocytosis*, defined as ingestion and destruction of foreign proteins. They are antigen-presenting cells, which means they assist other cells with the recognition of injurious agents.

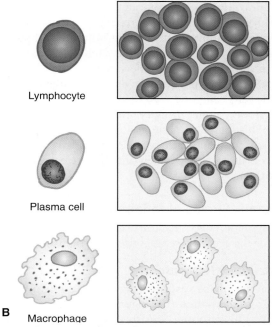

B Macrophage

Figure 2–8   B. Mononuclear granulocytes. Lymphocytes, plasma cells, and macrophages.

Macrophages are also responsible for the production of various *cytokines* and growth factors necessary for wound repair. Macrophages are activated and deactivated as needed in the inflammatory process.

2. *Lymphocytes* include T cells, B cells, and natural killer (NK) cells. They can be recognized by their large, central, strongly basophilic nucleus with scant cytoplasm. Characteristically, they are seen in the chronic inflammatory response as well as in autoimmune disease (discussed in Chapter 4).

3. *Plasma cells* are B lymphocytes that specialize in the production of antibodies. They can be seen in great numbers in chronic inflammatory processes in the oral mucosa.

Table 2.5	Function of Macrophages in the Inflammatory Response

Removal of dead/dying cells and tissue to promote wound healing

Contain, engulf, and/or remove particulate foreign material (phagocytosis)

Production of cytokines and growth factors

Present antigens to other cells of the inflammatory response for processing

Platelets (Fig 2-8C) make an important contribution in injury, inflammation, and repair by playing a role in activating complement, binding immune complexes, enhancing vascular permeability, and participating in the coagulation cascade. They are not cells but rather small fragments of cytoplasm derived from larger precursor cells called *megakaryocytes.* As they circulate in the blood, their primary function is hemostasis through adherence to the site of vascular injury, where they form a hemostatic plug. Platelets have a lifespan of 5 to 9 days, during which time they release multiple growth factors.

Systemic Effects of Inflammation

Two systemic effects that can occur during inflammation include the acute phase response and lymphadenopathy.

Acute Phase Response

The **acute phase response** occurs when severe injury causes inflammation that may result in a systemic reaction. This response consists of a rapid physiological reaction generated to deal with tissue damage caused by the inflammatory response. Some signs of acute phase response are discussed below.

Fever

Pyrogens are fever-producing substances circulating in the blood produced by cells within the body, such as leukocytes, or by agents of external origin, such as microorganisms. Fever can be a positive defense mechanism for the body. For example, some bacteria are sensitive to even slightly increased body temperature; therefore, fever is sometimes capable of killing them.

Increased Cortisol Levels

Cortisol is a steroid hormone, also called glucocorticoid or corticosteroid, that is produced by the adrenal gland in response to stress. Its primary functions are to increase blood glucose, suppress the immune system, and aid in fat, protein, and carbohydrate metabolism. Serum cortisol levels increase soon after the onset of inflammation stresses the body. Corticosteroids counteract the effects of the inflammatory response.

Leukocytosis

Leukocytosis is an increase in the circulating leukocyte count in the blood due to the additional release of neutrophils from the bone marrow. The white cell count typically reaches 15,000 or 20,000 per mm^3 but may reach levels of 40,000 to 100,000 per mm^3.

Lymphadenopathy

Lymphadenopathy is a term that refers to swollen or enlarged lymph nodes (Fig. 2-9). When the cause of lymph node swelling is the inflammatory response, the inflamed lymph nodes are referred to as **lymphadenitis**. The enlargement is due to an influx of inflammatory cells in response to the inflammatory disorder. The lymph nodes closest to the site of the injury are often the first to become enlarged. This is referred to as *regional lymphadenopathy.*

Clinical Implications

Inflammatory disorders of the head and neck often cause cervical lymphadenopathy that is detectable during the head and neck examination. It is improper to refer to enlarged lymph nodes as "swollen glands" because lymph nodes are not glandular organs.

Postinflammatory Tissue Healing

The final outcome for injured tissue that has gone through the inflammatory response is healing and

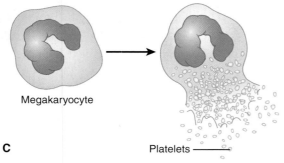

C

Figure 2–8   **C.** Platelets.

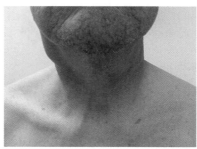

Figure 2–9   **Cervical lymphadenopathy.** Lymphadenopathy refers to swollen or enlarged lymph nodes. (From Taber's Cyclopedic Medical Dictionary, ed. 21. F.A. Davis, Philadelphia, 2009, p 1376.)

restoration. In some cases, the process results in complete restoration to the pre-wound state. This is known as *regeneration*. On the other hand, *repair* occurs when complete restoration is not possible and the damaged area is simply restored to the best state possible.

Granulation Tissue

Granulation tissue forms at the site of an injury as the body starts to rebuild. Whenever there is an injury, the natural response is for granulation tissue to form (Fig. 2-10A). Granulation tissue acts as a scaffold upon which new tissue will develop. Granulation tissue, no matter where it is found, is composed mainly of chronic inflammatory cells, fibroblasts, and angioblasts (Fig. 2-10B). Fibroblasts produce an extracellular matrix that serves as a foundation upon which new tissue will develop to repair the wound. Angioblasts form tiny new vascular channels to aid in reconstruction, a process called *neovascularization*. If the source of the injury is not removed or if the injured site becomes secondarily traumatized, there may be an excess buildup of granulation tissue in response to the continuous damage. The body will continually attempt to complete the repair, but it is impeded by continued assault via the injurious agent. If inflammation is resolved quickly, little additional tissue injury results; however, if inflammation persists, excessive tissue injury can occur. The resultant chronic inflammation can produce additional problems, such as joint destruction, as seen in rheumatoid arthritis, or bone loss around teeth, as seen in periodontitis.

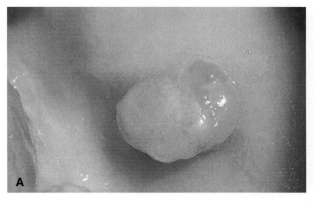

A

Fibroblast   Angioblast

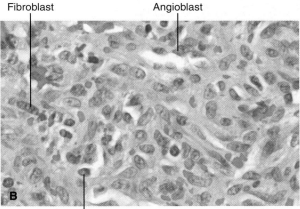

B

Chronic inflammatory cell

Figure 2–10   Granulation tissue. A. Exuberant granulation tissue response to injury of buccal mucosa. **B.** Chronic inflammatory cells, fibroblasts, and angioblasts make up granulation tissue.

Clinical Implications

A common example of inability of the body to proceed with completion of its repair function is the so-called *pyogenic granuloma*, incorrectly named because it is neither pyogenic (pus-producing) nor granulomatous (see Figs. 2-10A and B). A pyogenic granuloma is simply a localized exuberant attempt at repair. Pyogenic granulomas are overgrowths of granulation tissue in response to a local injury that is not resolved. Although pyogenic granulomas can occur anywhere on any skin or mucosal surface, they are common in the oral cavity. The most common location in the oral cavity is the gingiva, where the injurious agent is typically calculus that acts as a persistent irritant. Scaling can help resolve these lesions, but occasionally the granulation tissue is so bulky that it must be removed surgically.

Healing

Healing associated with physical tissue trauma is classified as healing by primary, secondary, or tertiary intention.

Primary Intention

Healing by *primary intention* occurs when wound edges can touch each other or can be held together by surgical staples, sutures, or tape. Examples are surgical incisions and injuries with minimal tissue loss, such as paper cuts. Complete regeneration is possible, and formation of lasting scar tissue is absent or minimal.

Secondary Intention

Wounds in which the edges cannot be closely opposed heal by *secondary intention*. Missing tissue limits the body's ability to restore pre-wound conditions. Surgical and trauma cases in which there is removal of significant portions of tissue result in this type of healing. The repair process often results in significant scarring.

Tertiary Intention

Healing by *tertiary intention* is similar to healing by secondary intention, with the exception that the wounds become infected with microorganisms. Formation of purulent exudate prolongs or delays healing and increases collateral tissue damage. This also results in the need for increased scar formation to cover or close large areas of injury.

CLINICAL FEATURES OF OROFACIAL SOFT TISSUE INJURY

The orofacial soft tissues encompass a wide range of oral structures that include the mucous membranes, gingiva, salivary glands, and dental pulp. These tissues are subject to trauma from various sources.

Injury to the Mucous Membranes

Mucous membranes that line the oral cavity vary in keratinization and therefore vary in resistance to injury. Nonkeratinized oral mucosa is more likely to be injured, but keratinized oral mucosa also may sustain injury.

Frictional Keratosis

Frictional keratosis is a benign reactive phenomenon that occurs when the mucous membranes are repeatedly irritated over a prolonged period of time. It represents a protective mechanism that increases the thickness of the surface epithelium in an attempt to protect the underlying tissues from persistent irritation. It can be seen in the oral cavity anywhere there is repeated mild trauma. Excess keratin that builds up on an epithelial surface is known as **hyperkeratosis**. When keratin collects moisture, it appears white (Fig. 2-11A). In hyperkeratosis, excess keratin is seen on the surface, and inflammatory cells may or may not be present in the underlying connective tissue (Fig. 2-11B). If the cause of the white hyperkeratotic area is a jagged tooth or rough restoration, the white lesion will be found on soft tissue adjacent to the irritating surface. Frictional keratosis in edentulous areas may be caused by mastication or rough foods (Fig. 2-12). Often the source of the irritation cannot be identified. If the irritating source can be removed, the lesion should regress on its own. See Table 2-6 for a summary of the most common forms of hyperkeratosis of the oral mucosa.

Clinical Implications

Frictional keratosis may appear identical to the premalignant changes that precede development of oral cancer. Often it is difficult to identify the source of irritation. Therefore, any white lesion for which no irritant can be identified, or one that does not regress with removal of the suspected source of irritation, should be removed. Figure 2-13 shows a plan to follow whenever a lesion appears to be reactive in nature.

Some specific types of frictional keratosis are defined here.

- **Linea alba** ("white line") is a specific form of frictional keratosis seen as a thin, slightly raised white keratotic line along the occlusal plane on the buccal mucosa, and it is often bilateral. Linea alba is considered to be a variation of normal anatomy but may become prominent in some individuals. (See Chapter 1.)
- *Morsicatio buccarum, linguarum,* and *labiorum* are forms of frictional keratosis caused by habitual chewing or nibbling of the cheek (morsicatio buccarum), tongue (morsicatio linguarum), and lip (morsicatio labiorum) (Fig. 2-14). Extra surface keratin builds up (hyperkeratosis) to minimize damage to the deeper tissues. The surface appears white and somewhat shredded. Cessation of the habit usually leads to regression of the lesion.
- *Snuff dippers keratosis* is seen in users of smokeless tobacco. White plaques develop in the vestibule where the tobacco comes into direct contact with the tissues. These lesions are characterized by thickened white mucosa that is typically wrinkled or corrugated (Fig. 2-15A). The clinical presentation may vary from an ill-defined area of white wrinkled thickening to deeply folded tissue with red patches (Fig. 2-15B). In addition to mucosal changes, gingival recession around the teeth may be pronounced. Caries in the gingival one-third of the tooth (Class V) may develop when sugar content of the smokeless tobacco is high. Treatment includes tobacco cessation, after which the mucosal effects may regress and disappear within a few weeks to months. If the keratosis does not regress or the patient declines cessation therapy, biopsy to rule out precancerous or cancerous change may be indicated. Long-term follow up is essential, and prognosis depends on behavioral changes of the patient and/or biopsy findings.

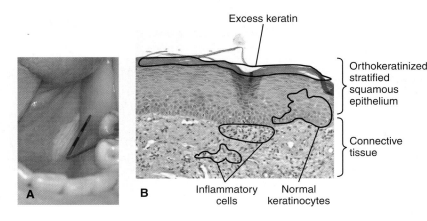

Excess keratin

Orthokeratinized stratified squamous epithelium

Connective tissue

Inflammatory cells

Normal keratinocytes

A

B

Figure 2–11 Frictional keratosis. A. Clinical photograph showing the site of injury. **B.** White appearance of hyperkeratosis due to buildup of excess orthokeratin, formed in response to chronic irritation.

Amalgam, Graphite, and Ethnic Tattoos

Amalgam tattoos are the result of accidental implantation of dental amalgam within the oral tissues (Fig. 2-16A). Injury to oral mucosa may permit amalgam debris to be introduced into tissue. Amalgam can be introduced into oral mucosa in several ways. It can occur during placement or removal of amalgam restorations or during crown preparation, when a *slurry* containing amalgam particles is produced within the gingival sulcus. Fracture of dental amalgams via trauma or tooth extraction may also leave residual amalgam within soft tissues. In addition, endodontic treatment that involved placing amalgam at the apex of the tooth can result in an amalgam tattoo.

Amalgam tattoos are often confirmed radiographically by detecting the presence of radiopaque amalgam fragments; however, not all amalgam tattoos produce radiographic findings. Amalgam tattoos may be produced by leaching of tiny silver particles into the underlying connective tissue rather than by deposition of larger particles (Fig. 2-16B). This means negative radiographic findings do not definitively rule out amalgam tattoos. A similar phenomenon can be seen in patients, especially children, who accidentally implant graphite from a lead pencil into the gingival tissues. Biopsy must be considered for any pigmented area in the oral cavity that cannot be confirmed radiographically to be an amalgam or graphite tattoo.

Clinical Implications

Occasionally, a patient with no amalgam restorations will present with what appears to be an amalgam tattoo in the premolar area. This generally represents an amalgam tattoo initiated at the time of extraction of a deciduous tooth containing an amalgam restoration (Fig. 2-16C). Another form of exogenous pigmentation referred to as *ethnic tattooing* is seen in cultures that use this as a decoration or status symbol (Fig. 2-17).

Hypermelanosis

Hypermelanosis is the result of excess melanin produced by melanocytes found in the basal layer of stratified squamous epithelium. Melanin is a protective pigment that can be produced in response to any injurious stimulus. It may be excessive in the oral cavity under several circumstances described below.

Post-inflammatory hypermelanosis or *postinflammatory hyperpigmentation* occurs after the skin or mucous membranes experience inflammatory events such as infection, allergic reaction, trauma, or other inflammatory diseases. Melanin is overproduced in an

Figure 2–12 Frictional keratosis. Thickening of surface in edentulous space due to rough foods.

Table 2.6	Types of Hyperkeratosis of the Oral Mucosa	
	Etiology	**Clinical Features**
Linea alba	Normal occlusal contact	Thin white line on buccal mucosa along line of occlusion
Frictional keratosis	Chronic rubbing	Thick white plaque that does not wipe off and contacts rough restoration or prosthesis; also from oral habits such as chewing on coarse foods
Morsicatio (buccarum, linguorum, labiorum)	Habitual chewing or nibbling of buccal mucosa, tongue, or labial mucosa	Thick white plaque that does not wipe off with a "shredded" surface texture
Snuff dippers keratosis	Direct contact of smokeless tobacco product	Wrinkled, corrugated, or folded pink, white to red; adjacent gingiva may show recession from teeth

attempt to protect the skin or mucous membranes from injury. This results from the release of prostaglandins and other inflammatory products stimulating melanocytes to increase synthesis of melanin. Melanin becomes trapped by macrophages, called *melanophages*, in the connective tissue, causing localized or diffuse black to brown pigmentation. Postinflammatory hyperpigmentation is more common in individuals with darker skin.

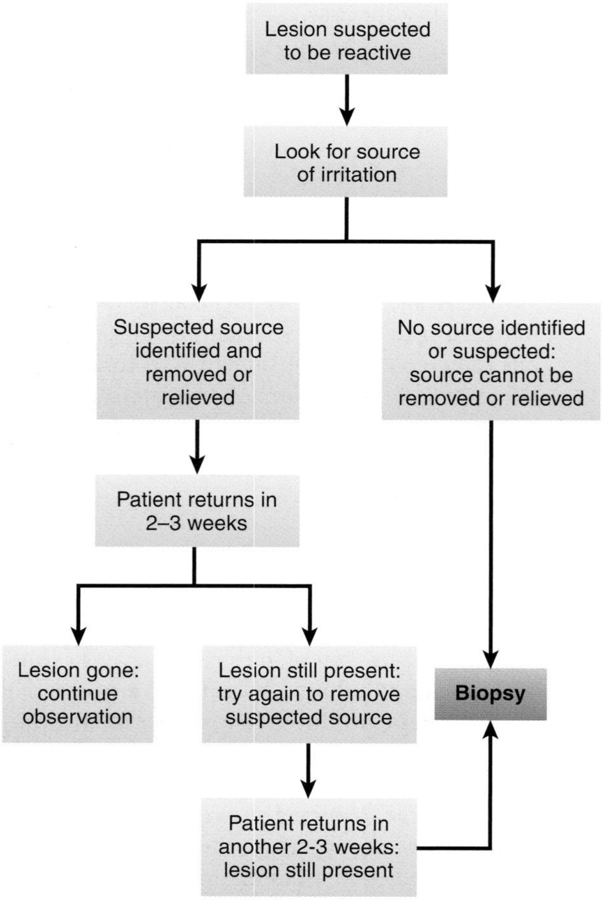

Oral postinflammatory pigmentation is associated with chronic inflammatory disorders such as oral lichen planus or pemphigoid (see Chapter 4) and can be seen following oral surgery. Lesions may be brief, disappearing shortly after the inflammatory process resolves. In other cases, the hypermelanosis may be present for many years (Fig. 2-18). These lesions cause concern because they may resemble early melanoma. In many cases, a biopsy and histological evaluation is the only way to differentiate between the two. Once confirmed, postinflammatory hyperpigmentation requires no treatment.

Oral melanotic macule most likely represents a form of post-inflammatory hyperpigmentation, although the precise etiology is unknown. It most often presents as a focal flat (macular) brown discoloration of the oral mucosa or the vermilion border of the lower lip, both sites that are readily traumatized. The buccal mucosa,

Figure 2–13   **Management of a lesion suspected to be reactive/traumatic.**

Lesion suspected to be reactive
↓
Look for source of irritation
↓
Suspected source identified and removed or relieved | No source identified or suspected: source cannot be removed or relieved
↓
Patient returns in 2–3 weeks
↓
Lesion gone: continue observation | Lesion still present: try again to remove suspected source → Biopsy
↓
Patient returns in another 2-3 weeks: lesion still present

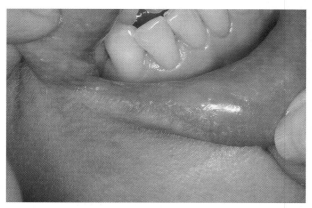

Figure 2–14   **Lip chewing.** Shredded appearance to labial mucosa results.

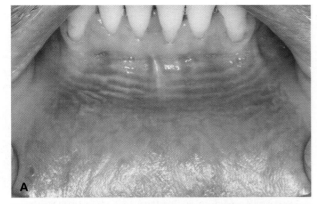

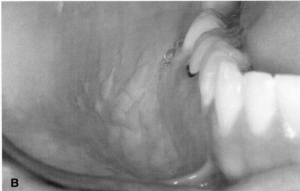

Figure 2–15   Snuff dippers keratosis. A. Corrugated tissue at site of tobacco placement. **B.** Thick red and white folded tissue at site of tobacco placement.

gingiva, and palate are common intraoral sites for oral melanotic macules. These lesions represent the intraoral equivalent of an *ephelis*, or common freckle, that appears on the skin.

Most oral melanotic macules are well-demarcated, uniformly tan to dark brown, asymptomatic, round or oval discolorations (Fig. 2-19). They rarely are larger than 7 mm in diameter. Although they tend to have an abrupt onset, the color and size stabilize over time and rarely demonstrate significant change. Because on rare occasion melanoma has been reported to develop in the site of an oral melanotic macule, any change in size, color, or texture should be viewed with suspicion, and steps should be taken to confirm the diagnosis with a biopsy.

Melanoacanthosis is a form of oral pigmentation seen almost exclusively in patients of African descent. Although its pathogenesis remains uncertain, its clinical behavior is suggestive of a reactive origin. The clinical appearance of oral melanoacanthosis is that of a flat, dark brown to black, well-defined area that arises alarmingly quickly following a traumatic event, often achieving a size of 2 to 3 cm. The most

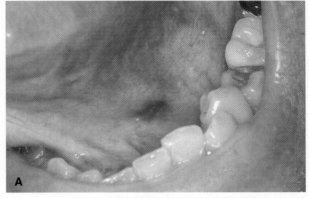

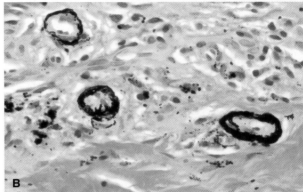

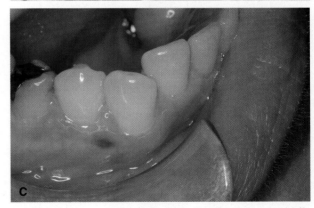

Figure 2–16   Amalgam tattoo. A. Amalgam traumatically implanted during dental procedure. **B.** Silver from amalgam stains the tissue. **C.** Amalgam tattoo created during extraction of deciduous tooth many years ago.

common locations are buccal mucosa, lip, palate, and gingiva (Fig. 2-20).

A biopsy is necessary to differentiate melanoacanthosis from other melanocytic lesions, including melanoma (Table 2-7). Melanoacanthosis may undergo spontaneous resolution rather quickly. When necessary, incisional biopsy is recommended because of the typically large size. The histopathologic appearance is quite characteristic. The spinous layer of the epithelium shows

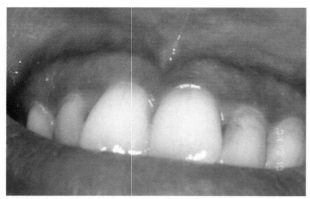

Figure 2–17   Ethnic tattoo. Young woman from Africa with tattoo placed as a status symbol.

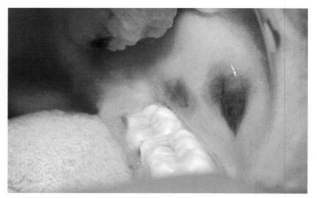

Figure 2–20   Melanoacanthosis. Flat, dark brown-to-black, well-defined area that arises suddenly following a traumatic event.

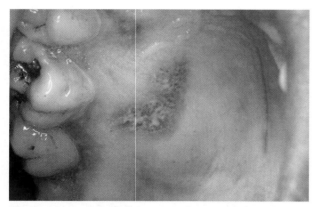

Figure 2–18   Post-inflammatory hyperpigmentation. Patient with chronic inflammation due to lichen planus, now with postinflammatory hyperpigmentation.

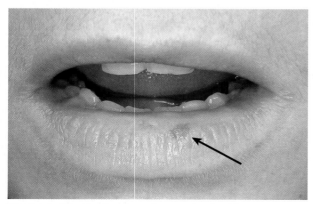

Figure 2–19   Oral melanotic macule. Oval brown discoloration of the lower lip of unknown etiology.

hyperplasia (acanthosis) and contains numerous dendritic melanocytes. Once the diagnosis has been established, no further treatment is necessary. Patients should be educated about the possible role that trauma can play in development of melanoacanthosis.

Smoker's melanosis is a condition of excessive melanin pigmentation found in the gingiva of about 20 percent of smokers and seen more frequently in females. Melanin deposition is considered a protective mechanism. Melanosis is thought to be an attempt by the body to protect itself from toxins and heat produced by smoking tobacco. Any mucosal surface can be affected, but melanosis is most commonly seen in the facial anterior gingiva and rarely in the molar areas (Fig. 2-21). Lesions appear as light to dark brown diffuse pigmentations and are seen most often in cigarette and pipe smokers. Cessation of smoking will result in gradual disappearance of the pigmentation over many months. A biopsy may be indicated to rule out other pigmented conditions if the pigmentation persists and/or does not resolve after cessation efforts.

Clinical Implications

Oral melanoma is rare. There are several non-neoplastic disorders of pigmentation that can mimic oral melanoma. The only way to achieve certainty about the diagnosis of unidentified pigmented lesions is to perform a biopsy. To prevent overlooking a developing melanoma, a good rule of thumb for pigmented lesions of the oral cavity is: *If a pigmented lesion cannot be identified and/or does not appear radiographically as an amalgam tattoo, biopsy it.*

Table 2.7	Nonneoplastic Pigmented Disorders of the Oral Cavity		
	Postinflammatory Hyperpigmentation	Oral Melanotic Macule	Melanoacanthosis
Etiology	Inflammatory cytokines stimulate melanocytes	Unknown; probably local trauma	Local trauma
Clinical Appearance	Diffuse, brown; fades over weeks or months	< 1 cm well-defined, brown; stable over time	> 1 cm large brown macules; fades within days or weeks

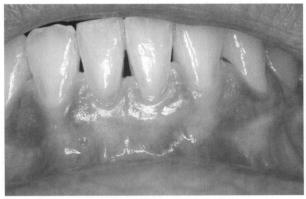

Figure 2–21   Smoker's melanosis. Woman with a 15-year smoking history shows diffuse brown pigmentation on anterior gingiva.

Traumatic Ulcers

An **ulcer** by definition is the loss of surface epithelium with exposure of the underlying connective tissues. Ulcers are one of the most common injuries to the human body. There are numerous forms of ulcers that result from destruction of the protective epithelium. Table 2-8 summarizes some of the most common oral ulcerations caused by trauma.

When trauma to the oral mucosa is severe enough to strip away surface epithelium, the result is a traumatic ulcer. Traumatic ulcers are almost always of acute onset, immediately following the traumatic event. The lateral border of the tongue (Fig. 2-22) and labial mucosa are the most common locations for traumatic ulcers. Lesions will appear as round to ovoid depressions with yellow necrotic centers and erythematous irregular borders. Patients complain of pain that slowly subsides as the lesion heals over 7 to 10 days. Topical analgesics, such as benzocaine to relieve pain, may be helpful. Topical corticosteroids are not used because they act to suppress the inflammatory response. If the inflammatory response is suppressed, then there will be delayed healing and the risk of secondary infection increases.

If trauma to the area is mild and repeated (chronic), a deep persistent ulceration may develop. Pain regresses and a build-up of granulation tissue develops to protect the underlying nerve endings. The term for these chronic traumatic ulcers is *traumatic ulcerative granuloma (with stromal eosinophilia)* or *TUGSE*. They are often slow to heal and develop a raised, rolled border filled with granulation tissue. TUGSEs often mimic oral cancer (Fig. 2-23). Surgical intervention is needed to remove the excess granulation tissue and promote healing.

Anesthetic necrosis is an unusual traumatic ulceration typically seen in patients who receive an injection in the greater palatine foramen for dental procedures on the maxillary teeth. It is believed that the epinephrine in the local anesthetic causes mild ischemia, leading to localized necrosis. Anesthetic necrosis appears as a well-defined tender-to-painful lesion at the injection site. The lesion heals without treatment in 7 to 10 days.

Burns to the oral mucous membranes destroy surface epithelium and are usually very painful. Burns can be thermal or chemical and are of acute onset following exposure to the source. *Thermal burns* can be induced by contact with hot foods or liquids. Hot foods that make contact with mucosa of the lips or oral cavity may result in acute tissue destruction. Palatal burns from eating hot pizza are a common example (Fig. 2-24). Occasionally, accidental contact with live electrical wires can cause deep burns to the face and/or oral cavity. *Electrical burns* of the lips and commissures can be seen in young children who accidentally chew or bite into electrical cords. Electrical burns to the lips are often severe, involving extensive tissue damage and requiring special reconstruction by a plastic surgeon.

Table 2.8	Traumatic Ulcerations of the Oral Mucosa	
	Etiology	**Clinical Features**
Traumatic ulcer	Physical injury such as biting the tongue or contact with sharp object	Usually single, well-defined area of erythema surrounding yellow fibrinopurulent membrane; slightly raised border; tender/painful; resolves in 7 to 10 days with removal of etiology
Traumatic ulcerative granuloma	Traumatic ulcer that receives persistent mild chronic trauma	Long duration; raised rolled border; crater with yellow fibrinopurulent membrane; nonpainful or mildly tender; slow to resolve with removal of etiology; often requires surgical excision and healing by primary intention
Denture ulcer	New denture with ill-adapted flange; prolonged denture wearing	Ovoid erythematous area with yellow necrotic center; contacts irregular area of denture; resolves with denture adjustment
Anesthetic necrosis	Ischemia from epinephrine in local anesthetic or trauma during injection	Usually on hard palate at injection site; painful well-defined intense red area with central necrosis; heals without treatment in 10 to 14 days
Thermal burn	Contact with hot foods such as pizza	Painful yellow to white zone of necrosis of surface mucosa of palate or buccal mucosa; tissue sloughs; patient reports etiologic event; resolve with no treatment
Electrical burn	Contact with live electrical cord or extension cord	Yellow to black painless area that gradually becomes edematous; sloughs and bleeds; usually on lips of children
Chemical burn	Contact with caustic medications, dental materials, improper use of analgesics, mouth rinses	Superficial white corrugated or "cracked" appearance; epithelium sloughs leaving red painful surface; resolves without treatment in 10 to 14 days

Chemical burns can result when caustic agents come in contact with the oral mucosa. Chemical burns may appear as thick, rough hyperkeratotic plaques with a corrugated or cratered surface and/or areas of ulceration. Patients may misuse acidic medications, such as

aspirin tablets or powders that contain acetylsalicylic acid (Fig. 2-25). Aspirin may cause a significant burn if placed adjacent to or over a painful tooth, rather than being swallowing. Patients may use strong agents, such as hypochlorite (bleach), to clean or disinfect

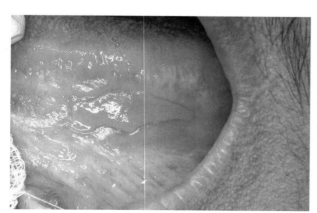

Figure 2–22 Traumatic ulcer. Large ulcer with yellow necrotic center and red halo.

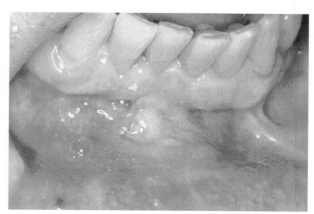

Figure 2–23 Traumatic ulcerative granuloma (with stromal eosinophilia) (TUGSE). Long-standing nonpainful ulcer that did not heal after 3 months.

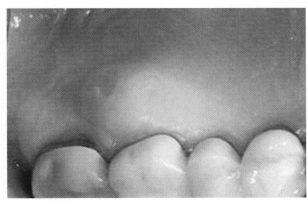

Figure 2–24 Burns. Burn on prominent bony exostosis after eating hot pizza.

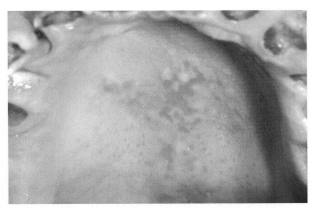

Figure 2–25 Aspirin powder burn. Patient with toothache in maxillary teeth, associated burn from aspirin powder placement.

complete dentures. Any residual chemical remaining from incomplete rinsing may also cause significant soft tissue burns.

Clinical Implications

Aspirin only works for a toothache when swallowed and introduced into the systemic circulation. Patients should be advised against placing aspirin tablets or powders on painful areas in the oral cavity because they may cause further injury to the soft tissues.

Iatrogenic (clinician-induced) burns may occur via accidental exposure to strong chemicals during dental treatment. Incompletely cured dental materials containing monomers and polymers that come in contact

with the oral mucosa may result in tissue burns and necrosis. Care must be taken when using disinfecting agents such as phenols and hypochlorite to avoid tissue contact. Chemical burns usually heal without treatment once the offending agent has been removed.

Clinical Implications

Over-the-counter (OTC) liquid toothache remedies often contain strong chemicals. When overused, they may cause burns of the oral mucosa that are more severe and painful than the original toothache. Patients may end up with both the toothache they were originally trying to treat and a nasty mucosal burn. Burns caused by liquids may appear diffuse and irregular, corresponding to uncontrolled flow of the liquid.

Nicotine Stomatitis

Nicotine stomatitis occurs in smokers and is the result of exposure of the palate to the smoke and heat of burning tobacco products. It generally appears as a thick, white plaque of the hard and soft palate, containing scattered, tiny, raised red (erythematous) dots. The erythematous dots represent irritated minor salivary gland ducts (Fig. 2-26). Nicotine stomatitis persists as long as the individual continues smoking. The lesion itself is benign and will regress upon smoking cessation.

Clinical Implications

Lesions similar to nicotine stomatitis have been observed in nonsmokers who habitually drink excessively hot liquids such as tea or coffee.

Geographic Tongue (Erythema Migrans)

Geographic tongue is a common condition that may produce mild to moderate discomfort but is usually asymptomatic. The etiology is unknown, but biopsy specimens show an abundance of both acute and chronic inflammatory cells. The condition is most often seen on the tongue, but any mucosal surface may be affected. On-the-tongue lesions are referred to as geographic tongue; on other mucosal surfaces, the lesions are referred to as *erythema migrans*. After the lesions develop, they most often spontaneously regress, followed weeks to months later by recurrence in the same or another location. Geographic tongue

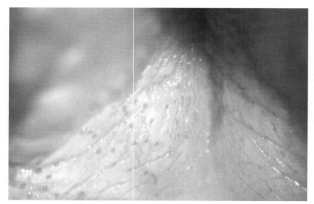

Figure 2–26   Nicotine stomatitis. Close-up view of dilated minor salivary ducts and hyperkeratosis of the palate in a smoker.

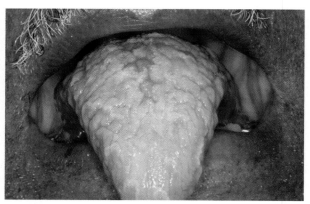

Figure 2–27   Geographic tongue. Characteristic asymmetrical well-demarcated areas of the erythematous mucosal atrophy, surrounded by circinate white or yellowish border.

presents as asymmetrical well-demarcated areas of erythematous mucosal atrophy, surrounded by white or yellowish circinate (circular or ring-shaped), slightly elevated borders (Fig. 2-27). Filiform papillae are absent inside these areas, which may appear as "bald" spots on the tongue. Patients may experience sensitivity to salty or acidic foods. This is due to dramatic thinning of the protective mucosa. Although the mucosa becomes atrophic and thin, no ulcerations develop. There is no treatment for geographic tongue. Patients may use palliative analgesic medications to control any sensitivity.

Clinical Implications

Many patients with geographic tongue wonder if their condition was precipitated by drinking hot coffee, resulting in scalding or burning, or by eating excessively spicy foods. In fact, the lesions of geographic tongue occur first, leaving an asymptomatic atrophic surface that is then vulnerable to irritation by heat or spices. Patients often only become aware of the lesions when something hot or spicy triggers a painful episode.

Hematoma

Hematoma is a form of submucosal hemorrhage. It presents as a red to dark blue elevated mass seen when a patient experiences minor trauma that causes rupture of blood vessels. During the traumatic event, blood escapes into the surrounding connective tissues, causing enlargement of the tissue as the blood fills the area. Additional predisposing causes for submucosal

hemorrhage include anticoagulant disorders (see Chapter 9) and infections (see Chapter 3).

Foreign Body Reaction

Foreign body reaction occurs when irritating foreign material is introduced into tissues and an inflammatory response is evoked. In addition to inflammation, scarring and/or encapsulation of foreign material may occur. Modified macrophages, called foreign body giant cells, form and attempt to digest and destroy the foreign material. If this attempt is unsuccessful, a granulomatous inflammatory response that walls off the foreign material occurs. Clinically, this produces a swelling that is firm and usually nonpainful. Treatment is excision of the granulomatous tissue. Foreign body reactions are often not suspected until the presence of foreign material is confirmed with a biopsy.

Clinical Implications

Foreign body gingivitis results from introduction of fine particles into abraded gingiva during dental procedures. These particles may be from pastes used in prophylaxis, or restorative materials that come in contact with abraded gingiva.

Keloid

Keloids are abnormal proliferations of scar tissue resulting from excess collagen production during healing. Individuals of African, Polynesian, and South Pacific descent, with darker skin colors, are at increased risk for developing these lesions. Keloids may appear as raised, hairless areas or fibrous nodules, varying from pink to flesh-colored or red to dark brown (Fig. 2-28). They often have a firm, rubbery texture and a smooth, shiny surface. Keloids may be accompanied by severe itchiness and pain as well as changes in texture. They may occur at the site of minor scratches and cuts, body piercings, severe acne, infected wounds, surgical incisions, or areas of repeated trauma. Treatment includes corticosteroids; however, the best treatment involves prevention whenever possible.

Body Piercing

Body piercing is currently in style in the United States; however, this form of body adornment has been practiced for thousands of years. Body piercing may occur anywhere on the body, including face, nose, ears, and lips. Piercings in the oral cavity, especially in adolescents and young adults, are seen most commonly on the tongue and lips. Complications of piercing such as pain, bleeding, swelling, foreign body reaction, and infection may occur. Damage to the lingual nerve may be experienced at the piercing site as well as infections. Contact between metal rings and/or studs that hit the teeth may result in chipped or fractured teeth. Tongue piercings have also been reported to contribute to gaps between the front teeth and altered periodontal status, including receding gingiva.

Proliferative Repair Responses

Proliferative repair responses occur whenever the normal healing process becomes exaggerated and overproduction of granulation tissue and other wound repair products result.

Pyogenic Granulomas

Pyogenic granulomas are exophytic lesions composed of an exuberant overgrowth of granulation tissue in response to minor chronic irritation. The name is inaccurate because they are not due to pyogenic (pus-producing) bacteria and are not granulomas. Although they can occur anywhere on the body, pyogenic granulomas frequently occur on the gingiva as a result of local irritation, such as calculus (Fig. 2-29) or orthodontic appliances. These lesions may be either sessile or pedunculated masses that bleed easily on gentle probing, due to large numbers of engorged capillaries that produce the bright red to deep purple coloration. As the granulation tissue matures, there is less bleeding and redness (Fig. 2-30). Although some lesions regress with removal of the irritant, many require surgical excision. They generally do not recur after removal unless the irritant remains. Although there is a female predilection, pyogenic granulomas also occur in males in response to local irritation.

> ### Clinical Implications
>
> Pyogenic granulomas in the oral cavity occur frequently in pregnant women. This may be related to hormonal changes and/or an increased responsiveness to local irritants. During pregnancy they are frequently called *pregnancy tumor*s or *granuloma gravidarum*. These terms are misnomers because they are not tumors. In many cases, they resolve or become fibroma-like after delivery of the baby.

Traumatic (Irritation) Fibroma

Traumatic (irritation) fibromas are benign lesions composed of dense, highly fibrous connective tissue, similar to a scar (Fig. 2-31). They are more appropriately called *focal fibrous hyperplasia* to denote a reactive

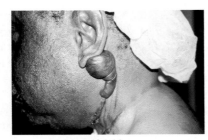

Keloids

Figure 2–28 Keloid scar. Man with keloid following trauma.

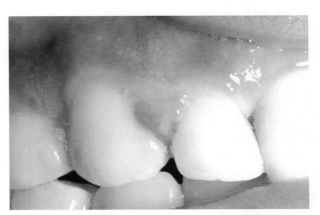

Figure 2–29 Pyogenic granuloma. Small pyogenic granuloma due to irritation of gingiva by subgingival calculus.

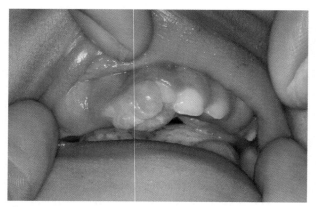

Figure 2–30 Pyogenic granuloma. Large pyogenic granuloma present for several months with decreased redness and bleeding.

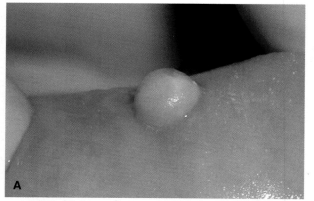

A

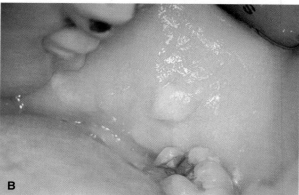

B

Figure 2–32 Traumatic fibromas. A. Pedunculated fibroma of lower lip. **B.** Secondary frictional keratosis can develop on the surface.

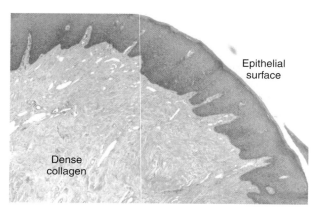

Epithelial surface

Dense collagen

Figure 2–31 Traumatic fibroma. Histologic appearance of a fibroma with surface epithelium and abundance of acellular dense fibrous scar-like collagen.

rather than neoplastic origin. They occur anywhere that persistent chronic tissue irritation occurs, most often along the line of occlusion, where repetitive trauma from biting may occur. They may be sessile or pedunculated with a pink smooth surface (Fig. 2-32A). Fibromas are usually several millimeters in diameter, but some may enlarge to 1 to 2 cm in diameter with repeated trauma. Secondary frictional keratosis can develop on the surface (Fig. 2-32B). Although fibromas are always benign, most are surgically removed to eliminate repeated trauma and/or rule out other lesions. Two lesions that must be ruled out are neurofibroma found in neurofibromatosis and mucosal neuroma found in multiple endocrine neoplasia (MEN) 2B (see Chapter 7). Fibromas usually do not recur once they are removed.

Traumatic Neuroma

Traumatic neuroma is an exuberant reactive non-neoplastic proliferation of nerve fibers occurring in response to traumatic or surgical transection of a portion of peripheral nerve. Traumatic neuromas appear as solitary smooth-surfaced nodules of normal, white or yellow soft tissue that is tender or painful. They are one of the few submucosal nodules that produce pain. They develop as the transected nerve attempts to regenerate and reestablish connection; however, this is prevented by the formation of scar tissue between ends of the transected fibers. Schwann cells grow through the scar, forming a disorganized nest of nerve endings. This extends into the surrounding soft tissue and forms an exophytic mass.

Traumatic neuromas may be found anywhere in the body. In the oral cavity they are most common at frequent sites of trauma, such as the mental foramen, lips, tongue and tooth extraction sites. Traumatic neuromas are unique among nerve sheath lesions in that involvement of the actual nerve ending leads to pain; most nerve sheath lesions are proliferations of Schwann cells without the nerve fiber. Treatment is surgical excision.

Verruciform Xanthoma

Verruciform xanthoma (VX) is a form of epithelial hyperplasia with a predilection for the oral cavity in middle-aged persons. It is an unusual lesion that is exceedingly rare in children under 10 years. The term *verruciform* means "wart-like," and the term *xanthoma* means "yellow tumor" or a subcutaneous collection of cholesterol. This is a misnomer because there is no cholesterol or fat present. The underlying connective tissue contains large vacuolated cells that appear to contain fat but are in fact large, foamy histiocytes. The clinical appearance is most commonly a solitary, well-defined, mildly exophytic, rough, white or yellow to reddish pink warty lesion less than 2 cm in diameter (Fig. 2-33). It is frequently misdiagnosed clinically as a papilloma, although human papillomavirus infection is not associated with VX. No definite etiology has been determined despite numerous investigations, but it is believed that verruciform xanthoma is an unusual reaction to mild epithelial trauma. Almost any part of the mouth can be involved, but the alveolar ridge and gingiva are the most common intraoral sites. Local surgical excision is almost always curative.

Injuries to the Gingiva

The term **epulis** is a nonspecific term used for tumors and tumor-like masses of the gingiva. There are numerous types of epuli (pl.), some of which are described here. Not all contain the word *epulis* in their name, and the term *peripheral* may be used to indicate that the lesion occurs in the soft tissues rather than within the bone.

Peripheral Ossifying Fibroma

Peripheral ossifying fibroma (POF) occurs on the gingiva and most often arises interproximally from the periodontal ligament space. The appearance is similar to a pyogenic granuloma because the surface is typically ulcerated and bleeds easily on probing. Microscopically, POFs contain small areas of dystrophic calcification, including osteoid or bone; hence the term *ossifying*. It is believed that these calcifications are deposited by osteoblasts associated with the periosteum of alveolar bone. Therefore, unlike pyogenic granulomas, these lesions are seen only in soft tissues overlying bone. The removal of POFs can be problematic, because the origin may be deep within the periodontal ligament space. Eradication may leave bony or soft tissue defects that need tissue augmentation. These lesions have a propensity to recur, especially if any residual cells remain following excision. Recurrent growth of this benign lesion may be quite rapid and worrisome.

Peripheral Giant Cell Granuloma

Peripheral giant cell granuloma (PGCG) appears to be a response to irritation or trauma of the gingiva or alveolar ridge. The lesions rarely reach a size greater than 2 cm and may be sessile or pedunculated. Clinically, they resemble pyogenic granulomas because they have an ulcerated surface and tend to bleed easily on probing. However, unlike pyogenic granulomas, they contain large numbers of giant cells of osteoclast origin and can occur only in soft tissues sites that cover bone. PGCGs contain areas of hemorrhage, which results in deposits of brownish hemosiderin pigment. This composition gives the lesion a blue to deep purple coloration. On occasion, PGCGs may produce resorption of the underlying bone, with a "cupped" pattern observed radiographically. PGCGs require complete excision and eradication of any stimulus. They rarely recur after excision (Fig. 2-34).

> ### Clinical Implications
>
> Pyogenic granuloma of the gingiva, peripheral ossifying fibroma, and peripheral giant cell granuloma all have a similar clinical appearance in the oral cavity. This can make them virtually impossible to tell apart. They are often referred to as *The Three P's.* A biopsy may be the only way to differentiate among these three lesions.

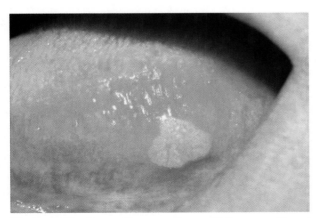

Figure 2–33   Verruciform xanthoma. Yellow wart-like appearance of verruciform xanthoma of lateral tongue.

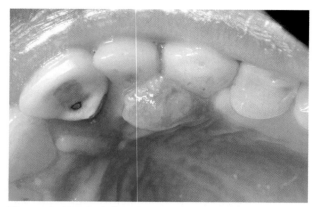

Figure 2–34 **Peripheral giant cell granuloma.** PGCG that bleeds easily on probing.

Localized Spongiotic Gingival Hyperplasia

Localized spongiotic gingival hyperplasia (LSGH) is a recently described condition first seen in children and adolescents but also found in adults. Lesions are often misinterpreted clinically as pyogenic granulomas because of their localized exophytic and erythematous appearance. The clinical presentation is a small, localized, papillary or velvety, bright red gingival overgrowth. They typically are located on the facial gingiva overlying the tooth root. Features that distinguish them clinically from pyogenic granulomas include a subtle papillary or finely granular surface not seen in pyogenic granulomas (Fig. 2-35). Unlike pyogenic granuloma, LSGH appears unrelated to plaque or calculus. It is refractory to conventional periodontal treatment and oral hygiene maintenance. Conservative surgical excision is generally curative, but recurrence is not rare.

Epulis Granulomatosum

Epulis granulomatosum is a postsurgical lesion that appears as a gingival mass extruding from a nonhealing socket following extraction (Fig. 2-36). This location is a pathognomonic feature for epulis granulomatosa. Under the microscope, they are identical to pyogenic granulomas. Epulis granulomatosum may be mistaken for a foreign body granuloma or a pyogenic granuloma. These lesions can be worrisome and may resemble cancer metastasis or lymphoma. Treatment is surgical excision with debridement of the socket.

Pericoronitis

Pericoronitis refers to inflammation of the gingival tissues around partially erupted teeth, most often third molars. Erupting molars are often partially covered by a flap or hood of fibrotic tissue known as an **operculum**. Bacteria and food debris become easily trapped under an operculum. Tissues become inflamed due to mechanical trauma from opposing dentition and/or poor oral hygiene (Fig. 2-37). Pain and swelling in pericoronitis can mimic more serious conditions. Treatment includes control of local infection, followed by debridement, and eventual removal of the tooth if it is impacted.

Drug-Induced Gingival Overgrowth (Drug-Induced Gingival Hyperplasia)

There are many causes for gingival overgrowth or hyperplasia. *Drug-induced gingival overgrowth* is considered a reactive phenomenon seen in patients taking medications that stimulate collagen growth or prevent its breakdown. It is well documented that phenytoin (Dilantin), cyclosporine, nifedipine, and other calcium

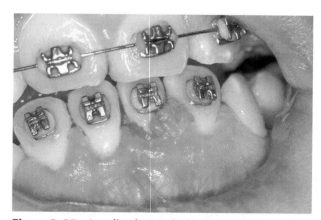

Figure 2–35 **Localized spongiotic gingival hyperplasia (LSGH).** Young orthodontic patient with localized reactive lesion that does not bleed on probing.

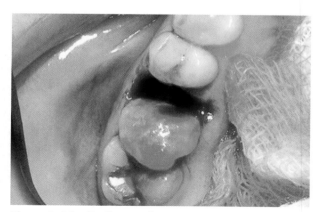

Figure 2–36 **Epulis granulomatosum.** Mass of granulation tissue arising in extraction site.

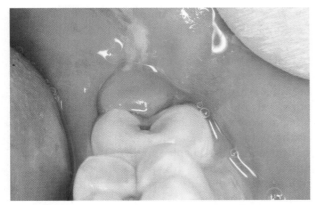

Figure 2–37 **Pericoronitis.** Flap of inflamed tissue over partially erupted third molar.

channel blockers may lead to gingival overgrowth (Fig. 2-38). Clinically, the lesions are similar and do not differ based on type of drug. Correlation with the patient's medical and medication history is essential in making this diagnosis. Treatment is gingivectomy. Drug discontinuation or substitution may be needed to control or prevent further overgrowth.

Traumatic Salivary Gland Disorders

Trauma to the salivary glands is not rare. Minor glands are more frequently involved than are major glands. This is most likely due to their close proximity to the oral mucosal surface, where the ducts can be more easily injured.

Mucous Retention and Extravasation Phenomena

Mucoceles result from trauma that severs, or cuts, a salivary gland excretory duct, resulting in spillage (extravasation)

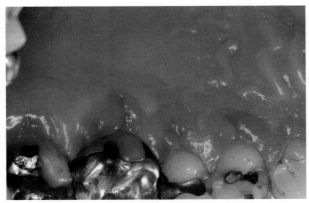

Figure 2–38 **Gingival overgrowth.** Patient on nifedipine for hypertension with drug-induced gingival enlargement.

of mucin into the surrounding soft tissues (Fig. 2-39). The spilled mucin then is surrounded by a layer of granulation tissue, which creates a localized fluctuant swelling. Mucoceles of minor salivary gland origin are also referred to as *mucous extravasation phenomenon* and *mucous escape reaction*. They are characterized by nontender, mobile, fluctuant dome-shaped enlargements with intact overlying epithelium. This may be present from a few days to months. Mucoceles close to the surface may have a bluish to translucent hue (Fig. 2-39), whereas deeper lesions are covered by normal-colored mucosa (Fig. 2-40). Mucoceles can be secondarily traumatized by biting and chewing. When this occurs, hyperkeratosis may result, giving the mucocele a white surface (Fig. 2-41). The most common location is the lower lip, but lesions can occur anywhere there are salivary glands. The patient may relate a history of trauma to the mouth or a habit of biting the lip; however, in many cases no injury can be identified.

 Clinical Implications

Mucoceles are rare on the upper lip. Therefore, any mass resembling a mucocele on the upper lip should be viewed with suspicion. The upper lip is a common location for minor salivary gland tumors. These may contain mucus that causes them to resemble a mucocele.

Ranulas

Ranulas are mucoceles that occur in the floor of the mouth within the submandibular or sublingual glands lateral to the midline. The name is derived from the appearance of the underbelly of a frog (Latin for frog = *rana*) (Fig. 2-42). *Oral ranulas* are mucus extravasation phenomena that lie superior to the mylohyoid muscle, whereas *cervical* or *plunging ranulas* lie below

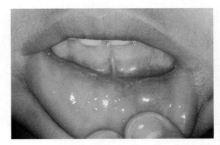

Figure 2–39 **Mucocele.** Lower lip of a child who fell.

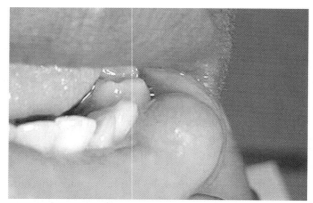

Figure 2–40 Mucocele. Deeper lesion covered by normal-colored mucosa.

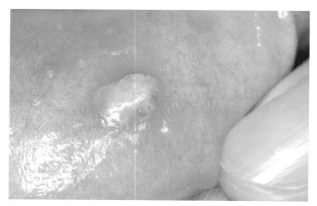

Figure 2–41 Mucocele with keratosis. Traumatized mucocele; biting or chewing resulted in white hyperkeratotic appearance.

the mylohyoid muscle. Trauma to the floor of the mouth or neck region may be associated with the development of a ranula. There may be a prior history of oral surgical procedures or treatment for a sialolith (salivary gland stone). Swelling of the floor of the mouth is usually painless. Oral ranulas may be large, unilateral, and blue-to-translucent and do not blanch on compression. Ranulas located in the deeper aspect of the floor of the mouth may not have the bluish translucent color. Displacement of the tongue by a ranula may interfere with speech, mastication, respiration, and swallowing. Surgical management is the preferred treatment.

Superficial Mucoceles

Superficial mucoceles involve minor gland ducts close to the mucosal surface and are caused by mucosal inflammation rather than blockage, dilatation, or rupture of the duct. They are typically tiny, clear, bubble-like lesions located in the soft palate, the retromolar region, and the posterior buccal mucosa (Fig. 2-43). Patients with xerostomia may experience them at a higher rate. They generally rupture spontaneously.

Salivary Gland Duct Cyst

Salivary gland duct cyst is a mucus retention phenomenon also called *mucus retention cyst* or *sialocyst*. It is clinically similar to a mucocele but is caused by blockage of the salivary duct rather than cutting of the duct. Mucoceles outnumber mucus retention cysts by a ratio of 15:1. The most common cause of blockage is a sialolith (salivary gland stone). Saliva backs up, causing expansion of the duct. These cysts are treated with conservative surgical excision. When they involve the

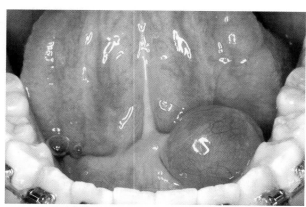

Figure 2–42 Ranula. Ranula (mucocele) in the floor of the mouth.

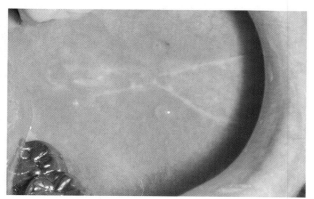

Figure 2–43 Superficial mucocele. Clear, bubble-like lesion in the buccal mucosa.

major glands, partial or total removal of the affected gland may be necessary.

Cysts of Blandin-Nuhn

Cysts of Blandin-Nuhn are either mucoceles or mucous duct cysts that form in the glands of Blandin and Nuhn. These mixed mucous and serous glands are embedded in the anterior ventral surface of the tongue. Although the lesions are similar to mucoceles, they tend to be pedunculated rather than sessile and dome-shaped (Fig. 2-44). Because of repeated trauma against the lower teeth, their surface may be red and white. Treatment is surgical excision.

> ### Clinical Implications
>
> Some mucoceles, mucous duct cysts, and ranulas resolve spontaneously, especially in young children. Surgical excision of the mucocele along with the adjacent associated minor salivary glands is recommended for lesions that persist. Unfortunately, surgery runs the risk of cutting another duct, causing what appears to be a recurrence of the lesion, when in fact a new one may have been created.

Necrotizing Sialometaplasia

Necrotizing sialometaplasia is a localized reactive lesion that often causes concern because of its clinical resemblance to a neoplasm. Seventy-five percent of all cases occur in the minor glands of the posterior hard palate, but the condition can be found in the minor glands of the retromolar pads, labial/buccal mucosa,

and tongue. The name of the lesion reflects the underlying necrosis of the minor salivary glands (*necrotizing sialo-*) and change in the ducts from cuboidal epithelium to stratified squamous epithelium (*metaplasia*). The etiology is believed to be vascular ischemia caused by trauma, vasoconstriction from dental injection, adjacent developing tumor, infection, or other ischemic events.

Necrotizing sialometaplasia most often is painless, but occasional discomfort or numbness has been reported. It initially appears as a single swelling or cluster of smaller swellings that eventually ulcerate, leaving a crater-like lesion with rounded borders (Fig. 2-45). Without treatment, these changes gradually return to normal in about 5 to 6 weeks.

> ### Clinical Implications
>
> Necrotizing sialometaplasia may resemble oral squamous cell carcinoma. Keep in mind that although the most common location for necrotizing sialometaplasia is the hard palate, this is a rare location for oral squamous cell carcinoma.

Sialolithiasis

Sialolithiasis refers to the formation of calcifications or "stones" in the salivary glands (stone in Latin = *lith*). Salivary gland stones are often seen in salivary glands affected by chronic infection and/or dehydration; however, in many cases the cause is unknown. Stones are most commonly found in the submandibular glands, where they can obstruct Wharton's duct (Fig. 2-46). Prior to and during meals, when salivation

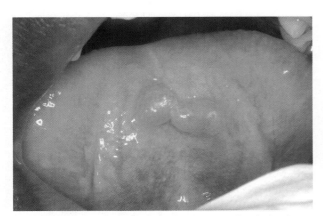

Figure 2-44   Cyst of Blandin-Nuhn. Glands of Blandin-Nuhn present either as a mucocele or mucous duct cyst.

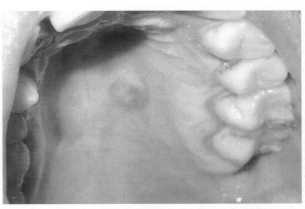

Figure 2-45   Necrotizing sialometaplasia. Painless swelling of minor salivary glands with rounded borders and necrotic center.

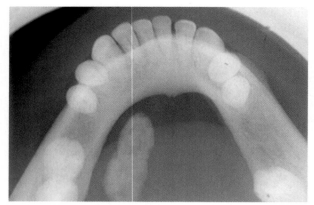

Figure 2–46 Sialolith. Sialoliths may be long and slender due to the shape of the duct in which they form.

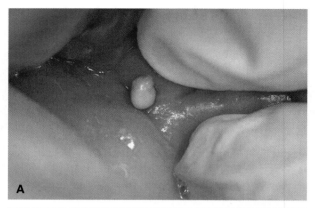

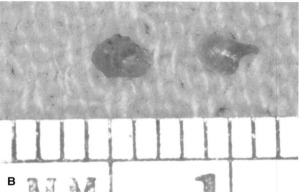

Figure 2–47 Sialolith. A. Clinical photo of sialolith. **B.** Sialoliths that have been surgically removed.

increases, pain may result from backup of the saliva into the affected gland. Diagnosis is made based on this characteristic history, plus physical and radiographic findings. Complications of persistent obstruction include risk of bacterial infection that requires antibiotic therapy. Small stones may go undetected radiographically, but the patient may experience symptoms consistent with sialolithiasis. Expulsion of sialoliths may occur with increased salivation associated with tart or sour foods (Fig. 2-47A and B). Surgical removal may be necessary for larger sialoliths or those located deep within the gland.

Sialadenosis

Sialadenosis is nonneoplastic, noninflammatory salivary gland enlargement, usually of the parotid gland. The cause is believed to be peripheral neuropathy of the autonomic nerve supply of the salivary glands, leading to disordered secretory activity in acinar cells. Patients experience a nonpainful, slowly enlarging, firm swelling of the face. In 50 percent of cases, the condition is associated with underlying systemic factors, including endocrine disorders such as diabetes, hypothyroidism, bulimia, malnutrition, alcohol abuse, and drugs. Patients who take certain antihypertensive or psychotropic drugs may experience **sialadenosis** as a side effect. Symptoms regress once the underlying cause is addressed.

Adenomatoid Hyperplasia

Adenomatoid hyperplasia is an increase in the size of minor salivary glands due to an increase in the number of gland acini. This creates a firm, nontender mass covered by normal mucosa often mimicking a minor salivary gland tumor. The most common location is the hard palate, but this can occur anywhere there is minor salivary gland tissue. The diagnosis is generally not suspected and only becomes apparent after surgical excision.

Denture and Prosthesis-Related Injury

Many patients wear prosthetic appliances to replace missing teeth or oral tissues. They are constructed of many different biocompatible materials but some patients may be allergic to them. Worn or broken dentures or partials may irritate the adjacent oral mucosa, leading to injury, inflammation, and repair. Selected specific forms of denture injury are discussed.

Denture Stomatitis

Denture stomatitis is a nonspecific term that refers to a number of different conditions that present as generalized inflammation of denture-bearing tissues. The mucosa may show erythema, edema, or reactive tissue hyperplasia. The most common cause of denture stomatitis is an ill-fitting denture that may lead to inflammation of the mucosa (Fig. 2-48). Other

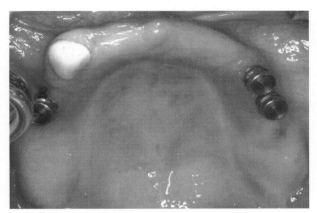

Figure 2–48 Denture stomatitis. Common result from an ill-fitting denture.

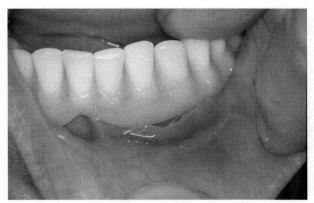

Figure 2–49 Epulis fissuratum. Firm excess tissue at the flange of the denture resembling "waves crashing on the shore."

causes of denture stomatitis include *Candida albicans* infection (see Chapter 3), allergy to denture acrylic (see Chapter 4), continuous wearing of the denture, and poor denture hygiene. The lesions are rarely symptomatic, but occasionally patients complain of mild burning. Replacement or adjustment of the prosthesis often leads to resolution of symptoms.

Epulis Fissuratum

Epulis fissuratum is a benign condition that occurs along the flange (edge) of an ill-fitting or loose denture. The most common location is the buccal or labial vestibules. The overgrowth of tissue represents a protective attempt to minimize or prevent displacement of the denture into adjacent delicate tissues. It is more frequent in the anterior oral cavity. Thick, hyperplastic folds of tissue form in response to biting forces. These folds surround denture flanges, sometimes resembling a "wave breaking on the shore" (Fig. 2-49).

 Clinical Implications

The hyperplastic tissues of epulis fissuratum perpetuate an unstable base for ill-fitting dentures in the oral cavity. Lesions are surgically removed prior to the fabrication of any new dental appliance.

Fibroepithelial Polyp

Fibroepithelial polyp also forms because of an ill-fitting denture. Instead of forming at the edge of the denture, this lesion forms on the palate under the denture. Characteristics include a flattened but pedunculated mass that usually has a serrated edge (Fig. 2-50). It sits

snugly into the palate, sometimes causing a cup-shaped deformity. Treatment is surgical excision before construction of a new denture.

Inflammatory Papillary Hyperplasia

Inflammatory papillary hyperplasia is a form of denture stomatitis that most frequently occurs on the hard palate under complete upper or partial dentures. It is asymptomatic and, as the name implies, is papillary or pebbly. Papillary hyperplasia is erythematous and velvety smooth to the touch (Fig. 2-51). The condition is thought to occur as a result of mild chronic irritation. It seems to occur with greater frequency in individuals who wear their dentures continuously or whose dentures are ill-fitting. Poor oral hygiene and denture cleanliness also have been implicated. Rarely, candidal microorganisms have been isolated in papillary hyperplasia but may be secondary to the condition. Inflammatory papillary hyperplasia has been observed in dentate patients with narrow, high-vaulted palates.

 Clinical Implications

Inflammatory papillary hyperplasia is most often diagnosed based on clinical features. Care must be taken not to mistake it for candidiasis (see Chapter 3). If it creates an unstable base for new denture fabrication, surgical removal may be indicated. Good denture and oral hygiene home care can help control this condition.

Denture Ulcer

Denture ulcers are caused by acute or chronic trauma at the flange (edge) of a prosthesis that is rough or ill fitting. The appearance is that of a traumatic ulcer,

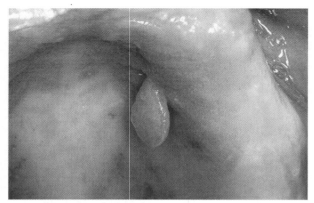

Figure 2–50   Fibroepithelial polyp. Lesion on the palate from an ill-fitting denture.

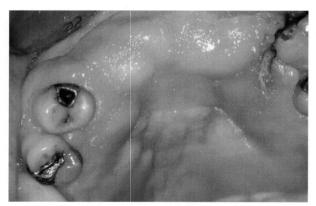

Figure 2–51   Inflammatory papillary hyperplasia. Bright red micropapillary tissue with velvety smooth texture under ill-fitting partial denture.

with a yellow necrotic center and erythematous border (Fig. 2-52). Inspection of the denture adjacent to the ulcer may reveal roughness or irregularity. Adjustment or smoothing of the denture and placement of a medicated tissue conditioner can bring relief.

Peri-implantitis

Peri-implantitis is the term for inflammation around dental implants. Inflammation may be confined to the soft tissues but can extend down to the bone tissue supporting the implant. Extension into bone may be a sign of impending implant failure. When supporting bone is involved, implant removal may be indicated.

Subpontine Hyperostosis

Subpontine hyperostosis is an overgrowth of bone occurring on the edentulous ridge underneath the pontic of a fixed bridge. Patients initially complain that they are no longer able to clean under the bridge with dental

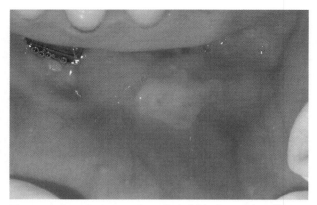

Figure 2–52   Denture ulcer. Painful lesion with yellow necrotic center and red halo where denture rubs continuously.

floss. Chronic irritation and functional stresses from the bridge are thought to be the cause. Treatment is surgical recontouring of the alveolar ridge to reduce impingement of bone overgrowth below the pontic (Fig. 2-53).

Pulpal Injury and Its Sequelae

Dental pulp can be injured in a number of ways. The resulting inflammatory response may extend to the periapical tissues, including the periodontal ligament and supporting bone. The tissues react to produce a variety of clinical signs and symptoms, which are summarized in Table 2-9.

Pulpitis

When injured, the dental pulp is susceptible to the same inflammatory changes seen in other soft tissues.

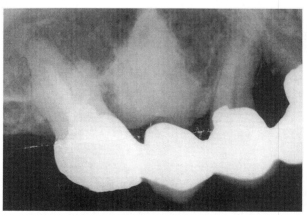

Figure 2–53   Subpontine hyperostosis. Well-defined radiopacity under pontic; patient complains of inability to floss beneath it.

Table 2.9	Sequelae of Pulpitis		
	Symptoms	**Tooth Vitality**	**Radiographic Features**
Apical Periodontitis (apical inflammation/ infection) a) acute or b) chronic (granuloma)	Symptomatic or Asymptomatic	+/-	None to slight widening of the PDL Ill to well-defined radiolucency
Apical Abscess a) acute or b) chronic	Symptomatic or Asymptomatic	-	None to well-defined radiolucency Sinus tract may form with chronic or long-standing infection
Apical Scar	None	-	Previous surgical endodontic treatment
Dystrophic Calcification/ Pulp stone	None	+/-	Radiopaque spherules within pulp
Condensing osteitis	None or history of mild trauma, caries and/or pain	+/-	Diffuse radiopacity that conforms to trabecular bone; no radiolucent rim

+ = vital
+/- = equivocal-positive to some tests but not others
- = nonvital
PDL = periodontal ligament

Diagnostic tests are often used to assess the health and vitality of the pulp. *Pulpitis* is inflammation of the pulp. A common symptom of pulpitis is increased sensitivity to heat or cold stimuli. Pulpitis may be due to bacterial invasion from the caries process or traumatic events. The fact that the pulp is encased within hard tooth structure (dentin) may contribute to symptoms of pulpitis commonly referred to as "toothache" or *odontalgia*. Inflammation of the pulp may be *reversible* or *irreversible*, depending on the extent of damage.

Chronic Hyperplastic Pulpitis (Pulp Polyp)

Chronic hyperplasic pulpitis is a dome-shaped growth of granulation tissue originating from the pulp. Often called a *pulp polyp*, it extrudes through the open occlusal surface of a carious or fractured tooth. Pulp polyps are most often seen in molars of children with immature root formation (open apical foramina). This is in contrast to adult teeth in which the foramen is more restricted (Fig. 2-54).

Apical Abscess

Apical abscess is an inflammatory response to bacterial infection and/or necrosis of the dental pulp. It is a form of liquefactive necrosis that involves the formation of purulent exudate (pus). Swelling, tissue edema, and pain are prominent features.

A drainage channel from the abscess to the epithelial or mucosal surface can occur over time, often over or near the root apex. These channels are known as *sinus tracts* (Fig. 2-55A). The terms *fistula* and *sinus tract* are often used interchangeably, which is incorrect. Strictly defined, an abnormal channel originating deep within tissues and extending to the epithelial or mucosal surface is known as a sinus tract. A dental abscess that drains from the apex of a tooth through bone to the oral mucosal surface is an example. In the oral cavity,

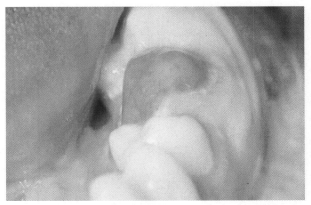

Figure 2–54 Pulp polyp. Young patient with necrotic pulp extruding from large carious lesion.

once the drainage tract reaches the oral mucosa, a mass of granulation tissue referred to as a **parulis** may form and be seen clinically. Strictly defined, fistulas are considered abnormal connections or pathways between two anatomic spaces or body cavities. An example is an orofacial fistula, in which infection from the oral cavity drains out through the skin surface (epithelium).

In some cases, dental abscess drainage may need to be established by the clinician. This can be achieved in two ways. The first is by establishing access through the crown of the tooth. The second is by a procedure known as incision and drainage (I & D), in which a small incision is made into the soft tissues to provide drainage (Fig. 2-55B). Irrigation with normal saline will assist in removal of purulent material. Then the patient's immune defenses, combined with dental treatment (and/or antibiotics), should resolve the problem.

Untreated dental abscesses can produce severe and life-threatening consequences. Infection can travel long distances along fascial planes and cause what are known as *space infections (cellulitis)*. In the maxilla, infection can spread to the cavernous sinus of the brain, where it can cause lethal thrombosis and blockage of cerebral vessels. This may result in cerebral infarction (stroke). Infection from the mandible can travel down fascial planes to enclose the throat. This can result in a life-threatening condition known as *Ludwig's angina*, in which breathing is severely compromised.

Radiolucent Periapical Pathology

Radiographically, lesions that affect the pulp and periapical tissues may present with radiolucent features if the disease process destroys the periapical bone.

Apical Granuloma (Chronic Apical Periodontitis)

Apical granuloma (chronic apical periodontitis) consists of a mass of granulation tissue comprised of fibroblasts and chronic inflammatory cells at the apex of a nonvital tooth caused by pulp necrosis. The tooth may be asymptomatic and the lesion discovered on routine radiographs. Excessive granulation tissue and inflammation result in bone loss at the apex, causing a radiolucency (Fig. 2-56). Lesions are treated by endodontic therapy that removes the source of the inflammation, which is bacterial contamination from a necrotic pulp. Endodontic treatment and host defenses lead to repair of the apical bone.

Apical Cyst and Lateral Radicular Cyst

Apical cysts develop around the apices of nonvital teeth. Mediators of inflammation stimulate the epithelial rests of Malassez to proliferate and form a cyst lining. A lumen or central cavity eventually forms that contains necrotic inflammatory debris. This debris attracts fluids by osmotic gradient into the lumen, which then causes the cyst to expand outward and increase in

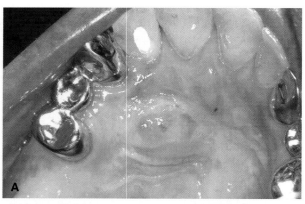

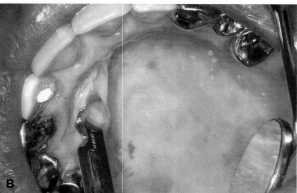

Figure 2–55 Apical abscess. A. Drainage channel (sinus tract). **B.** Incision performed to allow purulent material to drain.

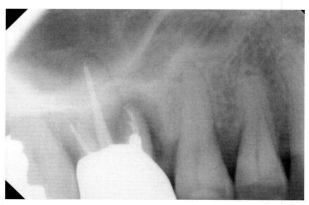

Figure 2–56 Chronic apical periodontitis (granuloma). Necrotic pulp treated with root canal therapy.

size. Resultant outward pressure destroys adjacent periapical bone, causing a radiolucent appearance (Fig. 2-57A). Cysts may develop along the tooth root in association with accessory lateral canals from the pulp. In this location they are called *lateral radicular cysts* (Fig. 2-57B).

Apical and lateral radicular cysts are most often indicative of pulp necrosis. The treatment is either endodontic therapy or extraction. If a tooth is extracted and the cyst or its lining is not completely removed, a *residual cyst* may result (Fig. 2-57C).

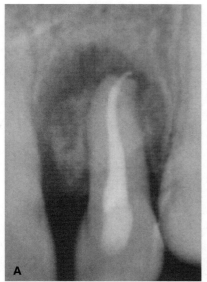

> ### Clinical Implications
>
> It is impossible to differentiate between chronic apical periodontitis and apical cyst on routine radiographs. Biopsy of the affected tissues with histopathologic evaluation is the only way to distinguish between them.

Apical Scar

Apical scars most often occur as radiolucent lesions around the apices of teeth with a history of prior surgical endodontic treatment (root end resection/root end fill). They are composed of dense fibrous connective tissue and sometimes residual chronic inflammation. Apical scars cannot be differentiated radiographically from apical cysts or granulomas. Diagnosis of an apical scar is made from excised apical tissues submitted for biopsy.

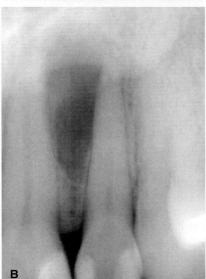

Internal Resorption

Resorption of dental hard tissues originating in the pulp is known as *internal resorption*. This can be seen in cases of trauma or injury but often the etiology is unknown. Radiographically, there is enlargement of the pulp chamber or canal, often with an irregular outline (Fig. 2-58). Occasionally, the crown of the tooth may appear reddish or pink, a condition referred to as "pink tooth of Mummery." This is caused by hyperplastic, highly vascular pulp tissue filling in areas that are resorbed. In many cases, the resorption is only detected radiographically and cannot be seen clinically. If left untreated, perforation through the root or crown may occur. Endodontic therapy can often stop this destructive process.

Radiopaque Periapical Pathology

Radiographically, lesions that affect the pulp and apical tissues may present with radiopaque features if the disease process causes tissues to calcify rather than undergo destruction.

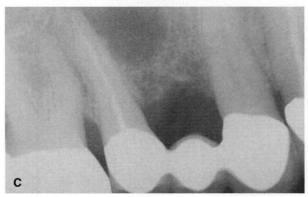

Figure 2–57   Apical cyst. A. Root canal therapy failed to resolve this apical cyst. **B.** Lateral radicular cyst. **C.** Residual cyst left behind after tooth extraction.

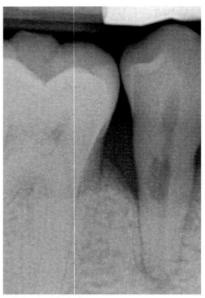

Figure 2–58 Internal resorption. Irregular enlargement of pulp canal of second premolar.

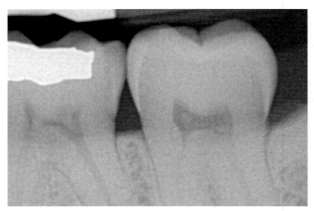

Figure 2–59 Pulp stones. Radiopaque flecks within pulp chamber of first and second molars.

Pulp Canal Obliteration and Pulp Stones

Pulp calcification often occurs due to chronic inflammation of the pulp. Total obliteration and calcification of the pulp chamber and canal can occur over time.

Pulp stones are an example of pathologic calcification that occurs within the dental pulp. Pulp stones are typically asymptomatic and found on routine radiographs (Fig. 2-59).

Usually associated with long-standing chronic pulpitis, pulp stones are believed to form around a nidus (center) of foreign material that may include necrotic bacteria or cell remnants. They may be solitary or multiple and may be free within the pulp or attached to the walls of the pulp chamber or root canal. Pulp stones may be of two types: those composed of dystrophic calcified material or those containing dentin with tubules and surrounded by odontoblasts. In the latter case, these are known as *denticles*. Incidence of pulp stones increases with age and is associated with some inherited disorders.

Condensing Osteitis

Condensing osteitis refers to localized areas of bone sclerosis or scarring. This is thought to represent a localized bony reaction to a low-grade inflammatory stimulus, such as from a diseased or necrotic pulp. The adjacent bone shows increased density. Condensing osteitis appears as a uniform zone of increased radiopacity

in bone adjacent to teeth with large caries or extensive restorations (Fig. 2-60). Typically, there is no expansion of alveolar bone. This disorder is seen most commonly near roots of posterior teeth. There is no radiolucent border around the area of increased bone density, a feature that helps to differentiate it from *focal cementoosseous dysplasia* (page 64). Lesions that remain following endodontic treatment or extraction are referred to as *bone scars* or *dense bone islands*.

Osteomyelitis

Osteomyelitis is a general term that refers to any inflammation of bone. It may result from trauma, dental infections, neoplastic conditions, radiation therapy, medications, and other etiologies. When dental infection in periapical bone becomes overwhelming, osteomyelitis may result. The process may involve the periosteum, resulting in both soft tissue swelling and bone expansion

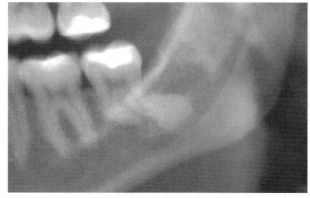

Figure 2–60 Condensing osteitis. Well-defined radiopacity developed following extraction of third molar.

(Fig. 2-61). If the periosteum is involved, the term *periostitis* is used.

Bony Sequestrum and Involucrum

Alveolar bone can fracture in cases of trauma and/or during tooth extraction. Fractured pieces of bone become necrotic when detached from their blood supply. These may appear radiopaque (Fig. 2-62A). A single fragment is called a *sequestrum*; multiple pieces are referred to as *sequestra*. Sequestra of bone can work their way through oral tissues to the surface, where they are lost. They often feel like a small, sharp, nonpainful sliver to the patient (Fig. 2-62B). If the bone spicule or fragment does not work its way out and is retained within and surrounded by vital bone, it is called an *involucrum* (pl., *involucra*).

Ankylosis

Ankylosis is solid fixation of cementum of tooth roots to alveolar bone caused by obliteration of the periodontal ligament. Without the periodontal ligament suspending the tooth in the socket, cementum fuses to alveolar bone, preventing the tooth from further eruption. The causes for ankylosis vary and include inflammation or infection, abnormal bone metabolism, excessive occlusal pressure, and physical trauma. It is primarily seen in children and deciduous teeth but may occur in adults (Fig. 2-63). Ankylosis can be recognized clinically by failure of a tooth to fully erupt. The occlusal surface of ankylosed teeth appears lower than adjacent teeth. Radiographically, there is lack of identifiable periodontal ligament around the tooth roots. Ankylosis makes tooth extraction difficult.

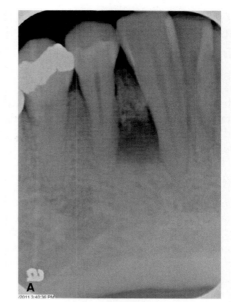

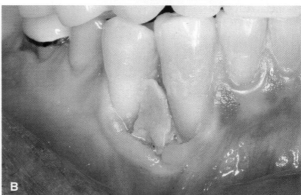

Figure 2–62   Sequestrum. A. Radiographic appearance of sequestrum. **B.** Sequestrum between canine and premolar.

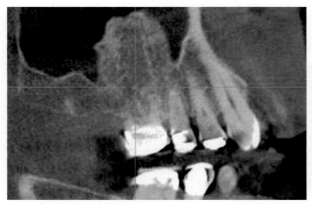

Figure 2–61   Osteomyelitis. Painful expansion of osteomyelitis into sinus space.

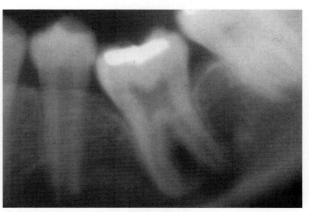

Figure 2–63   Ankylosis. Mandibular first molar failed to erupt and lies below the occlusal table.

CLINICAL AND RADIOGRAPHIC FEATURES OF ORAL HARD TISSUE INJURY

Bone Injury

Although we think of bone as hard and impervious, it is a vital living tissue that is subject to injury. The cells in the bone (osteoblasts, osteocytes, and osteoclasts) are metabolically active and can attempt to repair injury and restore the effects of disease. These processes produce changes that can be seen radiographically.

Cemento-osseous Dysplasia

Cemento-osseous dysplasia (COD) is a reactive disorder of bone that exclusively affects the tooth-bearing areas of the jaws. It is believed to arise from fibroblasts of the periodontal ligament but may represent a defect in bone remodeling. The condition was once called *cementoma*, but this term is no longer used. It represents a series of alterations in normal bone in which bone fails to mature properly (dysplasia). COD is more commonly seen in

females in the fourth to sixth decades of life, although males are also affected. CODs most often appear in the bone surrounding the roots of teeth; however, this is *not* related to pulpal pathology.

Lesions develop in three stages, each with unique radiographic appearances. The first is the *osteolytic stage.* This is characterized by replacement of normal bone with loose fibrous connective tissue. Radiographically, this presents as a well-defined radiolucency around the roots of a tooth or teeth (Fig. 2-64A). Early lesions often mimic periapical pathology but differ in that the teeth are vital. After the radiolucent fibrous tissue forms, the second stage, the *osteoblastic stage*, begins with calcification of the fibrous connective tissue. Small droplet calcifications form and coalesce. During this stage, the radiographic features become mixed radiolucent/radiopaque with a radiolucent border (Fig. 2-64B). This process is progressive, with the oldest, most calcified portion in the center and the newer, more fibrous portion at the periphery. The final stage, the *maturation*

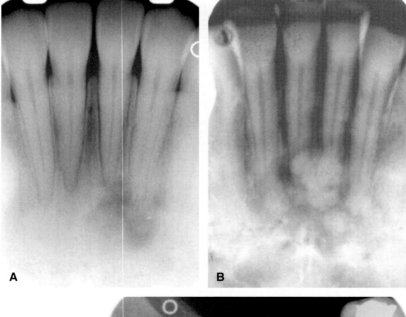

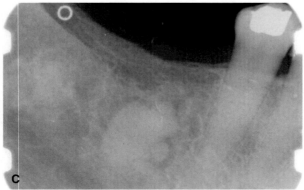

Figure 2–64 **Three stages of cemento-osseous dysplasia (COD). A.** Stage 1: Osteolytic stage. Radiograph showing well-defined radiolucency around the roots. **B.** Stage 2: Osteoblastic stage. Mixed radiolucent-radiopaque lesions, no bony expansion. **C.** Stage 3: Maturation/end stage. Solid radiopaque mass with distinct radiolucent rim.

stage, is characterized by uniformly radiopaque appearance with a radiolucent rim. This is also referred to as *end-stage COD* (Fig. 2-64C). New bone is poorly formed and less vascular than the bone it replaced. There is no soft tissue swelling or bone expansion and the majority of lesions remain asymptomatic.

There are three clinical variants of cemento-osseous dysplasia. The main difference is in their clinical distribution (Table 2-10).

1. *Focal cemento-osseous dysplasia* (FCOD) is defined as COD that is confined to one quadrant. Depending on the stage of development at discovery, FCOD may be radiolucent, mixed radiolucent/radiopaque, or radiopaque with a radiolucent border. Lesions rarely measure more than 1.5 cm in diameter (Fig. 2-65). FCOD lesions most often are misinterpreted as periapical pathology related to tooth vitality. If teeth in the area have not been injured or are not diseased, they should be vital on pulp testing. No swelling or tenderness to palpation and no draining sinus tracts are present. Serial radiographs over time will demonstrate gradual progression from a radiolucent to a solid radiopaque lesion. Lesions do not respond to endodontic therapy because they are *not* caused by pulpal pathology. Once the diagnosis is confirmed, no treatment is necessary for focal cement-osseous dysplasia.

2. *Periapical cemental dysplasia* (PCOD) is a form of COD that is confined to the bone around the roots of the mandibular anterior teeth. Multiple tooth involvement from canine to canine may occur. Other than location, the radiographic features, as well as the signs, symptoms, and management, are identical to those of FCOD.

3. *Florid cemento-osseous dysplasia* (FICOD) is defined as COD involving two or more quadrants. This is

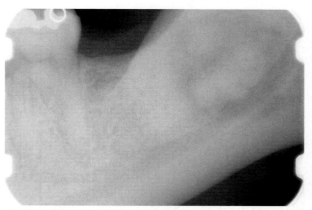

Figure 2–65 Focal cemento-osseous dysplasia (FCOD). Confined to one quadrant and rarely measuring more than 1.5 cm in diameter. Mixed radiolucent-radiopaque mass; no expansion of jaw.

not simply a large COD lesion but is a much more serious disorder with possible serious health consequences. FlCOD is more commonly observed in middle-aged patients of African descent. It appears as diffuse mixed radiolucent/radiopaque "moth-eaten" changes of the jaws that can resemble bone cancer. Lesions may be several centimeters in dimension (Fig. 2-66). As with other CODs, newly formed bone is poorly developed and relatively avascular. This has serious clinical implications. Due to poor vascular supply, the body cannot mount a typical inflammatory response when bacteria are present within FlCOD lesions. This can occur as a result of injury, caries, or periodontal disease. Antibiotics may not be especially helpful because there is compromised blood flow transporting them to the affected area. As a consequence, osteomyelitis may develop and

Table 2.10	Cemento-Osseous Dysplasia (COD)			
	Location (all in tooth-bearing areas)	**Radiographic Appearance**	**Clinical Features**	**Management**
Focal COD	Any area	Solitary mixed RL/RP with RL border	Teeth in area vital; asymptomatic, no jaw swelling	Biopsy to confirm; no treatment
Periapical COD	Confined to mandibular anterior teeth	Multiple discrete lesions; mixed RP/RL with RL border	Teeth vital; asymptomatic, no jaw swelling	Biopsy to confirm; no treatment
Florid COD	Two or more quadrants	Diffuse mixed RL/RP lesions with RL border	Teeth vital; will not resorb in edentulous areas; mild jaw swelling is rare	To prevent osteomyelitis: Do not biopsy! Confirm on radiographic and clinical features ALONE

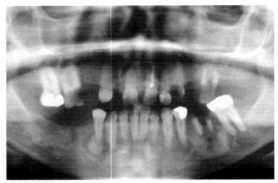

Figure 2–66 **Florid cemento-osseous dysplasia (FICOD).** Involves two or more quadrants. Lesions can be several centimeters in diameter. Diffuse radiolucent-radiopaque lesions in various stages of ossification. The noncarious teeth are vital, and there is no expansion of the jaw.

infected bone may become necrotic (osteonecrosis). Surgical removal of large portions of the jaw may be needed to control the spread of infection. This is not a problem with small lesions of FCOD that can rely on the healthy blood supply in adjacent normal bone to provide nutrients needed during healing after trauma.

Clinical Implications

Recognition of FICOD and prevention of bone infection are extremely important. Patients must be educated on how dental disease affects FICOD and how FICOD affects dental treatment. Preventing periapical pathology, periodontal disease, and tooth loss, along with early detection and clinical management, are critical.

Drug-Associated Osteonecrosis of the Jaw

Bisphosphonate-associated osteonecrosis of the jaw (BRONJ) is a recently discovered disorder found in patients who have received intravenous and/or oral forms of bisphosphonate therapy for bone-related conditions such as Paget disease, multiple myeloma, cancer that has metastasized to bone, and osteoporosis. Bisphosphonates attempt to preserve bone remodeling by interfering with osteoclasts that normally resorb old bone. Patients on intravenous medications are at higher risk for this disorder than those taking oral medications for osteoporosis. Table 2-11 lists some of the drugs implicated in BRONJ. BRONJ can occur following accidental or surgical trauma to the jaw bone, such as with tooth extraction; however, many cases occur spontaneously without preceding dental treatment. BRONJ

Table 2.11	Drugs Associated With Osteonecrosis of the Jaws	
Intravenous Bisphosphonates	**Trade Name**	**Indications**
Pamidronate	Aredia	Metastasis of cancer to bone; multiple myeloma
Zoledronic acid	Zometa	Metastasis of cancer to bone
Zoledronic acid	Reclast (once annually)	Osteoporosis
Ibandronate	Boniva (every 3 months)	Osteoporosis
Oral Bisphosphonates		
Alendronate	Fosamax	Osteoporosis
Ibandronate	Boniva	Osteoporosis
Risedronate	Actonel	Osteoporosis
Monoclonal Antibodies		
Denosumab	Prolia	Metastasis of cancer to bone; multiple myeloma; osteoporosis
Bevacizumab	Avastin	Breast cancer relapse; prostate cancer metastasis

manifests as exposed, nonvital bone commonly on the mylohyoid ridge, in extraction sites (Fig. 2-67A), and on palatal tori (Fig. 2-67B). Clinically, there is exposed, painful or painless nonvital bone surrounded by erythematous soft tissues. The best treatment for this disorder is prevention. Antimicrobial rinses and antibiotics have been used to control or prevent infections. Surgical intervention may be advisable only in advanced cases.

Similar cases of bone necrosis have been seen in patients taking non-bisphosphonate drugs that affect osteoclast function such as denosumab. Research is continuing into the cause and prevention of this serious problem.

Clinical Implications

Patients taking bisphosphonates or other drugs that affect osteoclast function should *not* avoid routine dental treatment. Most routine dental procedures are safe; however, consultation with the physician should be obtained prior to any *invasive procedures*. Minor areas of exposed bone often respond to routine rinses with the germicidal mouth rinse chlorhexidine gluconate that reduces microorganisms in the oral cavity as well as helps control inflammation.

Paget Disease of Bone

Paget disease of bone is seen most commonly in Caucasian patients older than age 40, predominantly males. The cause of Paget disease remains unknown, although several factors, such as genetics, endocrinopathies, and viral infection, have been implicated. It represents an abnormality of the bone remodeling process, leading to weak and distorted bone. The abnormal resorption and deposition of bone causes a classic radiographic pattern described as "cotton wool" or "cotton balls" (Fig. 2-68). Patients may initially be asymptomatic, but over time bone pain and enlargement occur. Most patients experience disease in more than one bone (polyostotic), with common involvement of the spine, pelvis, and femur. If a weight-bearing bone is affected, it may become bowed or fractured. If the skull is involved, the patient may report that his or her hat size has increased. Impingement on cranial nerves may lead to deafness or blindness.

If the jaws are affected, patients may complain that their dentures no longer fit (Fig. 2-69) or spacing between teeth has increased. Teeth may demonstrate hypercementosis (a buildup of cementum). Enlargement of the jaw may give the initial impression of bone tumor development, but this is not a neoplastic process. However, patients with Paget disease are at

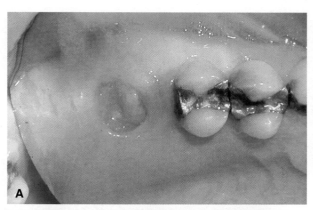

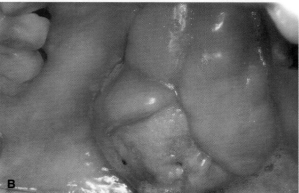

Figure 2–67   Bisphosphonate-associated osteonecrosis of the jaw (BRONJ). A. Non-healing extraction site of a patient taking intravenous bisphosphonates for breast cancer. **B.** Patient on oral bisphosphonates for osteoporosis, history of trauma to torus.

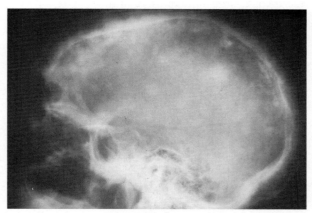

Figure 2–68   Radiograph of Paget disease. Cephalometric radiograph of patient with Paget disease with distinct "cotton ball" appearance to the bone.

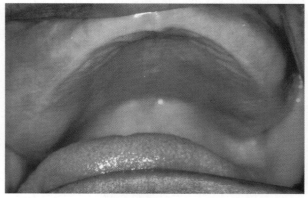

Figure 2–69   Paget disease. Patient can no longer wear denture, due to enlargement of the maxilla.

increased risk for developing malignant bone tumors later in life.

Diagnosis is based on clinical and radiographic features as well as biopsy of the affected bone. Elevated levels of alkaline phosphatase in the blood and hydroxyproline in the urine occur, both indicators of increased bone turnover. Treatment is based on reducing bone turnover. This may be accomplished with drugs such as calcitonin or systemic bisphosphonates. When abnormal bone turnover is reduced, bones regain strength and risk of fracture is reduced.

Central Giant Cell Granuloma

Central giant cell granuloma (CGCG) is a nonneoplastic growth of bone. This is seen in a wide variety of patients, although the majority involve the anterior mandible of females in the third decade of life. The etiology remains unknown. The name of the lesion is derived from the microscopic rather than clinical appearance. Under the microscope, large numbers of multinucleated giant cells of osteoclast origin are seen. The lesions can cause a rather dramatic enlargement of the affected bone. CGCG is *not* related to *peripheral giant cell granuloma* but represents a different disease process.

Clinical behavior of CGCG may vary from patient to patient (see page 51), with some CGCGs more aggressive than others. They most often cause few symptoms, grow slowly, and do not affect the teeth. However, in some individuals they grow more rapidly, are more aggressive, cause dramatic jaw swelling (Fig. 2-70A), perforate the outer cortex of the bone, and result in loosening of teeth (Fig. 2-70B). Radiographically, they are unilocular or multilocular, well-corticated, purely radiolucent lesions. They may cross the midline and reach several centimeters in size. Teeth are often displaced or malposed (Fig. 2-71). Biopsy of CGCG will have the identical histopathologic features as cherubism (see Chapter 6) and hyperparathyroidism (see Chapter 9), which also show a large number of multinucleated giant cells. Clinical assessment is important in differentiating between conditions that contain abundant multinucleated giant cells (Table 2-12).

Treatment for CGCG varies, with smaller less aggressive lesions curetted from the bone. Intralesional injections of corticosteroids or other **immunomodulary** drugs may help reverse some CGCGs. Calcitonin has been shown to be helpful in stopping or reducing bone destruction by lesions too large for surgery. Close follow-up after treatment is warranted, because CGCGs are known to recur.

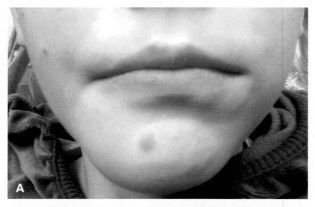

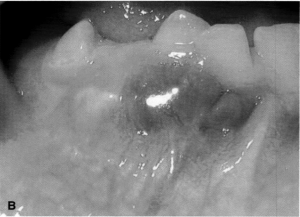

Figure 2–70 **Central giant cell carcinoma (CGCG).** **A.** Dramatic jaw swelling. **B.** Loosening of teeth.

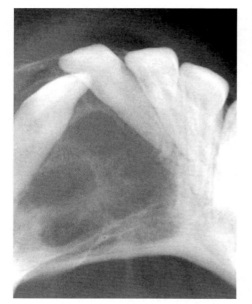

Figure 2–71 **Central giant cell granuloma.** Radiograph showing teeth displaced by multilocular radiolucency.

Table 2.12	**Giant Cell Granuloma-Like Lesions of the Jaws**		
	Distinguishing Features		
	Demographics	**Radiographs**	**Other**
Central Giant Cell Granuloma	Any age, favors younger than 30 years	1 quadrant, but may cross the midline	No underlying disease
Cherubism (Chapter 6)	Children age 2–5	Involves 2–4 quadrants	Inherited autosomal dominant
Brown Tumor of Hyperparathyroidism (Chapter 9)	Adults; Renal dialysis patients	Loss of lamina dura	Elevated serum PTH

PTH = parathyroid hormone

Renal Osteodystrophy

Renal osteodystrophy is a serious condition seen in patients with end-stage kidney disease and patients on renal dialysis. The diseased kidneys are unable to regulate proper blood levels of calcium and phosphorus. As a result, the blood becomes calcium deficient, increasing extraction of calcium from the bones. This makes the bones weak and brittle, leading to fractures and joint pain. Bony changes in renal osteodystrophy can begin many years before signs and symptoms occur. Diagnosis is made based on kidney function and blood tests and, in some cases, a bone biopsy.

Renal osteodystrophy may produce diffuse involvement of the jaws. Marked jaw enlargement results in severe malocclusion. Radiographic findings include bone resorption with loss of cortical bone and lamina dura. Condensation of bone trabeculae produces a "ground-glass" appearance, closely resembling fibrous dysplasia (see Chapter 6). Renal osteodystrophy can be distinguished from fibrous dysplasia because renal osteostrophy is associated with kidney failure and/or renal dialysis. Jaw enlargement eventually may cease with treatment, but in some cases surgical intervention is necessary.

Post-surgical Hyperostosis

Post-surgical hyperostosis is an unusual condition caused by stimulation of the osteoblasts in the periosteum during periodontal surgery. Osteoblasts begin to form new bone, resulting in a tumor-like growth at the surgical site (Fig. 2-72). The lesion is composed of normal, vital bone and has the same consistency as a torus. The treatment is to reduce the mass without further stimulating the osteoblasts of periosteum.

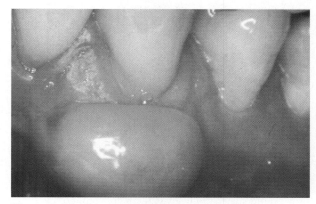

Figure 2–72   Postsurgical hyperostosis. Patient with history of periodontal surgery, now with bony enlargement.

Traumatic Bone Cavity (Simple Bone Cavity)

Traumatic bone cavity, previously known as *traumatic bone cyst,* is not a true cyst because it does not have an epithelial lining. The lesion is most often diagnosed in young patients in the mandible. Clinically, the lesion is asymptomatic and is discovered on routine radiographic examination. A unilocular radiolucent area that scallops between tooth roots (Fig. 2-73A) is typical. The etiology is unknown, but a history of trauma is sometimes elicited. It is hypothesized that the blood clot formed after a traumatic injury is destroyed, leaving an empty cavity. The definitive diagnosis is made at surgery when an empty unlined cavity is found (Fig. 2-73B).

Aneurysmal Bone Cyst

Aneurysmal bone cyst (ABC) is a destructive bony lesion caused by increased venous pressure with resultant dilation and rupture of the local vascular network.

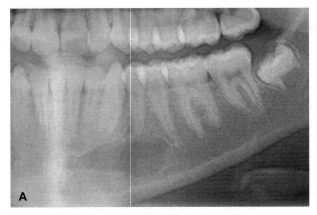

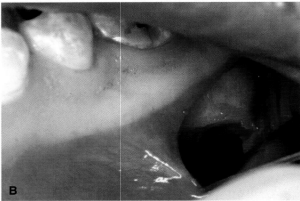

Figure 2–73   Traumatic bone cavity. A. Radiograph shows unilocular radiolucency; teeth are vital; no expansion of jaw. **B.** At surgery, an empty cavity is found.

At the time of surgery, the tissue has been reported to resemble a blood-soaked sponge. It is not epithelial-lined, so it does not represent a true cyst. Recent studies suggest that it actually represents a neoplasm. It generally arises in a pre-existing bone lesion, such as fibrous dysplasia. Whether it is reactive or neoplastic, it can be quite destructive because it deforms the bone and may cause fractures. ABCs may cause pain and swelling. Radiographically, they appear as large unilocular or multilocular radiolucent lesions that expand the bone. If they occur in the maxilla, they may bulge into the sinus. If they occur in the mandible, they may cause swelling of the ramus.

External Injuries to Teeth

Injuries to tooth hard tissues may occur as a result of normal mastication, caries, oral habits, and ingestion of caustic agents (Table 2-13).

Attrition

Attrition is wear that occurs as a result of tooth-to-tooth contact. This includes occlusal and incisal surfaces as well as interproximal contacts. Some amount of attrition is considered within normal limits. The wear usually continues throughout the life of the teeth, so long as they make contact. However, attrition can be exacerbated by grinding or clenching habits (**bruxism**). Because attrition is a gradual process, pulp exposure is rare (Fig. 2-74).

Abrasion

Abrasion is the loss of tooth structure as a result of an externally applied force. The most common type is due to tooth brushing with a hard-bristle brush and abrasive toothpaste. Repetitive back-and-forth motion at the cemento-enamel junction where enamel is thin and softer cementum and dentin are more vulnerable to wear, leads to notching and grooving that may extend deep into the dentin. Abrasion can be exacerbated by the ingestion of abrasive components in the diet or occupational exposures to grit or dust such as in farming. Because abrasion is a gradual process, pulp exposure is rare (Fig. 2-75).

Abfraction

Abfraction is wedge-shaped notching in the cervical region, unrelated to toothbrush abrasion. This appears to be caused by flexing pressures on the tooth, which manifest at the crown and root interface. The defects of abfraction are noncarious cervical lesions that result in hard tissue breakdown. Dentin is exposed, which is then vulnerable to abrasion and erosion (Fig. 2-76).

Erosion

Erosion is the loss of tooth hard tissue due to chemical exposure. The pH at which the hard tissues begin to lose mineralization is around 5.0 to 5.5. Erosion may occur as a result of ingesting low pH acidic foods, such as carbonated beverages and sports drinks, or sucking on lemons or citric acid–containing lozenges. Erosion from ingested acidic foods is seen primarily on the facial surfaces of the anterior teeth (Fig. 2-77) and sometimes the buccal surfaces of the posterior teeth where food contacts the enamel.

Chronic vomiting of stomach acid is another cause of erosion. This may occur with gastrointestinal reflux, vomiting during pregnancy, or self-induced vomiting in patients with an eating disorder such as bulimia. Because the pH of stomach acid is 1.0, hard tissue loss with regurgitation occurs quickly, often

Table 2.13	Chronic Injuries to Teeth		
Injury	**Etiology**	**Source**	**Clinical Features**
Attrition	Tooth-to-tooth contact	Bruxism; malocclusion	Short clinical crowns
Abrasion	Mechanical wear	Tooth brushing; abrasive dentifrice; oral habits	Well-defined grooves and notches on involved teeth, usually near CEJ
Abfraction	Tooth flexion and physical stress	Occlusal restorations; fixed prostheses	Smooth V-shaped notches at the CEJ in teeth with restorations
Erosion	Nonbacterial acids	Acidic foods; citrus foods; soft drinks; chronic regurgitation due to acid reflux or bulimia	Smooth cup-shaped depressions, often extending into the dentin

CEJ = cementoenamel junction

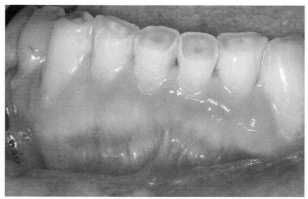

Figure 2–74   Attrition. Wear on the teeth from grinding, clenching, or other form of tooth-to-tooth contact (i.e., bruxism).

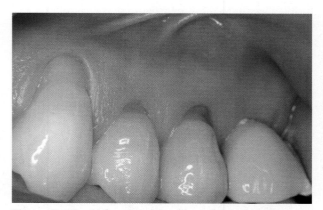

Figure 2–76   Abfraction. Notching of the cervical area due to occlusal disharmony.

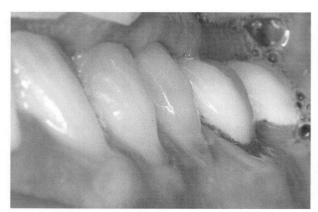

Figure 2–75   Abrasion. Wearing away of tooth due to excessive tooth brushing.

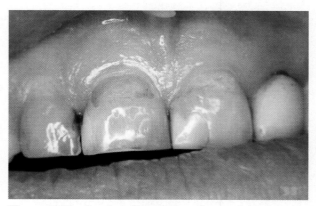

Figure 2–77   Erosion. Dissolution of enamel due to lemon sucking.

within weeks. Patterns of hard tissue loss provide clues to problems with regurgitation. On posterior teeth, amalgams appear to rise up above the tooth surface, and adjacent hard tissues appear to have washed away (Fig. 2-78A). On anterior teeth, hard tissue loss is most often seen on lingual surfaces, where vomited stomach contents and acid contact the palatal surfaces of the teeth (Fig. 2-78B).

External Resorption

External resorption is a condition in which root structure adjacent to the periodontal ligament is lost. External resorption may be initiated by chronic inflammation induced by trauma, infection, or reimplantation of an avulsed tooth. In some cases, the etiology is unknown. External resorption is occasionally seen in patients undergoing orthodontic treatment due to mechanical forces applied on the teeth. Cysts and tumors adjacent to teeth may cause pressure that results in external resorption. External resorption is thought to occur when undifferentiated cells of the periodontal

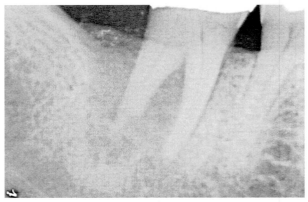

Figure 2–79   Idiopathic external resorption. Distal root of second molar.

ligament are stimulated to become "odontoclasts." Radiographically, the external surface of the tooth appears "moth-eaten" along the portions of the root (Fig. 2-79). Endodontic therapy is not effective in resolving external resorption because the cells of the dental pulp are not involved.

Fracture of a tooth can occur as a result of sudden blow to the face, excessive occlussal forces, or biting a hard object. The result is a sharp edge to the tooth that may injure adjacent soft tissue. Fractures also may impinge upon the dental pulp and lead to pulpitis and pulpal necrosis.

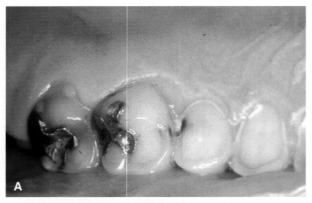

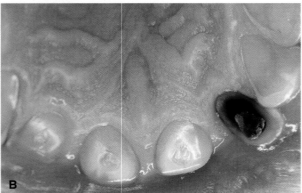

Figure 2–78   Erosion from gastro-esophageal reflux disease (GERD). A. Patient with chronic reflux disorder; amalgams appear to be protruding. **B.** Palatal surfaces of anterior teeth from chronic reflux disorder.

Critical Thinking Questions

Case 2-1:   Your patient has a chief complaint of pain in the floor of the mouth. On palpation, you feel a firm swelling, and he complains of tenderness as you palpate. He says it gets worse when he eats, especially sour or spicy foods.

• • •

What condition is your patient most likely suffering from?

What procedures can be undertaken to evaluate the cause of his condition?

Case 2-2:   You take a panoramic radiograph on your 45-year-old female African American patient. You notice a diffuse mixed radiolucent/radiopaque appearance to her entire mandible. Her jaw is normal size with no enlargement, and she has no dental complaints. All her teeth test vital.

• • •

What condition does she most likely have in her mandible?

In your role as a patient educator, what will you teach this patient about the relationship of her condition to good oral health care? What are the possible consequences of this patient undergoing invasive dental procedures or dental surgery?

Case 2-3: Your patient presents with a thick white lesion on the right retromolar pad and buccal mucosa. It does not wipe off. She is a long-term two-pack-a-day smoker, and she has no interest in quitting. You also notice a rough amalgam filling in the area.

• • •

Describe the management plan for this lesion. Please include details about the timeline that should be followed.

Case 2-4: Your patient presents with a darkly pigmented lesion on the facial gingiva in the area of number 22. She does not recall any trauma to the area. There are no amalgams in any of the teeth in this quadrant. The lesion is flat and homogeneously brown.

• • •

List three possible reasons that this area has become darkly pigmented.

What is the first step in the process to determine what this lesion is?

What is the "rule of thumb" for dealing with pigmented lesions in the oral cavity?

Case 2-5: Your patient has a full upper denture. On clinical inspection, you notice that since her last appointment she has developed thick folds of tissue along the flanges of the denture. When the denture is removed, the palate appears bright red and feels velvety smooth to the touch. The patient reports no symptoms but says that her denture has not fit well lately. She does not like to take it out at night.

• • •

What two denture injuries does this patient have?

How are these two injuries similar to each other? How are they different?

How will the dentist most likely treat your patient?

What advice will you give your patient to help prevent this from occurring in the future?

Case 2-6: Your 19-year-old patient returns for her 6-month prophylaxis visit after returning home from her first semester away at college. During your examination, you notice that the palatal surfaces of the maxillary central incisors are extremely smooth and the enamel is extremely thin so that some areas of dentin are exposed. She reports that these teeth have become sensitive to cold lately. You do not observe any caries.

• • •

List two possible explanations for the change in her teeth.

On further questioning, she reports that she has increased her intake of sports drinks recently. Do you think that this is contributing to her problem?

Case 2-7: Your 51-year-old male patient presents with the chief complaint, "There is a bump growing on my gums, and I can't floss around it anymore." On clinical inspection, you notice a 5- to 6-mm ovoid exophytic mass protruding from the interproximal space between teeth 28 and 29. When you examine it with your explorer, it bleeds slightly.

• • •

Name three possible diagnoses for this mass. What is the etiology of each? How are they similar and how are they different?

How will the lesion be treated?

What information can you give your patient about his condition that can help him prevent this from happening again?

1. **Which one of the following is NOT an indication of Paget disease of bone?**
   A. Elevated serum alkaline phosphatase
   B. Hypercementosis
   C. Onset of new spacing between teeth
   D. All are indications of Paget disease.

2. **The most common location for a sialolith is the**
   A. submandibular gland.
   B. parotid gland.
   C. sublingual gland.
   D. minor glands of the lower lip.

3. **Which of the following is NOT considered an etiologic factor in the development of necrotizing sialometaplasia?**
   A. Allergy to dentifrices
   B. Recent dental work in the area which included local anesthesia
   C. Development of a tumor in the area
   D. Trauma to the area

4. **An example of reversible cell injury is**
   A. necrosis.
   B. ischemia.
   C. hyperplasia.
   D. calcification.

5. **Free radicals are removed from the body by**
   A. macrophages.
   B. apoptosis.
   C. antioxidants.
   D. vasoactive amines.

6. **Tissue damage as a result of ischemia is termed**
   A. hypertrophy.
   B. atrophy.
   C. infarction.
   D. caseous necrosis.

7. **Which of the following is NOT a basic type of inflammation?**
   A. Acute
   B. Chronic
   C. Granulomatous
   D. Pyogenic

8. **All of the following are considered to be cardinal signs of inflammation EXCEPT**
   A. heat.
   B. redness.
   C. swelling.
   D. exudation.

9. **Chemotaxis is**
   A. recruitment of phagocytic white blood cells to an area of inflammation.
   B. destruction of worn red blood cells.
   C. destruction of target foreign proteins.
   D. formation of antibodies by plasma cells.

10. **Which of the following is NOT a granulocyte?**
    A. Lymphocyte
    B. Neutrophil
    C. Eosinophil
    D. Basophil

11. **A macrophage found within connective tissue proper is termed a**
    A. basophil.
    B. histiocyte.
    C. phagocyte.
    D. plasma cell.

12. **Which of the following is NOT considered to be part of the acute phase response?**
    A. Fever
    B. Increased cortisol levels in the blood
    C. Leukocytosis
    D. Lymphadenopathy

13. **A scaffold for tissue repair that is composed of chronic inflammatory cells, fibroblasts, collagen, and endothelial cells describes**
    A. granulation tissue.
    B. granulomatous inflammation.
    C. metastatic calcification.
    D. hyperplasia.

14. **Wounds in which edges cannot be closely opposed undergo healing by**
    A. primary intention.
    B. secondary intention.
    C. tertiary intention.
    D. scar tissue.

15. **Which of the following does NOT present as a white patch in the mouth?**
    A. Frictional keratosis
    B. Morsicatio buccarum
    C. Hypermelanosis
    D. Linea alba

16. **If a pigmented lesion does not appear radiographically as iatrogenically implanted dental amalgam**
    A. the patient most likely has cancer.
    B. the lesion should be removed and examined under the microscope (biopsy).
    C. no further treatment is required.
    D. it should be radiographed again in 6 months.

17. **The loss of surface epithelium with exposure of the underlying connective tissue describes**
    A. geographic tongue.
    B. an ulcer.
    C. hematoma.
    D. external resorption.

18. **An exuberant growth of granulation tissue in response to a minor irritant is termed**
    A. traumatic ulcer.
    B. traumatic neuroma.
    C. pyogenic granuloma.
    D. traumatic fibroma.

19. **The term *epulis* means that the lesion is**
    A. found on the gingiva.
    B. causing swelling.
    C. expressing pus when pressure is applied.
    D. seen as radiolucency on a periapical radiograph.

20. **Which of the following medications has NOT been associated with drug-induced gingival overgrowth?**
    A. Phenytoin (Dilantin)
    B. Nifedipine (Procardia)
    C. Cyclosporine
    D. Carbamezine (Tegretol)

21. **When a salivary gland duct is severed and mucin spills into the surrounding submucosa, this produces a swelling called a(n)**
    A. mucocele.
    B. mucous duct cyst.
    C. necrotizing sialometaplasia.
    D. adenomatoid hyperplasia.

22. **Which form of denture stomatitis appears as folds of tissue that look like "waves crashing on the shore" against the denture flange?**
    A. Candidiasis
    B. Inflammatory papillary hyperplasia
    C. Epulis fissuratum
    D. Fibroepithelial polyp

23. **Which of the following will NOT appear as an apical radiolucency?**
    A. Condensing osteitis
    B. Periapical cyst
    C. Chronic apical periodontitis (granuloma)
    D. Apical scar

24. **Florid osseous dysplasia is a potentially serious disease because patients are at risk for**
    A. bone cancer.
    B. jaw fracture.
    C. a serious jaw infection if they have a tooth extracted.
    D. rampant caries.

25. **Loss of dental hard tissue due to exposure to chemical agents is termed**
    A. abfraction.
    B. erosion.
    C. attrition.
    D. abrasion.

SUGGESTED READINGS

Books

Dawson, W, Willoughby, D: Inflammation – mechanisms and mediators. In: Lombardino, J (ed): Non-Steroidal Anti-Inflammatory Drugs. Wiley, New York, 1985, pp 76–101.

Eisen, D, Lynch, D: The Mouth, ed. 1. Mosby, St. Louis, 1998.

Fantone, J: Basic concepts in inflammation. In: Leadbetter, W et al (eds): Sports-Induced Inflammation. American Academy of Orthopaedic Surgery, Chicago, 1990.

Gallin, J, Goldstein, I, Snyderman, R: Inflammation: Basic Principles and Clinical Correlates. Raven Press, New York, 1992.

Neville, B, Damm, DD, Allen, CM, Bouquot, J: Oral and Maxillofacial Pathology, ed. 3. Saunders, St. Louis, 2009.

Neville, B, Damm, D, White, D: Color Atlas of Clinical Oral Pathology, ed. 2. Williams and Wilkins, Baltimore, 1999.

Regezi, J, Sciubba, J, Jordan, R: Oral Pathology: Clinical Pathologic Correlations, ed. 4. Saunders, Philadelphia, 2007.

Rubin, E, Reisner, H: Essential Pathology, ed. 5. Lippincott, Williams and Wilkins, Philadelphia, 2008.

Sigal, L, Ron, Y: Immunology and Inflammation – Basic Mechanisms and Clinical Consequences. McGraw-Hill, New York, 1994.

Trowbridge, H, Emling, R: Inflammation: A review of the Process. Quintessence Books, Chicago, 1997.

Journal Articles

Arduino, PG, Carrozzo, M, Pentenero, M, Bertolusso, G, Gandolfo, S: Non-neoplastic salivary gland diseases. Minerva Stomatologica 55(5):249–270, May 2006.

Damm, DD, Neville, BW, McKenna, S, Jones, AC, Freedman, PD, Anderson, WR, Allen, CM: Macrognathia of renal osteodystrophy in dialysis patients. Oral Surgery, Oral Medicine, Oral Pathology, Oral Radiology and Endodontology 83(4):489–495, April 1997.

Ellies, M, Laskawi, R: Diseases of the salivary glands in infants and adolescents. Head & Face Medicine 6:1, February 2010.

Eversole, R, Su, L, Elmofty, S: Benign fibro-osseous lesions of the craniofacial complex. A review. Head and Neck Pathology 2(3):177–202, September 2008.

Falchetti, A, Masi, L, Brandi, ML: Paget's disease of bone: There's more than the affected skeleton—A clinical review and suggestions for the clinical practice. Current Opinion in Rheumatology 22(4):410–423, July 2010.

Giovanni, M, Ergun, S, Vescovi, P, Mete, O, Tanyeri, H, Meleti, M: Oral postinflammatory pigmentation: An analysis of 7 cases. Medicina Oral Patologia Oral y Cirugia Bucal 11–14, January 2011.

Imbery, TA, Edwards, PA: Necrotizing sialometaplasia: Literature review and case reports. Journal of the American Dental Association 127(7):1087–1092, July 1996.

Lee, EJ, Calcaterra, TC, Zuckerbraun, L: Traumatic neuromas of the head and neck. Ear Nose Throat Journal 77:670–674, August 1998.

Neville, B: The verruciform xanthoma. A review and report of eight new cases. American Journal of Dermatopathology 8:247–253, June 1986.

Pape, SA, MacLeod, RI, McLean, NR, Soames, JV: Sialadenosis of the salivary glands. British Journal of Plastic Surgery 48:419–422, September 1995.

Reid, IR, Hosking, DJ: Bisphosphonates in Paget's disease. Bone 49(1):89–94, July 2011.

Rice, DH: Noninflammatory, non-neoplastic disorders of the salivary glands. Otolaryngologic Clinics of North America 32(5):835–843, October 1999.

Su, L, Weathers, DR, Waldron, CA: Distinguishing features of focal cemento-osseous dysplasias and cemento-ossifying fibromas: I. A pathologic spectrum of 316 cases. Oral Surgery, Oral Medicine, Oral Pathology, Oral Radiology and Endodontology 84(3): 301–309, September 1997.

Summerlin, DJ, Tomich, CE: Focal cemento-osseous dysplasia: A clinicopathologic study of 221 cases. Oral Surgery, Oral Medicine, Oral Pathology, Oral Radiology and Endodontology 78(5): 611–620, November 1994.

Thomas, BL, Brown, JE, McGurk, M: Salivary gland disease. Frontiers of Oral Biology 14:129–146, April 20, 2010.

Tomich, CE, Zunt, SL: Melanoacanthosis (melanoacanthoma) of the oral mucosa. Journal of Dermatologic Surgery and Oncology 16(3):231–236, March 1990.

3

Infectious Diseases

Basic Principles of Infectious Diseases
Pathogenic Microorganisms and Infectious Disease
Microorganisms
Infection and Transmission
Clinical Signs and Symptoms of Infection
Disease Control

Oral Manifestations of Infectious Diseases
Bacterial Infections
Fungal Infections
Protozoal Infections
Viral Infections

● Learning Outcomes

At the end of this chapter, the student will be able to:

3.1. Explain the causative microorganism and route of transmission for each infectious disease presented.

3.2. Explain the concept of indigenous microflora and how they may either prevent or cause disease.

3.3. Recognize infections associated with skin rashes.

3.4. Give examples of infectious diseases that may be harmful to a developing fetus.

3.5. Distinguish between clinical and pathologic features of latent versus active tuberculosis.

3.6. Outline the steps in the clinical progression of untreated syphilis.

3.7. Recognize and explain clinical manifestations of various forms of oral candidiasis and their treatment.

3.8. Describe the pathogenesis of primary, latent, and recurrent herpes simplex infection; recognize its stages; provide appropriate education to a patient with herpes simplex infection of the lips or oral cavity.

3.9. Compare and contrast the etiology and clinical manifestations of herpangina and hand-foot-and-mouth disease.

3.10. Give examples of the five oral manifestations strongly associated with HIV infection.

3.11. Distinguish among the various human papillomavirus infections that can affect the oral cavity.

BASIC PRINCIPLES OF INFECTIOUS DISEASES

Pathogenic Microorganisms and Infectious Disease

Infectious diseases are caused by **microorganisms** too small to be viewed by the unaided eye. Broad categories of microorganisms include bacteria, viruses, fungi, prions, protozoa, helminthes, and arthropods. Not all microorganisms are **pathogenic**. Maladies caused by pathogenic microorganisms are termed **infectious diseases**. Infectious diseases are responsible for more than 20 percent of deaths globally and are a major health burden in underdeveloped countries, particularly among young children. Despite medical advances and an increasing knowledge of microbiology, **antibiotic resistance** and increased air travel continue to facilitate the transmission of infectious diseases. Microorganisms also evolve at a much faster rate than the host, requiring constant development of new antimicrobial therapies. Emergence of new infections (e.g., methicillin-resistant *Staphylococcus aureus* [MRSA]) and resurgences of old infections (e.g., tuberculosis) are killing increasing numbers in both resource-poor and resource-rich countries. Additionally, certain infections are now being implicated in aberrant host reactions that may cause chronic immune-mediated diseases or malignancies.

The specific microorganism that causes disease is referred to as the **etiologic agent** or **infectious agent**. For example, the etiologic agent of tuberculosis is the bacterium *Mycobacterium tuberculosis*. Although some infectious diseases are the result of specific exogenous pathogens, infections may also be caused by **indigenous microflora**. Indigenous microflora is present at birth. The external and internal exposed surfaces of the body become colonized by organisms that establish the resident microflora (mostly bacteria). These microorganisms are usually protective but may become pathogenic with a change in host environment or immunity. For example, colonization of the intestine normally prevents infection by other microorganisms due to lack of available living space. However, systemic antibiotic therapy may inadvertently eliminate some of the protective microflora, allowing overgrowth of other bacteria that in small numbers are of low pathogenicity. The result can be antibiotic-associated diarrhea.

The most common infectious agents in the oral cavity are periodontal pathogens and cariogenic microorganisms. These agents are not discussed in this text because they typically comprise a separate topic of study within the dental hygiene curriculum. Many other infectious agents cause diseases with oral, skin, or **constitutional symptoms** that dental hygienists must be able to recognize in their patients. Constitutional symptoms, including fever and malaise, indicate that a disease is systemic. Although many diseases discussed here can be considered "rare," the dental hygienist must be aware that new immigrant populations as well as immunocompromised patients may present with infectious diseases seldom seen in the general population.

Opportunistic Infection

An **opportunistic infection** is caused by microorganisms that usually do not produce disease in a person with a healthy immune system. When the immune system is compromised in some way, and the host's natural defenses against the pathogen are reduced or eliminated, these microorganisms may cause disease. In other words, the microorganisms wait for an "opportunity" to thrive and cause disease. Some of the "opportunities" that allow for infection in an otherwise healthy host include immunosuppressive drugs, such as corticosteroids, or drugs given to transplant patients to prevent organ rejections; cancer chemotherapy; administration of antibiotics; damage to the skin or mucosal barriers; emotional or physical stress; malnutrition; pregnancy; and some genetic diseases. Opportunistic infections are especially common in patients with immunosuppressive conditions such as AIDS. Once the immune system is restored and the infection is treated, the patient generally recovers; however, in some cases the opportunistic infection may cause death. For example, patients with AIDS generally do not succumb to the HIV virus but to an opportunistic infection or other disorder that their immune system cannot control.

Carrier State

When a person comes into contact with an infectious agent, the healthy immune system may eliminate the agent so the person may not even know they were infected. However, if the immune system cannot eliminate the agent, the person will most likely become ill. Some individuals' immune systems neither eliminate the agent nor become ill. In this case, the person becomes a **carrier.** A carrier can transmit the microorganism to someone else who becomes ill. Specific types of carriers are the *incubator carrier*, a person who is infected but is not yet showing clinical signs (prodromal period), or a *convalescent carrier* who has passed the clinical stage of the disease but can still transmit it.

The classic case of a carrier state is the legendary *Typhoid Mary*. Typhoid Mary carried the bacterium

Salmonella typhi, though she was not ill herself. She worked as a cook and infected more than 100 people, killing several of them, before she was prohibited from working.

Microorganisms

Most infections are caused by bacteria, fungi, and viruses. **Bacteria** are single-celled microorganisms that contain DNA but no nucleus. The three basic shapes of bacterial organisms are cocci (spheres), bacilli (rods), or spirochetes (helical) (Fig. 3-1). Bacteria are classified as Gram positive or Gram negative based on the staining characteristics of their cell wall, which is intricately involved in the morphology, metabolism, and pathogenicity of the organism. The bacterial cell wall is primarily constructed of peptidoglycan molecules. Gram-positive bacteria have a thick peptidoglycan layer, whereas Gram-negative bacteria have a thin peptidoglycan layer with a surrounding lipopolysaccharide and lipoprotein outer membrane. Clinically, it is important to determine if bacteria are Gram positive or Gram negative because the illnesses they cause often require different treatment protocols.

Viruses are noncellular microorganisms that contain DNA or RNA within a protein capsid, which determines each virus' ability to survive in the outside world (Fig. 3-2). Unlike bacterial organisms, viruses can replicate only after entering and infecting a host cell. Upon entry to a host cell, some viruses replicate and cause the cell to undergo cell destruction called *lysis*. Lysis releases new viral particles that spread the infectious agent to other cells. Alternatively, an infected cell may not be lysed but release new viral particles at a slow rate. Some viruses become inactive or *latent* until a later point in time when replication is stimulated. Other viruses, such as Epstein-Barr virus and some subtypes of human papillomavirus, are *oncogenic*, which means the DNA or RNA of the virus enters the nucleus

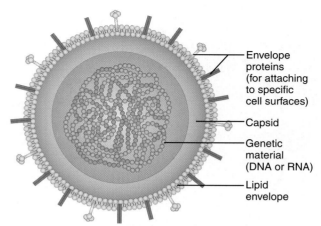

Figure 3–2   Virus. Viruses have multiple surface proteins that facilitate attachment and entry into host cells.

of a healthy cell and transforms it into a cancerous cell. When the cell divides, it begins the process of forming a tumor mass.

Fungi are microorganisms that exist as either single-celled yeasts, multicellular branching hyphae, or both (dimorphic) (Fig. 3-3). Fungal infections called *mycoses* or *mycotic infections* cause either mild, superficial disease, such as candidiasis spread by direct contact to nails, hair, skin, mouth, and vagina; or they may invade deeply into tissues, usually from inhalation of spores from the environment. Deep mycotic infections, such as histoplasmosis, are generally opportunistic infections that occur in immunocompromised patients.

Protozoa are single-celled organisms that are either free-living or parasitic. Protozoa have complex strategies for avoiding immune recognition and can occur in both intracellular and extracellular locations. Most infections are transmitted through contaminated food and water or by insects. The most significant protozoal infection is malaria, which, according to the Centers for Disease Control and Prevention (CDC), kills between 700,000 and 1,000,000 people per year worldwide. Protozoal infections in the oral cavity are very rare and typically represent disseminated disease in immunocompromised individuals. They are more commonly encountered in patients who emigrate from endemic areas.

Infection and Transmission

Microorganisms cause infection by attaching to the body and/or penetrating its surfaces. Sites of potential entry include the respiratory tract, gastrointestinal tract, urogenital tract, and skin. Intact skin is normally

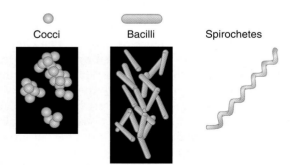

Cocci   Bacilli   Spirochetes

Figure 3–1   Bacteria. Cocci, bacilli, and spirochetes are the three most common bacterial shapes.

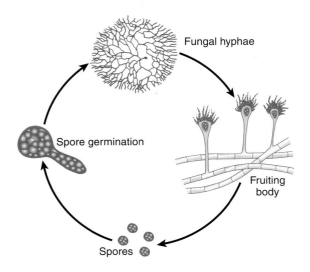

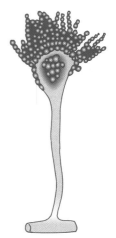

Figure 3–3   Fungi. Fungal life cycle.

protective; however, wounds and burns that open the skin can allow entry of microorganisms (Fig. 3-4). Some microorganisms multiply in epithelial cells at the site of entry without further spread and become *local infections.* Others spread from the site of entry into the lymph or blood and become *systemic infections.*

Globally, the most common infections are transmitted from one human to another through three main routes: 1) respiratory/salivary, 2) fecal-oral, or 3) venereal (sexual). Respiratory infections spread easily in crowded, indoor environments through coughing and sneezing, which release respiratory droplets containing infectious particles that may be inhaled by others. Infections transmitted by the fecal-oral route are common in young children, particularly in the setting of poor hygiene and insufficient public health sanitation. Urogenital tract infections spread by direct mucosal contact during sexual activity are referred to as **venereal** or *sexually transmitted diseases (STDs).*

Disease transmission of some microorganisms from animals to humans is possible. A disease that normally exists in animals but that can infect humans is referred to as a **zoonotic infection**. An example is Lyme disease. A **vector** is an animal that transfers an infective agent from one host to another. Arthropods, including blood-sucking insects, ticks, and mites, are the most common vectors and deliver diseases by piercing the skin while they feed. Ingestion of contaminated shellfish or meat is another zoonotic route. Domestic pets may also carry a number of pathogens that may be spread by bites, scratches, or handling contaminated feces, such as toxoplasmosis.

Pathogenicity is the ability of a microorganism to produce pathologic changes or disease. The clinical outcome of infection is determined by a complex interplay between the organism, host defenses, and the local environment (Fig. 3-5). A given microorganism seldom causes the same clinical picture in all individuals who are infected by it. Some infections may be totally asymptomatic in immunocompetent people but severe in the immunocompromised. In any given immunocompetent population, those who develop clinically evident disease may display a wide range in severity of

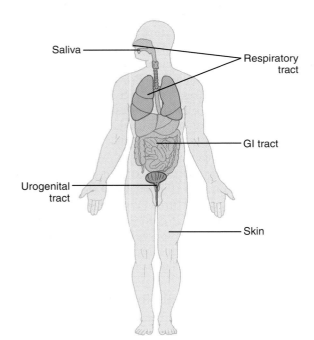

Figure 3–4   Pathways of entry. Pathways of infection; potential routes of entry for microorganisms.

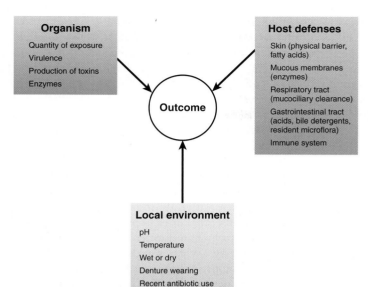

Organism

Quantity of exposure
Virulence
Production of toxins
Enzymes

Host defenses

Skin (physical barrier, fatty acids)

Mucous membranes (enzymes)

Respiratory tract (mucociliary clearance)

Gastrointestinal tract (acids, bile detergents, resident microflora)

Immune system

Outcome

Local environment

pH
Temperature
Wet or dry
Denture wearing
Recent antibiotic use

Figure 3–5 Variables affecting outcome of exposure to infectious agent. Multiple factors related to the organism, local environment, and host interact to determine the outcome of infection in a given individual.

symptoms. For example, the common cold may produce few symptoms in some individuals but cause others to be bedridden for several days. Other infections cause significant disease regardless of the immune status of the host.

Clinical Signs and Symptoms of Infection

A **sign** is an objective measurable assessment of disease, as opposed to a **symptom**, which is the subjective assessment perceived by the patient. Signs and symptoms of infection may be caused by the organism directly (e.g., by bacteria secreting *exotoxins*) or by the host response to being infected. Infections may be localized, systemic, or disseminated, so there is a wide variety of clinical signs of infection. Localized infections tend to cause pain in a specific part of the body. For example, if a cut on the skin is infected with bacteria, pain will occur at the site of the infection. The lesion will show redness, swelling, heat, edema, possibly a foul odor, and some form of exudate, such as pus. Systemic and disseminated infections tend to show extreme fatigue, weight loss, low-grade or spiking fever, night sweats and chills, and generalized body aches. Specific signs and symptoms of infections are discussed in this chapter.

Diagnostic Procedures

Accurate diagnosis is paramount to treatment outcome. One of the functions of microbiological testing is to generate information to help determine the appropriate treatment by using the appropriate antimicrobial agents. For some infections, a strong presumptive diagnosis may be made based on the clinical features alone. Others require additional testing to confirm the etiologic microbial agent. The diagnosis may be enhanced by: 1) isolation and culture of microorganisms, 2) identification of microbial products, or 3) detection of the patient's antibodies specific to a pathogen.

Microbiology laboratories examine infected specimens to identify the presence or absence of microbes. Bacteria and fungi can be "cultured," a method of multiplying microbial organisms by allowing them to reproduce in special nutrient media, usually in a Petri dish, under controlled laboratory conditions. Culture techniques depend on multiplication of the organism resulting in visible colonies and may require at least 24 hours for a preliminary result. Samples of the colonies are examined under the microscope to visualize and identify specific organisms. Viruses are difficult to grow under routine laboratory conditions. To test for a suspected virus, material thought to contain the virus is placed in a medium that contains cells that the suspected virus can infect. This is called a *tissue culture*. If the cells show changes, known as *cytopathic effects*, then a culture is positive. Another faster method for detecting viral infections is serologic testing, in which the patient's blood serum is examined for the presence of antibodies produced against a virus (see Chapter 4). If the antibodies are found, the infection can be confirmed.

Examination of a patient's tissue by cytology and light microscopy are other techniques that may be useful in the diagnosis of infectious diseases. Fungi and some bacterial organisms can be seen by special staining techniques (Fig. 3-6). Due to their extremely small size, viruses cannot be seen at the light microscopic level, but visualization of cellular changes resulting from infection, such as giant cells in herpes virus infections, is possible (Fig. 3-7). Electron microscopy can detect virus particles but is rarely used in the pathology laboratory.

Disease Control

Vaccines are used whenever possible to prevent infectious diseases within a population. The most successful vaccines are generally those containing live attenuated microorganisms. Attenuation takes a living microbial agent and alters it so that it becomes harmless but still recognizable by the body. The body then can make antibodies against it. Other types of vaccines use killed organisms or their fragments. The objective of immunization is to prime the host so that a quick, effective immune response will be generated upon subsequent exposure to the organism. This requires both B and T lymphocytes to form immunologic memory (see Chapter 4).

Antimicrobial drugs are used to treat infections in individuals who have contracted the infection. Antimicrobials include *antibiotics* for bacterial infections, *antivirals* for viral infections, and *antifungals* for fungal infections. Appropriate antimicrobial use and selection is important because antibiotics do not have any effect on viruses, antivirals do not have any effect on fungal infections, etc. For example, the common practice of administering antibiotics for the common cold that is caused by a virus serves no useful purpose. Overuse or inappropriate use of antibacterials contributes to the natural selection of drug-resistant bacterial strains. This type of antibacterial misapplication has led to the rapid development of resistant bacteria through either random mutation or genes acquired from other microorganisms.

The goal of all antimicrobial therapy is *selective toxicity*, which means that the drug should affect the microbe but not the host. Antibiotics are generally the most successful antimicrobial drugs because bacterial cells have many features that can be targeted without affecting human cells. Different classes of antibacterial drugs target different bacterial properties, such as metabolic pathways, nucleic acids, proteins, or the cell wall. Antibacterial drugs may be bactericidal (kill bacteria) or bacteriostatic (inhibit growth of bacteria). Bacteriostatic drugs ultimately rely on host immunity to resolve the infection and therefore may not be the best choice for immunocompromised patients.

Compared to bacteria, fungi have more cellular features in common with humans, making selective toxicity difficult to achieve. Consequently, the number of available antifungal drugs is extremely limited and treatment can be very challenging. Most antifungals target intracellular membranes in fungi. Drug resistance is increasing and deep fungal infections are a major cause of death and disease among immunosuppressed patients. The search for safer, more effective antifungals is a high priority.

Viruses are difficult to target due to their intracellular lifestyle. Antiviral drugs must enter host cells and selectively damage the virus but not the host. All currently available antivirals are virustatic, which means they target viral enzymes involved in

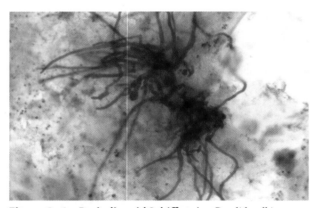

Figure 3–6   Periodic acid Schiff stain. *Candida albicans* smear taken from the oral cavity.

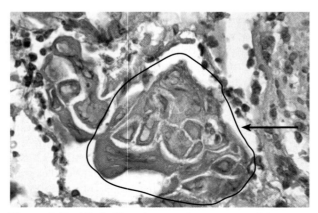

Figure 3–7   Viral effect: herpes. A smear containing keratinocytes infected with herpes simplex virus; note enlargement of the nucleus caused by the virus.

nucleic acid or protein synthesis and stop viral replication. Over the past 15 years, the number of available antivirals has increased dramatically, with most of these being used in the treatment of HIV-infected individuals.

ORAL MANIFESTATIONS OF INFECTIOUS DISEASES

The dental hygienist is expected to recognize the oral manifestations of infectious diseases in order to prevent the inadvertent transmission of the disease to himself or herself, as well as to other patients. Some infectious diseases do not have oral manifestations but can be recognized by signs and symptoms that may present during a dental hygiene appointment. Awareness of these diseases may help reduce the risk of transmission in the dental office and assist in making the proper referral for treatment.

Bacterial Infections

Bacteria may be beneficial, harmless, or pathogenic. They range from beneficial bacteria in the gut and harmless flora on the skin to pathogenic foodborne, airborne, and sexually transmitted bacteria. Some of the most common bacterial infections with oral manifestations are discussed here, as well as some rare bacterial infections of interest to health-care providers.

Necrotizing Ulcerative Gingivitis

Necrotizing ulcerative gingivitis (NUG) is a well-known, painful gingival disease of acute onset that characteristically develops in the setting of emotional stress. It was given the nickname *trench mouth*, as it was common among military servicemen during wartime. Another synonym for this condition, *Vincent's infection*, is named for the French physician who identified the relationship between NUG and unique fusiform and spirochete bacterial forms. More advanced techniques have now identified *Treponema* and *Fusobacterium* species, *Prevotella intermedia*, and *Porphyromonas gingivalis* as the most likely etiologic agents responsible for NUG. These microorganisms are usually components of the resident microflora that become proliferative and invasive during a change in nutrient availability. Additional predisposing factors, such as smoking, poor hygiene and nutrition, and recent illness, suggest that decreased immunity plays an important role in the etiology of NUG. In immunocompromised patients, NUG may

sometimes lead to *noma* (discussed next). Although the disease has been called ANUG (acute necrotizing ulcerative gingivitis) in the past, the preceding word "acute" has fallen out of favor because no chronic form of the disease exists.

NUG is most often seen in teenagers and young to middle-aged adults. Although the clinical distribution varies, the anterior gingiva is involved more often than posterior sites. The interdental papillae become swollen, hemorrhagic, and ulcerated, imparting a blunted, "punched out" appearance (Fig. 3-8A). The gingival surface is covered by a pathognomonic gray *pseudomembrane* composed of necrotic debris (Fig. 3-8B), accompanied by intense pain and foul odor. Despite severity of symptoms, no gingival attachment loss is seen. NUG usually resolves quickly after removal of the offending bacteria. Gingival debridement, usually with anesthesia, is the most important therapeutic measure. Analgesics and

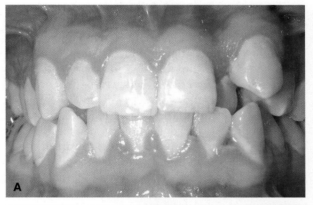

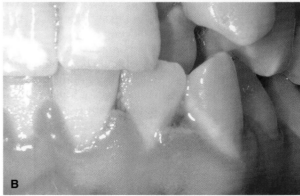

Figure 3–8   **NUG. A.** Early NUG: Swelling and erythema; note blunting of the gingival papillae between the mandibular left canine and incisors in a heavy-smoking adult male. **B.** Ulcerated and punched-out appearance of the interdental papillae.

chlorhexidine or warm salt water rinses can be useful adjuncts. Systemic penicillin or metronidazole may also be helpful.

Clinical Implications

Early cases of NUG may be subtle, with ulceration involving only the very tips of the interdental papillae. Affected areas are extremely tender to periodontal probing. Early recognition can prevent a great deal of discomfort for the patient. NUG may sometimes lead to **necrotizing ulcerative periodontitis** or **noma** if the patient is immunocompromised.

Noma (Cancrum oris)

Noma is a destructive opportunistic infection whose name comes from the Greek word *nomein*, which means "to devour." The etiologic microorganisms are components of the patient's normal resident oral microflora that become pathogenic when immunity is compromised. Noma classically develops after measles or another significant acute illness. Most experts believe the disease begins as NUG and represents extension of the infection into the surrounding oral soft tissues. Noma usually progresses rapidly. The mucous membranes of the mouth develop ulcers, after which rapid, painless tissue degeneration can destroy the bones in the face. Anatomic barriers to spread of the infection are violated and involved tissue develops black discoloration and yellow necrosis. Patients present with large areas of facial and oral tissues destroyed with exposure of the oral and sometimes nasal and sinus cavities. Additional clinical features include malodor, pain, fever, and lymphadenopathy.

Noma is extremely rare in developed countries. The population most affected is malnourished young children in sub-Saharan Africa, but it can occur in adults with an underlying debilitating disease in any demographic location. The mortality rate is still significant and survivors suffer major facial disfigurement.

Impetigo

Impetigo is a very contagious superficial skin infection caused by *Streptococcus pyogenes* and/or *Staphylococcus aureus*. Most cases develop in an area of skin damage such as a cut, scrape, or insect bite, and can spread rapidly. Impetigo tends to be most prevalent in regions with warm, humid climates. Two main clinical patterns exist: nonbullous and bullous impetigo.

Nonbullous impetigo is the more common form and typically develops in school-aged children. It is also referred to as *impetigo contagiosa* because it is easily spread from one person to another. Although the legs are the most common site of involvement, the facial skin may be affected, particularly around the mouth and nose. The lesions begin as red papules, which later form blisters that rupture and become covered by a thick, amber-colored crust (Fig. 3-9). These areas are nonpainful but *pruritic* (itchy). Regional lymphadenopathy is common. Treatment for limited nonbullous impetigo involves applying a topical antibiotic ointment such as mupirocin after carefully removing the overlying crusts with a warm, wet washcloth.

Bullous impetigo, sometimes called *staphylococcal scalded skin syndrome*, usually occurs in infants and newborns, most often affecting the extremities, trunk, and skin of the face and perioral area. *S. aureus* is the primary etiologic agent. Involved areas develop large bullae that become purulent and then rupture to become covered by a thin, brown crust. (See Chapter 4 for a description of *bullae*.) Systemic symptoms such as fever, malaise, and diarrhea may be present. Bullous impetigo is treated with systemic antibiotics and may require hospitalization to prevent dehydration and electrolyte imbalance.

Erysipelas

Erysipelas is a skin infection caused by *Streptococcus* bacteria affecting the deep epidermis with extension into the lymphatic system. It is seen most frequently in patients who have immune deficiency, diabetes, alcoholism, skin ulceration, fungal infections, and impaired lymphatic drainage following surgery. The face is involved in 20 percent of cases. It may be present in dental patients

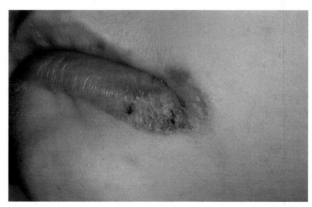

Figure 3–9   Impetigo. Dermatitis associated with superficial infection of the skin caused by *Staphylococcus aureus*.

who also complain of leg involvement. Blisters, fever, chills, as well as painful, very red, swollen, and warm skin underneath the lesions, can be seen on the cheeks and bridge of the nose. The erythematous skin lesions enlarge rapidly and have a sharply demarcated raised edge, which distinguishes them from cellulitis related to a dental infection (Fig. 3-10). The cervical lymph nodes may be swollen and palpable during the head and neck examination. Occasionally, a red streak extending to the lymph node may be seen. Antibiotics such as penicillin are used to eliminate the infection. Patients experiencing repeated episodes of erysipelas may require long-term antibiotics.

Streptococcal Pharyngitis and Tonsillitis

Although most cases of *pharyngitis* are the result of viruses, group A β-hemolytic streptococci are responsible for up to 30 percent of acute cases in children. Streptoccocal pharyngitis, also called strep throat, is most common in children ages 5 to 15, and is usually spread by direct contact. Adults may be affected, especially parents of young children, or anyone in close contact with an infected person. Symptoms include sore throat, **dysphagia** (difficulty swallowing), cervical lymphadenopathy, and fever. Erythema and swelling of the uvula and tonsils are noted clinically (Fig. 3-11). A yellowish exudate may be seen in the tonsillar crypts.

Without treatment, streptococcal pharyngitis usually resolves in 3 to 4 days; however, antibiotic therapy reduces patient morbidity and prevents potential complications such as scarlet fever, rheumatic fever, *glomerulonephritis*, and peritonsillar abscess. Penicillin is prescribed only after a diagnosis of streptococcal infection is confirmed by rapid antigen detection in the laboratory.

Clinical Implications

The presence of yellow-white material in a patient's tonsillar crypts does not necessarily imply an acute infection. *Tonsillar concretions* are foul-smelling masses of food debris, superficial epithelial cells, and bacteria that commonly form in these invaginations. In contrast to tonsillitis, the patient is asymptomatic and the surrounding tonsillar tissue is not inflamed.

Scarlet Fever

Scarlet fever is a systemic infection that most often occurs secondary to streptococcal pharyngitis. The characteristic oral clinical features are white coating

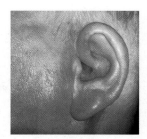

Figure 3–10   Erysipelas. Warm, swollen erythema with sharp border caused by superficial infection of *Streptococcus pyogenes*. (From Taber's Cyclopedic Medical Dictionary, ed. 21. F.A. Davis, Philadelphia, p 83.)

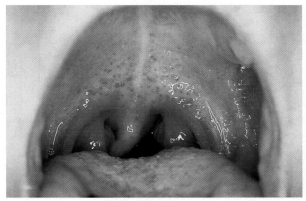

Figure 3–11   Strep throat. Inflammation of the oropharynx and petechiae of the soft palate caused by strep throat. (From Tamparo, CD: Diseases of the Human Body, ed. 5. F.A. Davis, Philadelphia, 2011, p 357.)

of the dorsal tongue during the first few days. The fungiform papillae become hyperplastic and can be seen through the coating—an appearance described as *white strawberry tongue*. By the fourth or fifth day of the infection, the white coating disappears to reveal an erythematous surface underneath known as *red strawberry tongue* (Fig. 3-12). The most diagnostic feature of scarlet fever is its classic skin rash, which develops within 2 to 4 days and is likened to "sunburn with goose bumps." The distribution of the rash is usually limited to the trunk and extremities, normally sparing the facial skin. After a week, scaling and desquamation of the skin begins and may last for several weeks. These clinical features are the result of a toxin produced by group A β-hemolytic streptococci, which preferentially attacks blood vessels rather than infection of the tissues themselves. A course of systemic antibiotics is recommended to prevent possible complications.

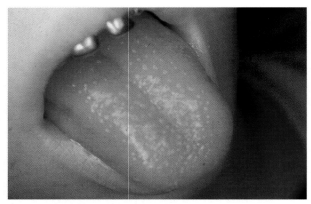

Figure 3–12   Red strawberry tongue. Smooth, erythematous appearance of the dorsal tongue with hyperplastic fungiform papillae.

Diphtheria

Diphtheria is a potentially fatal infection caused by *Corynebacterium diphtheria*. The organism is transmitted through direct contact and produces a deadly exotoxin that results in a spreading tissue necrosis. Vaccination against diphtheria has been universal since the 1920s. Cases are extremely uncommon in the United States and are usually seen in immunosuppressed patients or persons who did not receive the full schedule of recommended booster vaccines. According to the CDC, no confirmed cases of diphtheria have been reported in the United States since 2003. However, the potential for cases to reemerge increases as more parents decline to have their children vaccinated.

Among the unvaccinated, symptoms of diphtheria include low-grade fever, sore throat, headache, and vomiting. Mucosal surfaces of the nose and throat are often affected. Intraorally, a thin yellowish exudate forms over the tonsils and evolves into an adherent necrotic membrane. Eventually, the pseudomembrane becomes green or black in color and may spread to the soft palate and larynx. Myocarditis, neuropathy, and airway obstruction are frequent potential complications. The presence of *C. diphtheria* is diagnosed by laboratory culture. Treatment consists of antibiotics and diphtheria antitoxin, which is available in the United States only through the CDC. The death rate from diphtheria has improved from 50% to 5% since the development of antitoxin.

Clinical Implications

Cutaneous diphtheria presents as nonhealing skin ulcers and can occur even in vaccinated patients. The diagnosis should be kept in mind for patients who have recently traveled to countries where diphtheria is endemic.

Actinomycosis

Actinomycosis is an opportunistic infection caused by *Actinomyces israelii*. About two-thirds of cases are diagnosed in the head and neck region, a condition called *cervicofacial actinomycosis*. The *Actinomyces* species are found ubiquitously in tonsillar crypts, carious lesions, oral biofilm, and calculus. They are members of the resident oral microflora that can cause disease upon access to areas they would not normally colonize. The organisms gain entry via an injury or break in local barrier, such as through an extraction socket, soft tissue trauma, nonvital tooth, or blow to the jaw. Unlike most infections, actinomycosis spreads by direct extension through tissues, ignoring the usual lymphatic and vascular channels.

The most common location for cervicofacial actinomycosis is the soft tissue overlying the angle of the mandible (Fig. 3-13). The process is usually chronic, slowly progressing, and nonpainful. A "wooden" area of fibrosis develops initially, followed by formation of a central abscess. The suppurative phase of the infection contains characteristic yellow flecks or particles called *sulfur granules*. The fibrotic nature of affected areas makes it difficult for antibiotics to

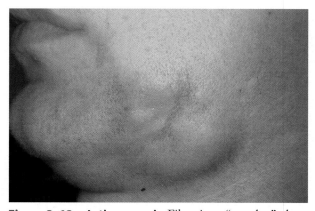

Figure 3–13   Actinomycosis. Fibrotic or "wooden" phase with erythema and swelling of the skin overlying the mandible.

penetrate the lesion. Patients usually require at least 6 weeks of antibiotic therapy in conjunction with surgical drainage.

Clinical Implications

Apical inflammatory lesions with actinomycotic colonization may be difficult to resolve with root canal therapy, but typically stay localized and do not require antibiotics.

Cat-Scratch Disease

Cat-scratch disease is a *self-limiting infection* that usually occurs after contact with a kitten. Cats are natural reservoirs of the causative organism *Bartonella henselae*. No person-to-person transmission has been documented. Cat-scratch disease is the most common cause of *regional lymphadenopathy* in children. The first presenting feature is a skin pustule that develops within 2 weeks in an area that was scratched, bitten, or licked by a cat. Regional lymphadenopathy develops around 3 weeks later and is the most important aspect of the infection (Fig. 3-14). Single or multiple lymph nodes may be enlarged, often accompanied by fever and malaise. Scratches located on the face most often result in submandibular lymphadenopathy.

A diagnosis of cat-scratch disease may be made based on the clinical history and features and then be confirmed by serological testing for antibodies to *Bartonella henselae*. The infection is self-limiting but long-lasting. Total resolution may take months and lymph node aspiration may be necessary for comfort. Antibiotics are reserved for immunocompromised patients or severe infections.

Clinical Implications

The initial site of skin trauma in cat-scratch disease is often resolved by the time lymphadenopathy develops. This may make clinical diagnosis challenging due to a low index of suspicion for contact with a cat. Presentation of lymphadenopathy adjacent to the mandible may be suggestive of a dental infection. Asking children or parents about contact with pets and looking for evidence of scratches may be helpful in the absence of dental disease.

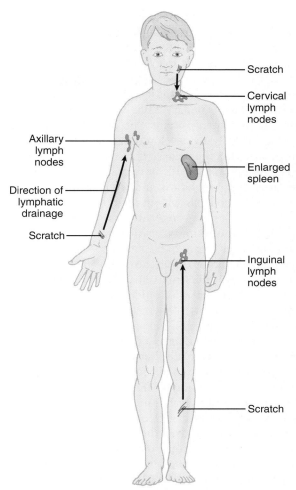

Figure 3–14 Cat-scratch disease. Bacterial infection introduced by a cat scratch drains to the nearest group of lymph nodes (regional lymph nodes) causing pain and swelling.

Tuberculosis

Tuberculosis (TB) is a potentially life-threatening infection caused by *Mycobacterium tuberculosis*. One-third of the world's population is infected with TB. Although the incidence of TB in the United States continues to decline every year, disproportionally high rates are occurring among minorities and foreign-born persons. The organism is acquired by inhalation of airborne droplets from someone with active disease. TB infection is not synonymous with active TB disease. A person's initial exposure to *M. tuberculosis* causes a localized, chronic inflammatory reaction in the lungs called *primary TB*. The body creates a physical, granulomatous barrier that successfully "walls off" the bacteria but is unable to destroy or remove the bacteria (*latent TB*). Individuals with latent TB do not become ill and cannot transmit the infection to others (Fig 3-15).

Active TB disease develops in only 5% to 10% of infected individuals. This usually occurs later in life as *secondary TB*. Secondary TB is a reactivation of the infection, usually in patients who become immunosuppressed, elderly, or develop other debilitating chronic diseases. AIDS is a major risk factor for active TB disease. Symptoms of TB develop slowly and include malaise, fever, weight loss, and productive cough. Chest pain and hemoptysis (bloody sputum) occur as the disease progresses. Lesions that occur outside the lungs, called **extrapulmonary lesions,** are possible and can develop in any organ. In the head and neck, the cervical lymph nodes are involved most often. Oral lesions are rare and usually present as a painless, nonhealing ulcer with rolled borders, not unlike an oral squamous cell carcinoma. Notably, 50 percent of AIDS patients with active TB have extrapulmonary involvement.

TB infection is diagnosed by purified protein derivative (PPD) skin test, but the test does not distinguish between latent and active disease. A chest x-ray is usually the next diagnostic step when an individual has a positive PPD test, followed by **sputum culture** if active TB is suspected. Treatment for active TB consists of multi-agent drug therapy owing to the organism's propensity toward developing resistance to a single medication. Combination drug therapy for active tuberculosis is usually 6 to 24 months. Compliance with drug therapy for this long time period may become problematic.

A vaccine for tuberculosis (BCG) is often given to children in countries with high rates of tuberculosis. Because the United States does not have a high incidence of tuberculosis, BCG vaccination is usually recommended only for certain health professionals and military personnel who may be exposed to TB carriers.

Clinical Implications

About 5% to 10% of the U.S. population will have a positive PPD skin test. Patients with a positive PPD and a negative chest x-ray pose no health risk to dental personnel. It is important for health-care providers to have a PPD annually and a chest x-ray if their PPD is positive. The potential to transmit infection to patients is only possible if the clinician has active untreated TB.

Syphilis

Syphilis is an infection caused by a spirochete bacterium called *Treponema pallidum*. The organism is transmitted mainly by sexual contact, but transmission from a pregnant woman to her developing fetus also may occur. Syphilis is five to ten times more common in African Americans than in Caucasians and continues to be a major health problem in urban areas and the southern United States. Following the emergence of penicillin in the 1940s, the incidence of syphilis in the United States declined gradually until the 2000s. According to the CDC, from 2001 to 2009, the rate of syphilis increased every year, mainly among men. Specifically, men who have sex with men (MSM) accounted for 63 percent of reported cases of primary and secondary syphilis in 2008. Oral sexual practices are being implicated in an increasing proportion of cases occurring in MSM.

Syphilis progresses through three clinical stages, referred to as primary, secondary, and tertiary stages. Patients are very contagious during the primary and secondary stages.

Primary syphilis occurs upon infection with *T. pallidum*. A painless ulcer called a **chancre** develops at the anatomic site of exposure (Fig. 3-16). This may occur anywhere from 3 days to 3 months after infection and is accompanied by regional lymphadenopathy. Although the vast majority of chancres develop on the genitalia and anus, the oral cavity is the second most common extragenital location, especially on the lips and tongue. Without treatment, a chancre heals gradually over a period of several weeks.

Secondary or disseminated syphilis may develop anywhere from 4 to 10 weeks after the primary infection, even before the chancre has resolved. This stage is characterized by a **maculopapular skin rash** that is distributed all over the body, including the palms and soles (Fig. 3-17A). Symptoms are nonspecific and include fever, headache, body aches, lymphadenopathy, and malaise. **Mucous patches** of the oral mucosa occur in about 30 percent of patients and appear as areas of tender white mucosa (Fig.3-17B). The signs and symptoms of secondary syphilis generally resolve within 3 to 12 weeks.

The next step is **latent** *syphilis*, a symptom-free and lesion-free period that may last anywhere from 1 to 30 years. With the exception of mother-to-fetus transmission, individuals are unlikely to infect others

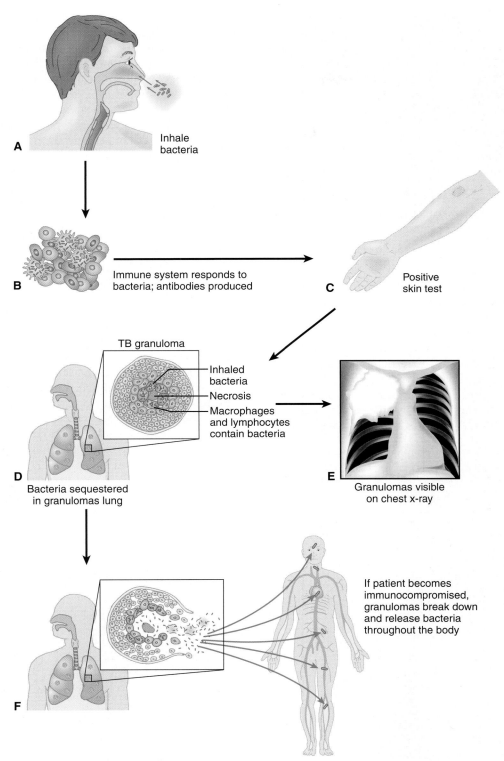

A   Inhale
     bacteria

B   Immune system responds to
     bacteria; antibodies produced

C   Positive
     skin test

TB granuloma

     Inhaled
     bacteria
     Necrosis
     Macrophages
     and lymphocytes
     contain bacteria

D   Bacteria sequestered
     in granulomas lung

E   Granulomas visible
     on chest x-ray

If patient becomes
immunocompromised,
granulomas break down
and release bacteria
throughout the body

F

Figure 3–15   Tuberculosis. Inhalation of *Mycobacterium tuberculosis* leading to primary and disseminated tuberculosis.

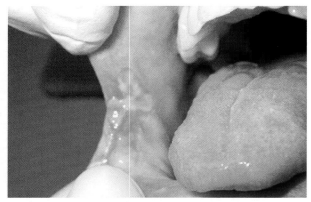

Figure 3–16   Chancre: labial mucosa. Primary syphilis; painless chancre at site of contact following 3-week incubation.

during the latent phase. About 30 percent of patients will progress to *tertiary syphilis*, the most serious stage. Complications of the vascular system, such as aortic aneurysm and congestive heart failure, are life-threatening. The central nervous system (CNS) is frequently affected and may manifest as paralysis, psychosis, or dementia. Active sites of granulomatous inflammation called **gummas** may cause significant tissue destruction and can be seen throughout the body. Intraoral gummas are seen most often on

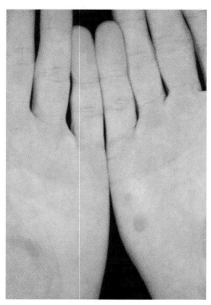

Figure 3–17   Secondary syphilis. Generalized nonpruritic red-brown macules and papules of palms.

the tongue or palate. Palatal lesions may cause perforation into the nasal cavity (Fig. 3-18).

Maternal transmission of *T. pallidum* to the fetus during primary or secondary syphilis usually results in miscarriage, stillbirth, or an infant with birth defects. Fetal infection during latent syphilis results in a child born with *congenital syphilis*. Untreated infants who survive develop tertiary syphilis, which affects the CNS, eyes, ears, bones, and teeth. Common stigmata include frontal bossing, high-arched palate, and saddle nose deformity. An English venereologist and pathologist named Sir Jonathan Hutchinson described three other features of congenital syphilis known collectively as **Hutchinson's triad** and include: 1) Hutchinson's incisors and mulberry molars, 2) ocular interstitial keratitis, and 3) eighth cranial nerve deafness. Although very few patients demonstrate all three components of Hutchinson's triad, the combination is considered to be pathognomonic for congenital syphilis. Hutchinson's teeth are the most common component of the triad, seen in greater than 60 percent of patients. *Hutchinson's incisors* are widest in the middle one-third of the crown and tapered toward the incisal edge, imparting a screwdriver-like appearance. Enamel hypoplasia is seen at the incisal edge, creating a characteristic notch. *Mulberry molars* also taper toward the occlusal surface and have irregular occlusal anatomy with multiple enamel projections that have been likened to a mulberry (Fig. 3-19).

Syphilis can be diagnosed by serological testing for antibodies or identification of the microorganisms

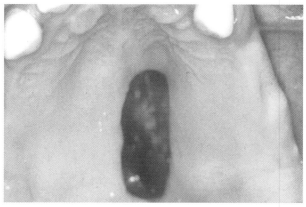

Figure 3–18   Tertiary syphilis (gumma). Untreated syphilis may lead gummas to erode into underlying tissue causing deformities as seen here on the palate.

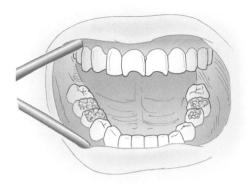

Figure 3–19   Congenital syphilis: oral manifestations. Hutchinson's incisors and mulberry molars.

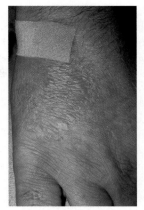

Figure 3–20   Leprosy. Tuberculoid form presents with maculopapular and hypopigmented skin lesions. (From Barankin, B: Derm Notes. F.A. Davis, Philadelphia, 2006, p 195.)

in a biopsy specimen. Syphilis is treated with intramuscular or intravenous penicillin. The formulation and dose schedule is tailored to the individual based on stage, immune status, and clinical features.

Leprosy

Leprosy (Hansen's disease) is a granulomatous infectious disease characterized by disfiguring skin lesions, nerve damage, upper respiratory mucosal lesions, and progressive debilitation. It is caused by the organism *Mycobacterium leprae*. Leprosy is not very contagious and has a long incubation period. The exact mode of transmission is unknown. Approximately 95 percent of people are naturally immune and do not contract the illness when exposed to the bacterium. Leprosy is common in temperate, tropical, and subtropical climates. Approximately 100 cases per year are diagnosed in the United States, mainly in the South, California, Hawaii, and U.S. island possessions.

Leprosy has two common forms, tuberculoid and lepromatous. Both forms produce skin lesions but the lepromatous form is most severe, producing large, disfiguring nodules. The skin becomes pale (Fig. 3-20) with gradually decreasing sensation to touch, heat, and pain. Repeated injury that cannot be felt may lead to loss of hands or feet. In the lepromatous form of the disease, large disfiguring nodules develop. In advanced stages, destruction of the nasal bridge is characteristic, resulting in a saddle-nose deformity. Antibiotics are used to treat leprosy

and infected individuals are no longer contagious after as few as 2 weeks of treatment.

Fungal Infections

Fungi are primitive vegetable forms that include mold and mildew. Fungi live in air, in soil, on plants, in water, and in the human body. Only about half of all types of fungi and their spores are harmful. Fungal spores may be inhaled or acquired on the skin and mucous membranes. As a result, fungal infections often start in the lungs, on the skin, or in the mouth. Fungal infections are more common in patients with a weakened immune system due to illness or immunosuppressive medications or in those taking antibiotics that alter normal oral flora.

Candidiasis

Candidiasis is the most common superficial fungal infection seen in the oral cavity. It also has been called *candidosis* and *moniliasis* in the past. Formerly, it was considered to be strictly an opportunistic infection, but it is often detected in otherwise healthy persons. Most cases of candidiasis are mild and localized, although it can disseminate and become life-threatening in an immunocompromised patient. There are more than 40 known species of *Candida*. The most common causative fungal organism, *Candida albicans*, is a part of the indigenous oral microflora in about half of the general population. In addition to *C. albicans*, species known to cause infection in the oral cavity include *C. krusei, C. glabrata, C. tropicalis, and C.*

dubliniensis. The risk of developing a clinical infection depends on the immune status of the patient, the local environment, and the virulence of the particular strain of *Candida.* Several clinical patterns of candidiasis have been identified and are discussed below.

Pseudomembranous Candidiasis

Pseudomembranous candidiasis is characterized by adherent, white "cottage cheese-like" plaques that consist of *C. albicans* organisms, superficial epithelial cells, and debris (Fig. 3-21). The plaques can be wiped off with dry gauze. Underlying mucosa may be erythematous but is intact. This clinical presentation is often referred to as *thrush.* The most common precipitating factors for developing thrush are use of broad-spectrum antibiotic therapy or immunosuppression either from underlying disease or therapeutic immunosuppression with corticosteroids or other immunomodulary medications. Use of steroid asthma inhalers is an increasingly common cause of oral candidiasis localized to the soft palate where the medication initially contacts the tissues (see Figs. 3-22 and 3-23). Infants whose immune systems have not fully developed are also susceptible. The lesions are commonly distributed on the buccal mucosa, palate, and dorsal tongue. Symptoms vary: patients may be completely asymptomatic, complain of an unpleasant taste, or experience oral burning.

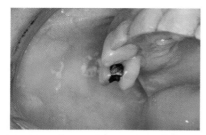

Figure 3–21   Pseudomembranous candidiasis. Multiple white plaques on the buccal mucosa.

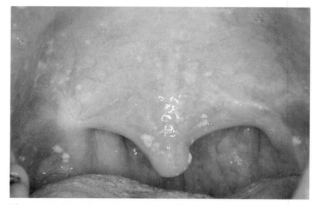

Figure 3–22   Pseudomembranous candidiasis. Patient with asthma developed pseudomembranous candidiasis of the uvula and tonsillar pillars after using corticosteroid-containing inhaler.

Clinical Implications

Coated tongue represents an increase in the thickness of keratin on the dorsal tongue that is often mistakenly attributed to candidal infection. Coated tongue is common among smokers and individuals with a soft diet, suggesting an etiology related to either increased production or decreased desquamation of keratin. Patients who have coated tongue but do not complain of oral burning or other symptoms most likely do not have candidiasis.

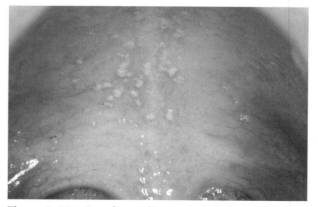

Figure 3–23   Pseudomembranous candidiasis. White-yellow plaques on the palate of a patient using inhaled corticosteroids to manage asthma.

Erythematous Candidiasis

Erythematous candidiasis is more common than pseudomembranous candidiasis, but may be more challenging to diagnose. *Acute atrophic candidiasis* is a symptomatic form of erythematous candidiasis characterized by diffuse atrophy of the filiform papillae on the dorsal tongue, creating a smooth, bald appearance (Fig. 3-24). This type of candidiasis tends to occur in xerostomic patients or those taking antibiotics. Patients normally complain that their tongue feels "scalded." More localized loss of the filiform papillae is called *central papillary atrophy,* also known as median rhomboid glossitis. The lesion is

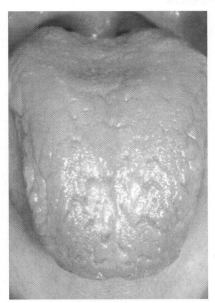

Figure 3–24 **Acute atrophic candidiasis.** Generalized erythema and atrophy of the dorsal tongue papillae.

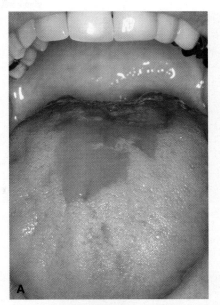

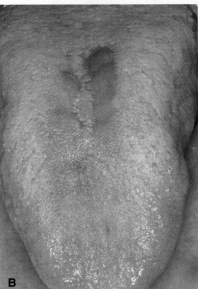

Figure 3–25 **Central papillary atrophy. A and B.** Smooth, bald appearance localized to the mid-dorsal tongue.

located on the posterior dorsal tongue at the midline and is usually asymptomatic (Fig. 3-25A and B). Erythematous candidiasis may also develop on the hard palate as a "kissing lesion" in contact with central papillary atrophy.

Denture stomatitis is the term used to describe erythema limited to denture-bearing areas of the oral mucosa (Figs. 3-26 and 3-27). Denture stomatitis is more likely to develop in patients who wear their dentures constantly and fail to remove them overnight. Expert opinions differ on whether denture stomatitis is a true candidal infection or simply a host inflammatory response to colonization of the denture by *C. albicans*.

Clinical Implications

A patient with denture stomatitis who complains of pain and tenderness should be tested for oral candidiasis. Table 3-1 describes how to perform a cytologic smear.

Angular Cheilitis

Angular cheilitis is a term used to describe redness and cracking at the corners of the mouth (Fig. 3-28). Contrary to popular belief, this problem is not related to vitamin deficiency, but caused by infection with *C. albicans* and/or *S. aureus*. Patients with reduced vertical dimension of occlusion due to loss of posterior teeth

or an inadequate vertical dimension of prosthesis are particularly prone to angular cheilitis due to the skin creases that develop near the corners of the mouth. Saliva wicks out into these folds, creating a constant, moist environment that predisposes the patient to candidal infection. More extensive involvement of the lip vermillion and perioral skin called *cheilocandidiasis* or *candidal cheilitis* can occur and is usually associated with thumb sucking or habitual lip licking (Fig. 3-29).

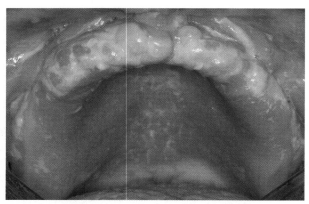

Figure 3–26 Denture stomatitis. Intense erythema of the denture-bearing mucosa with thick white plaques of Candida albicans.

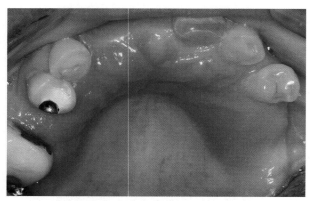

Figure 3–27 Denture stomatitis. Atrophic candidiasis on the palate in a patient wearing an ill-fitting denture.

Treatment often involves a combination of antifungal and anti-inflammatory agents.

Chronic Hyperplastic Candidiasis

Chronic hyperplastic candidiasis is an uncommon type of oral candidiasis with unique clinical features. The classic presentation is a white or speckled red/white lesion on the anterior buccal or labial mucosa just inside the commissure that cannot be scraped off (Fig. 3-30A and B). It is often seen in immunocompromised patients (Fig. 3-31). Some experts feel that this condition is simply candidiasis superimposed on a pre-existing keratotic lesion. If the lesion does not resolve after 2 weeks of therapy, it should be biopsied.

A diagnosis of candidiasis may be made based on clinical appearance, culture, cytology, or biopsy. The most commonly prescribed antifungal medications include oral dissolvable clotrimazole troches, Nystatin oral suspension, and systemic fluconazole. Several factors may be considered in determining the best treatment for each patient. Topical medications include dissolvable lozenges (troches) and liquid. In order for them to be effective, they must contact the affected mucosal surfaces. Clotrimazole troches must be dissolved on the tongue five times per day for 10 to 14 days. Nystatin suspension is heavily sweetened to disguise the unpleasant taste and therefore may be a poor choice for patients with a high caries risk. It must also be used four to five times per day, making compliance a problem. Neither is practical for denture patients who must remove the prosthesis to use

Table 3.1	How to Perform a Cytologic Smear
Procedural Step	**Armamentarium**
1. Do NOT wipe or otherwise disturb the area to be sampled.	
2. Write the patient's name in PENCIL (not pen) on the frosted end of the glass slide.	

Table 3.1	How to Perform a Cytologic Smear—cont'd

Procedural Step	Armamentarium
3. If the patient has a very dry mouth, have them rinse gently with a few drops of water before the specimen is collected.	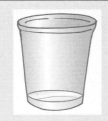
4. Using a damp (not soaked) wooden tongue blade, firmly wipe the area. Use enough strokes to collect a visible accumulation of oral fluids.	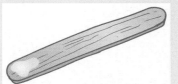
5.Transfer the fluids to a clean, dry glass slide. Smear the sample across the slide to make a thin coat.	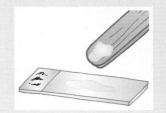
6. Hold the glass slide up to the light. If you can see the sample on the slide, you have enough. Do not overload the slide. Repeat in another area, if necessary, to obtain an adequate sample.	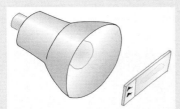
7. Spray Cytofix or alcohol-based hair spray on the slide from a distance of about 1 foot. DO NOT spray too closely to prevent rinsing the cells off the slide. Do not overspray; one or two swipes should be enough.	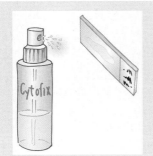
8. Allow the slide to dry for a few minutes and place the slide in the slide container.	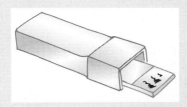

Continued

Table 3.1 How to Perform a Cytologic Smear—cont'd	
Procedural Step	**Armamentarium**
9. Send to a pathology laboratory for diagnosis.	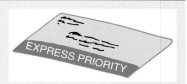

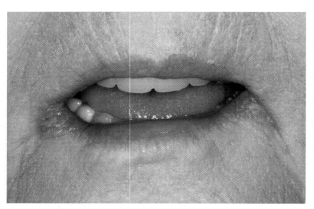

Figure 3–28   Angular cheilitis. Erythema, cracking, and subtle white plaques at the corners of the mouth in a patient with reduced vertical dimension of occlusion.

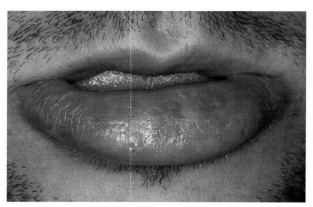

Figure 3–29   Cheilocandidiasis. Surface erosions and prominent swelling of the lower lip of a habitual lip balm user, which seals in moisture and can worsen the problem.

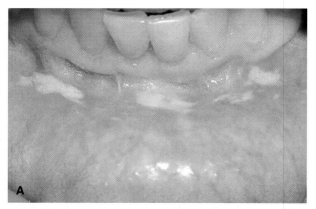

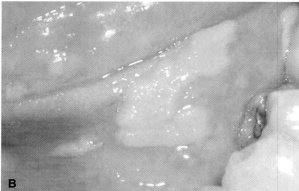

Figure 3–30   Hyperplastic candidiasis. A and B. Patient with autoimmune disease on immunosuppressive therapy presents with thick white adherent plaque of the floor of the mouth and labial vestibule.

Histoplasmosis

Histoplasmosis is a systemic fungal infection common in humid geographic locations. The etiologic agent *Histoplasma capsulatum* exists in the environment as spores, which become airborne and are inhaled into the lungs. It is commonly found in bird and bat droppings and can be contracted by hunters and others who live in **endemic** areas. Person-to-person transmission does not occur. It is the most common systemic fungal

the medication. Fluconazole is taken orally for 2 weeks. It requires the least amount of patient compliance but may be contraindicated with other medications. A bioadhesive disc is now available that adheres to the maxillary or mandibular vestibule and releases miconazole continuously for 12 hours. It may be used in both dentate and edentulous patients.

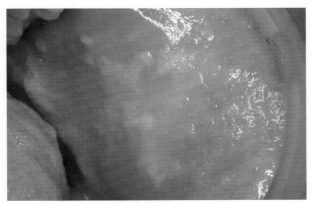

Figure 3–31   Hyperplastic candidiasis. Patient on systemic corticosteroid therapy with thick white adherent plaque of buccal mucosa.

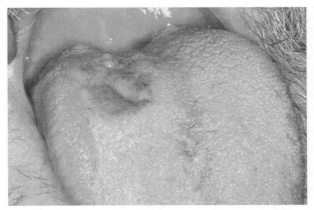

Figure 3–32   Disseminated histoplasmosis: tongue. Irregular ulceration and cratering of the dorsal tongue.

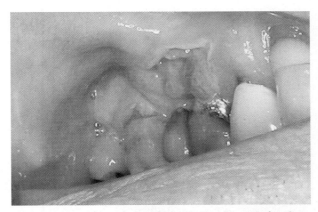

Figure 3–33   Disseminated histoplasmosis: periodontium. Histoplasmosis in an immunocompromised patient.

infection in the United States and is endemic to the Ohio and Mississippi River valleys. Nearly 80 percent of the population living in these areas has been infected and will have a positive *histoplasmin* skin test similar to that used in detecting tuberculosis. The severity of infection is variable and depends mainly on the amount of spores inhaled and the immune status of the patient. Most cases that occur in healthy patients are mild or totally asymptomatic. Immunocompromised patients are at higher risk for infection.

Acute histoplasmosis is a flu-like infection of the lungs that usually occurs in people who are exposed to a large quantity of spores. The disease is self-limiting and resolves in about 2 weeks. The host immune system may destroy the yeasts or contain them inside macrophages with the potential for reactivation later in life if the patient becomes immunocompromised. *Chronic histoplasmosis* is less common than the acute form and typically develops in elderly patients with emphysema. The clinical presentation is similar to pulmonary TB.

Disseminated histoplasmosis is the least common type of infection and is generally limited to immunocompromised or debilitated patients. Disseminated histoplasmosis is characterized by extrapulmonary spread and may affect any organ system. Oral lesions are usually a manifestation of disseminated disease and appear as a solitary, nonhealing ulcerated area (Fig. 3-32) or local tissue destruction (Fig 3-33). The lesion is often firm to palpation and mimics oral cancer. Disseminated histoplasmosis is usually fatal if not treated and requires intravenous antifungal drugs.

Rarely, inhaled spores can become entrapped within the oral tissues and produce a localized reaction. *Gingival histoplasmosis* may present as a recalcitrant gingivitis (Fig. 3-34) or severe periodontitis. The organisms can be highlighted in biopsy specimens with special tissue staining techniques (Fig. 3-35).

Mucormycosis (Zygomycosis)

Mucormycosis is an uncommon opportunistic infection caused by fungal organisms of the genera *Mucor* or *Rhizopus*. The organisms grow on decaying organic debris and are released into the air as spores. Mucormycosis affects immunocompromised patients, particularly insulin-dependent diabetics who are poorly controlled and develop ketoacidosis. Ketoacidosis results in increased serum iron levels, which enhances the growth of these fungi. These large organisms tend to invade blood vessels, causing infarction and extensive necrosis (Fig. 3-36). The following discussion is limited to the form most relevant to the dental profession.

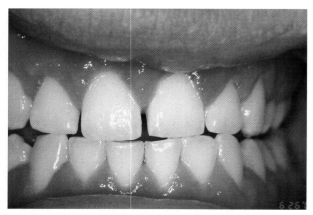

Figure 3–34 Localized gingival histoplasmosis. Child with environmental exposure to *Histoplasma capsulatum* and no systemic disease.

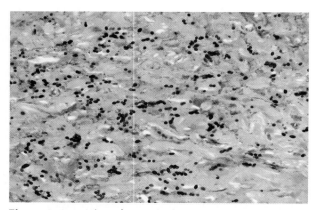

Figure 3–35 Histoplasmosis. Numerous *Histoplasma capsulatum* spores in an oral biopsy of an HIV-positive patient are highlighted by Grocott-Gomori methenamine silver stain.

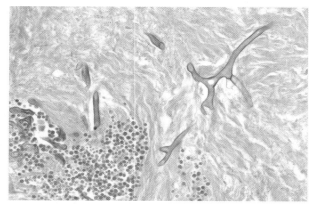

Figure 3–36 Mucormycosis. Large, branching *Mucor hyphae* tend to occlude small blood vessels.

Rhinocerebral mucormycosis involves the nose and sinuses with potential spread to the brain. It often presents with facial pain, headache, fever, and orbital cellulitis. Cranial nerve involvement can occur and may manifest as loss of vision, pupil dilation, seizures, or altered mental state. Nasal obstruction and discharge are also common. Infection of the maxillary sinus may present as swelling and ulceration of the palate or maxillary alveolus. Tissue surfaces involved by mucormycosis are characteristically black and necrotic. Imaging studies show significant destruction of normal tissues and opacification of the sinuses. Radical surgical debridement and high-dose intravenous amphotericin B is the recommended treatment for mucormycosis. Control of the patient's predisposing condition is also important, but even with appropriate treatment rhinocerebral mucormycosis is fatal in more than half of affected patients.

Aspergillosis

Aspergillosis is a fungal infection that primarily affects the respiratory tract. *Aspergillus fumigatus* is extremely common in the environment and is responsible for most cases. *Aspergillus* can be found in soil, dust, plants, and building materials and is an occupational hazard for construction workers in the setting of building construction, which can stir up *Aspergillus* spores from the soil.

Aspergillosis occurs in noninvasive and invasive forms. *Noninvasive aspergillosis* is a superficial disease that affects the respiratory tracts of otherwise healthy patients. It may present as either allergic fungal sinusitis or a tangled mass of organisms in the sinus called an aspergilloma. Healthy patients with noninvasive aspergillosis are treated with surgical debridement. *Invasive aspergillosis* is a common opportunistic infection and is usually limited to immunosuppressed patients. Most patients with invasive aspergillosis have pulmonary involvement. Patients often acquire aspergillosis as a **nosocomial** infection while in the hospital. Aggressive surgical debridement and systemic antifungal therapy is indicated for invasive aspergillosis, which is uniformly fatal if untreated.

Clinical Implications

Extraction or endodontic treatment of a maxillary molar tooth may cause minor damage to the maxillary sinus lining and predispose a patient to developing oral aspergillosis. The gingival sulcus has been suggested as the most likely route of entry. Clinical features include painful gingival ulceration surrounded by swollen, red-purple mucosa which becomes necrotic if untreated.

Blastomycosis

Blastomycosis has an overlapping geographic distribution with histoplasmosis but is much less common. Males with outdoor occupations or hobbies are at risk. Pulmonary blastomycosis may become disseminated, especially to the skin and mucous membranes of the mouth. Unlike most systemic fungal infections, blastomycosis is not seen with increased frequency among immunocompromised patients.

Coccidioidomycosis

Coccidiodomycosis is caused by *Coccidioides immitis* and *C. posadasii*, which are endemic to the southwestern United States and Mexico. About 40 percent of infected persons will have respiratory symptoms and a hypersensitivity reaction known as *valley fever*. Disseminated disease may develop weeks, months, or years after the primary infection and is usually seen in immunocompromised patients. The skin of the head, neck, and chest are most often involved with nodules, papules, pustules, verrucous lesions, abscesses, or ulcerations. Cervical lymph nodes that are infected may become necrotic, ulcerate, or drain.

Cryptococcosis

Cryptococcosis is a fungal infection caused by C*ryptococcus neoformans*, an encapsulated yeast that can live in both plants and animals. Disease occurs primarily in immunosuppressed patients. The organism usually affects the CNS, causing *meningitis* in the majority of cases. Cryptococcosis is a major cause of death in AIDS patients who are not receiving appropriate treatment.

Protozoal Infections

Protozoa are one-celled organisms that move about by means of appendages known as cilia or flagella. *Protozoal infections* are most common in rural areas of underdeveloped countries in Africa, Asia, and South America. They are relatively rare in the United States and other industrialized nations, but do occur among Western travelers to developing countries. One protozoal infection seen in the United States is *toxoplasmosis*, caused by *Toxoplasma gondii*. The organisms are present in cat feces and may be ingested by other animals or accidentally by humans who have close contact with infected cats. Lymphadenopathy of the buccal or submental nodes in the head and neck with an unknown etiology may be toxoplasmosis in a susceptible individual. Toxoplasmosis rarely causes problems in healthy patients,

but it is important for a pregnant patient to receive attention for this disorder. Transmission to the developing fetus can occur, causing *congenital toxoplasmosis*, which can lead to blindness and intellectual disabilities. To reduce the likelihood of infection, women should avoid cleaning a cat's litter box or handling raw meat during pregnancy (Fig. 3-37).

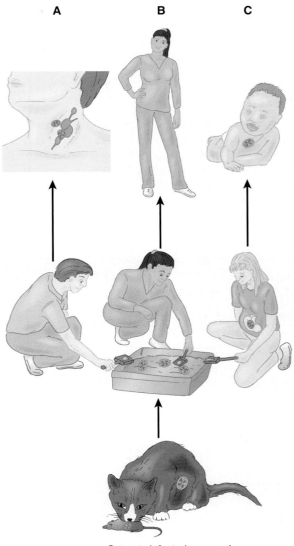

Cat eats infected prey and passes protozoa to litter box

Figure 3–37   Toxoplasmosis. A. Person with compromised immune system develops toxoplasmosis seen in cervical lymph nodes. **B.** Person with normal immune system with no signs of toxoplasmosis. **C.** Pregnant woman passes disease to child who is born with congenital toxoplasmosis.

Viral Infections

Although bacteria and viruses are both too small to be seen without a microscope, they are structurally very different. Bacteria are relatively complex, single-celled organisms, whereas viruses are not cells. They are composed of a protein coat and a core of genetic material, either RNA or DNA. They cannot survive without a host and must take over a cell to use its proteins to reproduce. Eventually, the cell ruptures and dies. Unlike bacteria, most viruses cause disease. Some of the most common viral infections seen in the oral cavity and tissues of the head and neck are discussed here.

Clinical Implications

Antibiotics do not kill viruses and are useless during a viral infection, such as the common cold. Only antiviral medications should be used to treat viral infections. Overuse of antibiotics for viral infections is promoting antibiotic resistance.

Herpes Virus Family

The human herpes viruses (HHV) are a large group of related DNA viruses endemic to humans, who are the only natural hosts. The HHV family is seen in Table 3-2. All the herpes viruses share a common theme of potential lifelong host infection. After the initial exposure to the virus, the virus is either completely or partially eliminated by host antibodies. When the virus is not eliminated, *latency* is established. Latency means the virus remains indefinitely to infect specific cells. Later in life, when immune conditions permit, the virus may be reactivated and cause clinical disease.

Herpes Simplex Virus

The two types of herpes simplex viruses, also called HSV-1 and HSV-2, or HHV-1 and HHV-2, have significant overlap in clinical disease presentation but they differ in anatomic distribution. HSV-1 predominantly affects the orofacial region and is transmitted through saliva or contact with active lesions. HSV-2, also known as genital herpes, is spread by sexual contact and affects the genitalia. Antibodies against one HSV type reduce

Table 3.2	Herpes Virus Family		
Type	**Eponym**	**Pathophysiology**	**Means of Transmission**
HHV-1	Herpes simplex virus-1 (HSV-1)	Oral and/or genital herpes (predominantly orofacial)	Close contact, including sexual contact
HHV-2	Herpes simplex virus-2 (HSV-2)	Oral and/or genital herpes (predominantly genital)	Close contact, primarily sexual contact
HHV-3	Varicella zoster virus (VZV)	Chickenpox and shingles	Respiratory and close contact, including sexual contact
HHV-4	Epstein-Barr virus (EBV)	Infectious mononucleosis, Burkitt's lymphoma, CNS lymphoma in AIDS patients, post-transplant lymphoproliferative syndrome (PTLD), nasopharyngeal carcinoma, HIV-associated hairy leukoplakia	Close contact, transfusions, tissue transplant, and congenital
HHV-5	Cytomegalovirus (CMV)	Infectious mononucleosis-like syndrome	Saliva
HHV-6	Roseolovirus, herpes lymphotropic virus	Roseola infantum	Respiratory and close contact
HHV-7	Roseolovirus	Roseola infantum	Respiratory and close contact
HHV-8	Kaposi's sarcoma-associated herpes virus (KSHV)	Kaposi's sarcoma	Close contact, including sexual contact

the chance of infection by the other type, but cannot be considered protective.

HSV-1 is **ubiquitous** worldwide and most adults will become infected by their 40s. Asymptomatic recurrences, where virus is released without any clinical signs or symptoms, occur frequently and are likely responsible for a large proportion of new primary HSV infections. The following discussion will focus on HSV-1 due to its clinical relevance to dental hygiene practice.

Primary HSV-1 Infection

Primary infections result from contact with a person who is actively shedding the virus. If the host mounts an effective immune response, HSV-1 primary infections are asymptomatic. However, in some individuals, usually children with developing immune systems, *acute herpetic gingivostomatitis* may occur. This form is characterized by fever, irritability, cervical lymphadenopathy, and painful oral lesions. The *stomatitis* suffix refers to tiny, fragile vesicles that develop on both the attached and unattached oral tissues and quickly rupture to form ulcers (Figs. 3-38 and 3-39). The *gingivo* prefix refers to painful, red, swollen gingiva that often ulcerates at the free gingival margin (see Fig. 3-38). Signs and symptoms resolve on their own within 1 week to 10 days, but antiviral medication such as acyclovir is beneficial if started during the first 3 days. Symptomatic primary HSV-1 infection that occurs in adulthood may present as **pharyngotonsillitis**. In this form, the lesions are localized to the throat and tonsils and accompanied by headache, fever, and sore throat. The clinical presentation may be difficult to distinguish from other forms of pharyngitis.

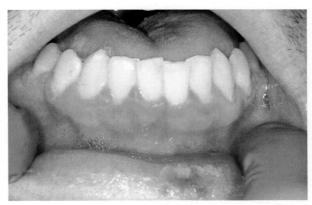

Figure 3–38 Primary herpetic gingivostomatitis in an adult. Ulcerations of the labial mucosa, tongue, and gingiva.

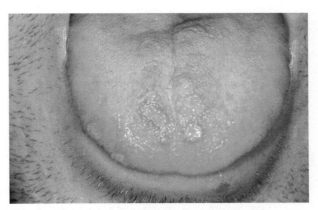

Figure 3–39 Primary herpetic gingivostomatitis. Painful ulcers of the dorsal tongue.

> ### Clinical Implications
>
> Recommended palliative care for children with acute herpetic gingivostomatitis includes non-aspirin analgesics, popsicles, and hydration. Aspirin should be avoided due to the association with Reye's syndrome when taken by children with a viral infection.

Recurrent HSV-1 Infection

After the primary infection, HSV-1 becomes latent in the trigeminal ganglion and may be reactivated in the future. Upon reactivation, lesions develop in any area of the skin or mucosa supplied by that nerve. The most common site of recurrence is the lip vermillion and perioral skin, known as *herpes labialis* (also known as cold sores or fever blisters) (Fig. 3-40). Recurrence of oral lesions is triggered by stimuli that can vary from person-to-person. Many patients can identify their triggers, such as exposure to sunlight, trauma, illness, emotional stress, or after manipulation of tissues during dental treatment. About 60 percent of patients report that the outbreak of the lesion is preceded by a *prodrome* of pain, tingling, burning, or itching in the area where a lesion will develop. The prodrome may precede the clinical lesion by up to 24 hours.

The initial presentation of herpes labialis is the development of a small cluster of vesicles that coalesce with each other to form larger vesicles that remain intact for up to 2 days (Fig. 3-41A). After 48 hours the vesicles rupture and leave tender, painful ulcers (Fig. 3-41B) that gradually form crusts (Fig. 3-41C). When crusting occurs, the virus can no longer be transmitted to another individual. Gradually, the

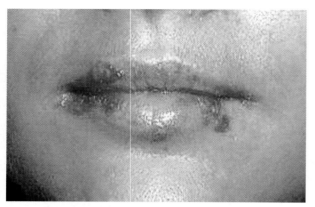

Figure 3–40   Herpes labialis. Widespread lesion of the lips.

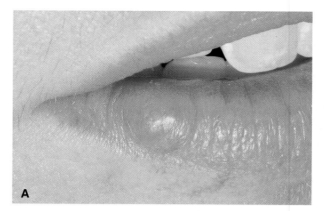

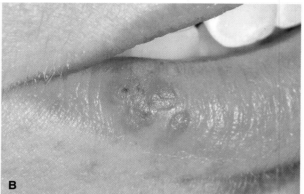

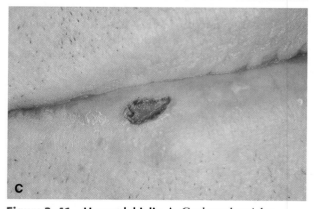

Figure 3–41   Herpes labialis. A. Coalesced vesicles. **B.** Same lesion 6 days later with ruptured vesicles and ulceration. **C.** Crust forms over the ulcer.

crust resolves and the skin returns to normal without scarring. Systemic antiviral medications may significantly reduce the discomfort and duration of herpes labialis, but have minimal effect if taken after the prodrome phase. Topical antivirals are less effective. Immunosuppressed patients generally show severe widespread lesions (Fig. 3-42).

> **Clinical Implications**
>
> Mechanical rupture of vesicles should be avoided, as this can cause spread of the virus to other areas. Accordingly, dental treatment should be postponed while patients are in the vesicle stage.

> **Clinical Implications**
>
> If dental treatment is a known trigger for a patient, then prophylactic antiviral therapy should be considered before dental appointments. Antiviral therapy given after the prodrome is not effective.

Recurrent Intraoral Herpes (Herpes Stomatitis)

Recurrent intraoral herpes or herpes stomatitis is a less common form of HSV-1. Lesions are limited to the keratinized attached mucosa of the gingiva or hard palate. Like herpes labialis, herpes stomatitis presents as a cluster of tiny vesicles that coalesce and then rupture to leave erosions or ulcerations rather than a crust (Fig. 3-43A, B, and C). Symptoms are usually less severe than herpes labialis; however, some outbreaks cause burning and pain, limiting the patient's ability to eat. Treatment is limited because there are few

medications that may be applied intraorally. Systemic medications administered after the outbreak begins are not effective.

Herpetic Whitlow

Herpetic whitlow is a painful herpes infection of the nail beds and fingers (Fig. 3-44). This was an occupational hazard among dental care providers before the advent

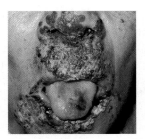

Figure 3–42 **Herpes simplex.** HIV-positive patient with severe orofacial lesions. (From Barankin, B: Derm Notes. F.A. Davis, Philadelphia, 2006, p 99.)

of universal precautions that include wearing gloves during treatment of all patients. Recurrences are painful and may lead to numbness and scarring, not to mention many days of missed work.

Herpetic Conjunctivitis

Herpetic conjunctivitis can also be a risk for dental care providers who do not wear eye protection. The virus may be carried to the eye when aerosols are created from a patient with an active HSV-1 lesion. Before the routine use of protective eyewear, this condition was common among dental personnel. Central nervous system involvement may also occur, where the virus causes life-threatening *herpes* **encephalitis**, predominantly in the elderly and immunocompromised.

Clinical Implications

Aphthous ulcers are often mistakenly diagnosed as a herpetic infection. Lesions of recurrent intraoral herpes are seen only on the keratinized attached tissues, whereas aphthous ulcers are usually limited to nonkeratinized moveable mucosa. Aphthous ulcers can be distinguished from ulcers of HSV-1 infection by their lack of a prodrome, absence of vesicles, and by their location. See Table 4-3 in Chapter 4 for comparison of recurrent aphthous ulcers and herpes simplex infection.

Varicella-Zoster Virus

Varicella-zoster virus (VZV or HHV-3) is spread through either direct contact or respiratory droplets. VZV is highly contagious and has a 10- to 20-day incubation period. Primary infection with VZV is usually symptomatic and causes *varicella*, or chickenpox. The incidence of varicella has decreased dramatically since the mid-1990s when an effective vaccine was

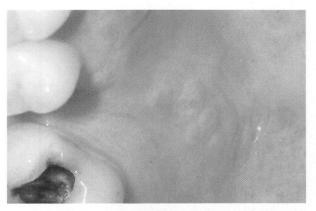

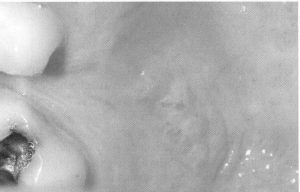

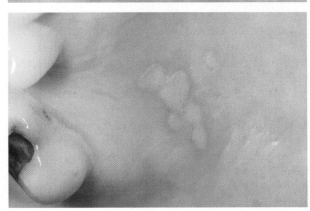

Figure 3–43 **Herpes: intraoral. A.** Cluster of vesicles on keratinized tissue of palatal gingiva. **B.** Vesicles coalesce and begin to rupture. **C.** Ulcers; intraoral lesions do not form a crust.

approved for use in the United States. Despite the vaccine, cases are still seen due to a national vaccination rate of only 85 percent.

Varicella usually affects school-age children and is characterized by rhinitis, or runny nose, sore throat, fever, and a **pruritic** skin rash often appearing in several crops. Skin lesions start as clear vesicles with a red base,

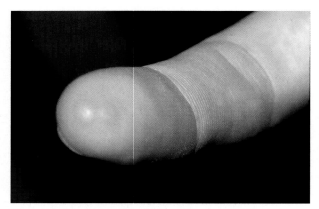

Figure 3–44 Herpetic whitlow. Herpes vesicles and ulcers on finger of dental health-care worker causing pain and scarring.

resembling "a dewdrop on a rose petal" (Fig. 3-45). These may progress to form **pustules** before crusting over. The rash develops first on the trunk and face and then spreads to the extremities. Oral involvement is common, especially on the lips and palate. Lesions are present for about 4 days. A person is considered contagious until all vesicles have crusted. Uncomplicated varicella in healthy children is usually treated symptomatically with non-aspirin analgesics and diphenhydramine (Benadryl). Varicella in adults tends to be much more severe and is associated with serious potential complications, such as varicella pneumonitis and encephalitis. Use of antiviral medications in adults may be helpful if started early.

VZV establishes latency in the dorsal root ganglia and may be reactivated later in life as *herpes zoster*, also called shingles. About 30 percent of the population suffers from shingles. Reactivation usually occurs only once and the risk increases with the increasing age of the patient. A prodrome of unilateral, intense pain typically precedes the clinical lesions and develops within the associated dermatome, which is an area of skin innervated

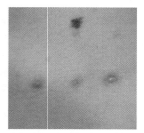

Figure 3–45 Chickenpox on skin. Pruritic erythematous vesicles resemble "dewdrops on rose petals." (From Barankin, B: Derm Notes. F.A. Davis, Philadelphia, 2006, p 75.)

by the infected nerve. Herpes zoster most often develops on the trunk, neck (Fig. 3-46), and face. The acute phase develops after 1 to 4 days and is characterized by clusters of small vesicles that collapse and crust over. The lesions are limited to the involved dermatome and therefore do not cross the midline. If the trigeminal nerve is affected, intraoral lesions (Fig. 3-47) are usually accompanied by involvement of the overlying facial skin (Fig. 3-48). If given promptly, systemic antivirals may reduce the duration and severity of the infection.

Clinical Implications

If the ophthalmic division of the trigeminal nerve is involved, the patient should be referred to an ophthalmologist immediately. Lesions present on the tip of the nose are an indication of potential ocular infection that can lead to blindness if left untreated.

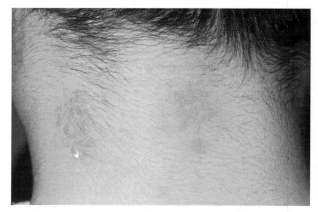

Figure 3–46 Herpes zoster. Neck of an adult.

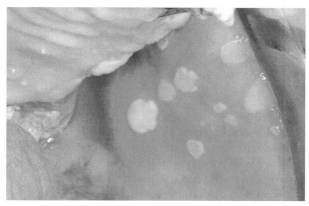

Figure 3–47 Herpes zoster. Painful ulcers of left buccal mucosa, confined to V2.

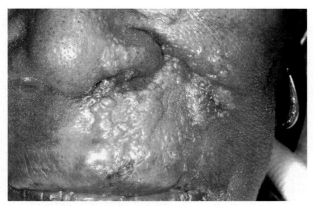

Figure 3–48   Herpes zoster. Lesions on face of the same patient, confined to V2.

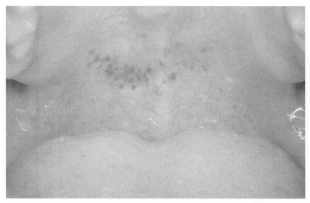

Figure 3–49   Infectious mononucleosis. Palatal petechiae in a young person with infectious mononucleosis.

The acute phase of herpes zoster resolves within 2 to 3 weeks; however, 15 percent of the population may experience continued pain known as *postherpetic* **neuralgia,** which is the chronic phase. Systemic antiviral medications given during the acute phase may decrease the likelihood of developing postherpetic neuralgia. Half of patients older than 60 years who develop zoster will progress to the chronic phase. Most cases of postherpetic neuralgia resolve within a year. Topical capsaicin provides relief for most patients. A vaccine called Zostavax is now available for people older than age 60 who had chickenpox as a child to help reduce the risk of zoster reactivation.

Epstein-Barr Virus

Epstein-Barr virus (EBV or HHV-4) is a member of the herpes virus family and one of the most common human viruses. As a herpes virus family member, it establishes a lifelong, persistent infection. As many as 95 percent of adults between 35 and 40 years of age have been infected.

Mononucleosis

Mononucleosis is caused by the Epstein-Barr virus (EBV). EBV is spread by direct contact with infected saliva, which has resulted in the common nickname "kissing disease." Young adults are prone to symptomatic primary infection characterized by a prodrome of prominent fatigue, followed by fever, sore throat, and lymphadenopathy. Hepatosplenomegaly may also be seen in some cases. Oral clinical features include swollen tonsils with a yellowish exudate. Palatal petechiae (Fig. 3-49) and NUG are also possible. The diagnosis of mononucleosis should be confirmed by blood studies. Most cases resolve within 4 to 6 weeks and supportive care with nonaspirin analgesics is recommended to manage symptoms.

Oral Hairy Leukoplakia

Oral hairy leukoplakia (OHL) is associated with the Epstein-Barr virus (EBV) mainly in people with HIV, both immunocompromised and immunocompetent. Among HIV-positive patients, the prevalence of OHL is higher in smokers and among homosexual males. It can affect patients who are HIV negative but are otherwise immunosuppressed. Cases are seen in those with acute lymphocytic leukemia, as well as heart, kidney, and bone marrow transplants.

OHL is often asymptomatic, with most patients unaware of its presence. Some patients experience symptoms including mild pain, **dysesthesia,** alteration of taste, and the psychological impact of its cosmetic appearance. OHL may appear and regress spontaneously. Unilateral or bilateral white lesions are classically seen on the lateral tongue (Fig. 3-50), but may also occur on the dorsal or ventral surfaces or on buccal mucosa. The lesions may vary in appearance from smooth, flat lesions to irregular and finely folded areas. There is no associated erythema or edema of the surrounding tissue. Unlike lesions caused by tongue chewing, also called morsicatio linguarum, that show horizontal folds of tissue, OHL often has vertical folds, thus distinguishing it from morsicatio linguarum.

As a benign lesion with low morbidity, OHL does not require specific treatment. Institution of highly active antiretroviral therapy (anti-HIV or HAART) in HIV and AIDS is useful in eliminating OHL.

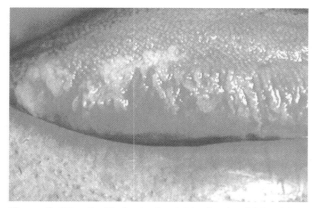

Figure 3–50 Oral hairy leukoplakia. Leukoplakia with vertical white striations along the lateral border of the tongue of an HIV-positive adult.

EBV-Related Cancer

EBV is also considered to be an oncogenic virus. It is associated with Burkitt's lymphoma and nasopharyngeal carcinoma, which are discussed in Chapter 7.

Cytomegalovirus

Cytomegalovirus (CMV or HHV-5) is a ubiquitous herpesvirus that typically causes symptomatic disease only in newborns and immunocompromised patients. Neonates may acquire it through the placenta, during delivery, or through breastfeeding. According to the CDC, about 1 out of every 150 children in the United States is born with CMV infection and 80 percent are asymptomatic. Symptomatic disease may be present at birth or develop around age 2. CMV infection during childhood manifests as hearing and vision loss or mental disability. Developmental tooth defects, typically enamel hypoplasia, are seen.

Most individuals will have contracted CMV by sometime in adulthood. The majority of primary CMV infections are asymptomatic in normal, healthy patients. The virus may remain latent in salivary ductal cells, endothelium, or chronic inflammatory cells. CMV is the most common opportunistic viral infection among AIDS patients. CMV co-infection is identified in 90 percent of *MSM* who are HIV-infected. Infection often manifests as CMV colitis, a bloody diarrhea; or *CMV chorioretinitis*, inflammation of the retina that can lead to blindness. Chronic oral ulcerations are seen frequently in AIDS patients and may be caused by co-infection with CMV and HSV.

Enteroviruses

Enteroviruses enter the body through the gastrointestinal tract. They represent a diverse group of RNA viruses that include echoviruses, coxsackievirus, polio viruses, and others. Infections can range from asymptomatic to life-threatening. Transmission occurs mainly through the fecal-oral route by ingestion, but saliva and respiratory droplets can be infectious during acute illness. Most symptomatic enterovirus infections are seen in young children and tend to occur in epidemics. Enteroviruses are extremely common and everyone is at risk. Individuals may become infected multiple times by different enterovirus strains. Most clinically evident infections are self-limiting, but the severity depends on the particular strain of virus.

Herpangina

Herpangina is usually caused by a coxsackievirus and is characterized by fever, sore throat, and oral lesions that develop on the soft palate, uvula, and tonsillar pillars. About 2 to 12 lesions are usually present and begin as small vesicles on nonkeratinized tissue that rupture to form shallow ulcers. Symptoms are fairly mild and lesions resolve within 1 week.

Clinical Implications

Herpangina may be confused with primary HSV-1 infection. However, herpangina does not occur on keratinized tissue, nor is the gingiva painful, red, or swollen.

Hand-Foot-and-Mouth Disease

Hand-foot-and-mouth disease is a common pediatric infection most often caused by coxsackievirus A16. Oral involvement precedes the skin rash and is accompanied by flu-like symptoms. Oral lesions are similar in appearance to that of herpangina but are more numerous and can affect almost any intraoral site (Fig. 3-51). Skin lesions that classically develop on the hands and feet begin as red macules that form tiny vesicles which heal without rupturing. The disease resolves within a week and symptomatic relief is the only treatment indicated.

Rubeola (Measles)

Measles is a disease caused by an extremely contagious paramyxovirus transmitted through respiratory droplets. Widespread use of the measles, mumps, and rubella (MMR) vaccine has led to more than a 99 percent reduction in the prevalence of measles in the United States

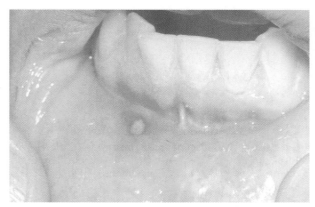

Figure 3–51   Hand-foot-and-mouth disease: oral.
Multiple small ulcers of the mandibular vestibule.

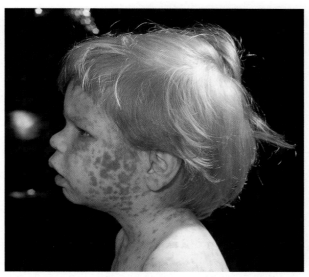

Figure 3–52   Measles. Diffuse, red, slightly elevated maculopapular rash in a child with a fever. (From Tamparo, CD: Diseases of the Human Body, ed. 5. F.A. Davis, Philadelphia, 2011.)

compared to the pre-vaccine era. However, measles continues to be common in other countries. Unvaccinated children and citizens traveling abroad have contributed to a resurgence of cases in recent years. The clinical features of infection classically progress through three stages, each lasting for about 3 days. The first stage is characterized by cough, runny nose, malaise, and low-grade fever. Multiple bluish-gray macules set on an erythematous background, called Koplik's spots, occur on the buccal and labial mucosa and are a pathognomonic oral manifestation of measles. The second stage is marked by a diffuse, red maculopapular skin rash that begins on the face (Fig. 3-52) then travels downward to affect the trunk and extremities. During the third and final stage, the fever and rash resolve, beginning with the skin that was involved first.

Potential complications such as otitis media, pneumonia, and encephalitis develop in about 20 percent of measles cases. Normal, healthy patients are treated symptomatically, but the infection can be devastating for immunosuppressed patients. The ideal therapy is prevention through vaccination.

Rubella (German measles)

Rubella (German measles) is caused by a togavirus that results in asymptomatic or mild infection in most individuals, but can cause serious harm to a developing fetus. The virus is spread through respiratory droplets and has a 2- to 3-week incubation period. Before the advent of the MMR vaccine in 1963, infections tended to occur in epidemics about every 6 to 9 years. The last major outbreak occurred in the early 1960s, during which over 12 million cases were reported in the United States.

Rubella is often completely asymptomatic. Infections are more likely to be symptomatic in teenagers and adults than in children. Features include lymphadenopathy and fever, followed by a measles-like skin rash. Although the rash lasts only for a few days, lymphadenopathy often takes weeks to resolve. Arthritis is a common complication.

Risk of transmission to the fetus is high if a woman becomes infected with rubella during the first trimester of pregnancy. The classic triad of features associated with *congenital rubella syndrome* includes deafness, heart disease, and cataracts. According to the CDC, during the epidemic in the 1960s, about 20,000 infants were born with congenital rubella syndrome in the United States. Due to widespread vaccination, rubella is no longer endemic to the United States.

Mumps (Epidemic parotitis)

Mumps is a paramyxovirus infection that causes inflammation and swelling of exocrine glands. The salivary glands are most commonly affected, but other tissues such as the testes, brain, pancreas, and ovaries may also be involved. The virus can be transmitted through saliva, urine, or respiratory droplets. Vaccination has resulted in a tremendous decrease in new cases; however, outbreaks continue to occur. This may be attributed to either inadequate vaccination or vaccine failure (the MMR vaccine is estimated to be 76% to 95% effective against mumps).

Infection occurs most often in children and teenagers and is usually symptomatic. Patients develop fever, headache, malaise, and body aches followed shortly thereafter by swelling and discomfort of the salivary glands. The parotid gland is most commonly affected and is bilateral in 75 percent of cases (Fig. 3-53). Pain is intensified by chewing and intake of saliva-stimulating foods. The most common complication is *orchitis*, a form of testicular inflammation, which develops in 20% to 30% of infected postpubertal males. The swelling associated with orchitis can be dramatic and very painful, but rarely causes permanent effects. Females may develop a similar condition of the ovaries called *oophoritis*.

Clinical Implications

Parotid enlargement usually begins on one side, followed by involvement of the contralateral gland. Poor oral hygiene may result from tenderness, lack of salivary flow, and limited opening.

Molluscum Contagiosum

Molluscum contagiosum is a common skin disease caused by a DNA poxvirus. Infection causes focal hyperplasia of the epidermis, resulting in multiple small papules on the skin (Fig. 3-54). The virus is spread through direct contact and is most often seen in children and young adults. The most frequent sites of involvement are the face, neck, trunk, and genitals. More widespread involvement occurs in immunocompromised patients. Individual lesions are 2 to 4 mm in diameter, red-pink, smooth-surfaced, and may be dimpled or have a whitish central core. The lesions resolve spontaneously within 6 to 12 months,

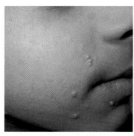

Figure 3–54 Molluscum contagiosum. Small flesh-colored, dome-shaped "pearly" papules. (From Barankin, B: Derm Notes. F.A. Davis, Philadelphia, 2006, p 121.)

but treatment is often recommended to prevent **autoinoculation** where the patient spreads the infection to other parts of the body, or transmission to others. Conservative surgical removal or cryotherapy is the most common treatment.

Human Immunodeficiency Virus

HIV is an RNA retrovirus that infects and destroys CD4+ T-lymphocytes, which are essential to helping the body fight diseases. When HIV enters a host cell, its RNA is converted into double-stranded DNA by an enzyme called reverse transcriptase. This newly formed viral DNA is then incorporated into the DNA of the lymphocyte. Eventually, this results in a decrease in the number of CD4+ T-lymphocytes and reduced immune function. HIV can be found in most body fluids of infected persons, but is usually spread through sexual contact, parenteral exposure to blood, or from mother to fetus.

Over one million people are estimated to be HIV-infected in the United States and up to 20 percent of these individuals may be unaware of their HIV positive

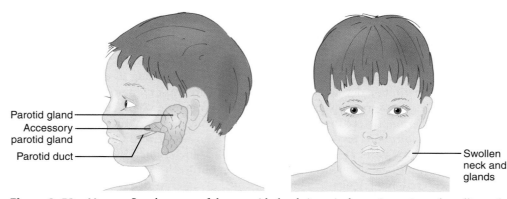

Parotid gland
Accessory parotid gland
Parotid duct

Swollen neck and glands

Figure 3–53 Mumps. Involvement of the parotid glands is typical, causing pain and swelling of the soft tissues of the posterior cheeks and neck.

status. Men having sex with men (MSM) is the single biggest risk factor for HIV infection and accounts for about half of all new infections.

Clinical Implications

Although occupational transmission to dental providers is rare, oral fluids can be infectious. The risk of HIV seroconversion after percutaneous skin puncture exposure with HIV-infected blood is 0.3 percent. If exposure does occur, a person's risk of infection can be further reduced by prompt initiation of post-exposure prophylaxis with antiviral medications.

A few weeks after initial exposure to HIV, more than half of patients develop the *acute viral syndrome*. The clinical features mimic mononucleosis and may include lymphadenopathy, fever, headache, sore throat, and malaise. The acute viral syndrome resolves after a few weeks, but some patients continue to have *persistent generalized lymphadenopathy* (PGL). PGL is usually the only potential sign of HIV infection during the asymptomatic phase of HIV, which follows the acute viral syndrome. People who are HIV-infected may appear and feel healthy for many years.

Acquired immunodeficiency syndrome (AIDS) is diagnosed when an HIV-infected person's CD4 count drops below 200 cells per microliter. The clinical presentation is variable but often includes weight loss, persistent diarrhea, and opportunistic infections. Many infections that are asymptomatic or mild in immunocompetent patients (such as HSV and CMV) can be devastating for AIDS patients. Pneumonia caused by *Pneumocystis jirovecii* (formerly *P. carinii)* is highly suggestive of AIDS and leads to the initial diagnosis in a significant percentage of cases. The following oral manifestations are considered to be strongly associated with HIV infection and will be discussed further.

- *Candidiasis.* Candidiasis is the most frequent oral sign of HIV infection. The two most common clinical patterns seen are *pseudomembranous* and *erythematous candidiasis* (discussed earlier in this chapter). Pseudomembranous candidiasis may be extensive and is more likely to develop when the patient's CD4 count drops below 200. Treatment of candidiasis in AIDS patients can be challenging. Topical treatments are associated with a high recurrence rate and systemic antifungals may interact with other medications. As a general guideline,

clotrimazole troches are the ideal choice if the patient is receiving antiretroviral treatment and has a CD4 count of at least 50. Systemic fluconazole is recommended for patients with a CD4 count under 50.

- *Oral hairy leukoplakia.* Oral hairy leukoplakia is an EBV infection that causes adherent white plaques that characteristically develop on the lateral tongue of HIV-infected patients. The clinical appearance may range from subtle white streaks to a shaggy keratotic plaque. The presence of oral hairy leukoplakia is often a sign of disease progression and should prompt referral for re-evaluation in an HIV-positive patient.

- *Periodontal diseases.* Three unusual clinical patterns of periodontal disease are seen in HIV-infected patients: linear gingival erythema, necrotizing ulcerative gingivitis, and necrotizing ulcerative periodontitis. *Linear gingival erythema* is limited to the free gingival margin and may represent an atypical presentation of oral candidiasis (Fig. 3-55). Because the clinical presentation is similar to marginal gingivitis, the diagnosis should only be made for erythema that is resistant to improved oral hygiene. The presentation of NUG in HIV-infected patients is similar to the appearance seen in immunocompetent patients. *Necrotizing ulcerative periodontitis (NUP)* is gingival necrosis accompanied by rapid, severe loss of supporting alveolar bone (Fig. 3-56). Focal defects are more likely to be seen than diffuse involvement. Treatment of NUG and NUP consists of irrigation and debridement of all necrotic tissue, followed by long-term use of prophylactic chlorhexidine rinse.

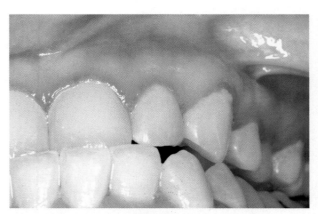

Figure 3–55 Linear gingival erythema. Prominent erythema at the gingival margin in an HIV-positive patient.

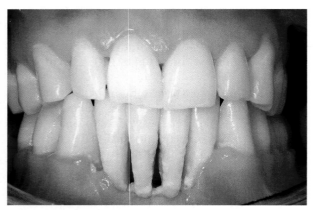

Figure 3–56   NUP. Extensive loss of periodontal support around the mandibular incisors in an HIV-positive patient.

■ *Kaposi's sarcoma.* Kaposi's sarcoma (KS) is a vascular neoplasm that develops in up to 20 percent of AIDS patients. Most experts believe KS to be caused by viral infection with HHV-8, also called Kaposi's sarcoma-associated herpesvirus (KSHV). KS is characterized by multiple red-purple macules on the skin and/or oral mucosa that eventually progress to raised plaques and nodules. Areas prone to trauma, such as the hard palate (Fig. 3-57), gingiva, and tongue, are the most commonly affected intraoral areas. KS tends to regress with antiretroviral therapy and disease control.

■ *Non-Hodgkin's lymphoma.* AIDS patients are 60 times more likely to develop non-Hodgkin's lymphoma (NHL) than the general population. Although the term NHL encompasses a wide spectrum of lymphoid malignancies, most cases in AIDS patients are aggressive and associated with a poor prognosis.

■ *HIV-salivary gland disease.* The epidemiology of HIV-salivary gland disease (HIV-SGD) suggests it is a viral opportunistic infection. This condition is more common in children and may be seen in up to 5 percent of HIV-positive patients. Some patients may experience parotid enlargement due to infection by cytomegalovirus or other viruses. HIV-infected individuals often present with peripheral lymphadenopathy, notably in cervical regions. This precedes by months the opportunistic infections and neoplasia of AIDS. Because lymphoid tissue becomes entrapped within the parotid during embryonic development, a form of lymphadenopathy termed *cystic lymphoid hyperplasia* may present in the parotid glands. Patients present with nontender bilateral swelling (Fig. 3-58) that is firm to palpation and xerostomia.

Clinical Implications

Patients who present with nontender bilateral parotid enlargement and xerostomia accompanied by cervical lymphadenopathy may be showing early signs of HIV infection.

HIV infection was considered to be uniformly fatal before the development of *highly active anti-retroviral therapy (HAART)*, which has significantly increased survival and the overall number of persons living with HIV and AIDS. HAART is a drug combination usually consisting of reverse transcriptase inhibitors and protease inhibitors. Although not a cure, HAART has resulted in dramatically reduced viral loads and the return of immunocompetence in many patients. Unfortunately,

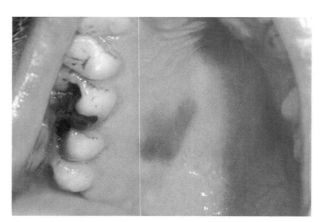

Figure 3–57   Kaposi's sarcoma. Discovered on routine dental examination.

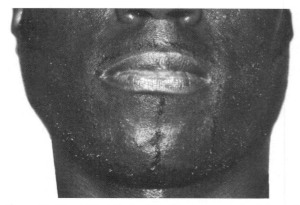

Figure 3–58   HIV sialadenitis. Firm, nontender bilateral swelling of the parotid glands in an HIV-positive patient.

HAART is very expensive and therefore not accessible for most HIV-infected patients in resource-poor countries. Additionally, it causes significant side effects and may not be effective in all patients.

Human Papillomavirus

There are more than 40 types of human papillomavirus (HPV) that may affect the genitals, oral cavity, and pharynx. Other HPV types cause infections of the skin. HPV infection is usually asymptomatic, and the virus is therefore unknowingly transmitted. Most HPV infections are cleared by the body's immune system within a period of about 2 years, but some may persist and cause a wide spectrum of clinically evident disease. Table 3-3 summarizes the clinical manifestations of the most common intraoral HPV lesions.

Squamous Papilloma

Squamous papilloma is a benign mucosal mass produced by HPV-6 and HPV-11. These types also cause skin warts but are not among those associated with malignancy or precancer. Squamous papilloma has an extremely low virulence and infectivity rate and is not considered contagious. Lesions are painless and may develop on any mucosal surface, with the tongue and soft palate affected frequently. Squamous papillomas occur singly and often are pedunculated. They are usually pink or white and may have long finger-like to cauliflower-like projections or short raspberry-like projections (Figs. 3-59 and 3-60).

Conservative surgical excision including the base of the lesion is adequate treatment and recurrence is unlikely. Lesions may go untreated for years with no change or spread to other parts of the body. There are no reports of transformation into malignancy.

Verruca Vulgaris

Verruca vulgaris (vulgaris = *common*) is an infection of the skin commonly known as a *wart* (Fig. 3-61), most often caused by the subtypes HPV-2, HPV-4, and HPV-40. The skin of the hands is the most common site. Verruca vulgaris is contagious and capable of spreading to other parts of an affected person's skin or mucous membranes through autoinoculation. Verruca vulgaris of the oral mucosa is typically seen on the vermilion border, labial mucosa, or anterior tongue (Fig. 3-62). The appearance of the lesion may be identical to a squamous papilloma, but it is often characterized by white pointed or *verruciform* surface projections and a broad base. They seldom are more than 5 mm in diameter.

Skin and intraoral verruca vulgaris lesions may be treated by conservative surgical excision or curettage down to the base of the lesion. Skin lesions are amenable to liquid nitrogen cryotherapy and topical application of salicylic acid or lactic acid. For obvious reasons, these agents should not be used in the mouth. Recurrence is seen in a small proportion of treated cases. Most will disappear spontaneously within 2 years. Lesions do not transform into cancer.

Condyloma acuminatum

Condyloma acuminatum is considered to be a *sexually transmitted disease (STD)* most commonly found on the genitalia. However, the lesions can also occur in the oral cavity at sites of sexual contact. They are caused by HPV-6 and HPV-11, but are often mixed with other HPV types. Nevertheless, they are classified as low-risk HPV types that are highly transmissible. The clinical appearance is a pink, papillary, exophytic mass that may be indistinguishable from squamous papilloma in the early stages (Fig. 3-63A), but some lesions enlarge and become confluent with other lesions over time, covering a large surface area (Fig. 3-63B).

Condyloma acuminatum can occur in healthy patients, but may also be one of many potential oral manifestations of HIV infection (Fig. 3-64). Treatment for genital lesions includes topical application of caustic medication that "burns" the lesions off. Oral lesions may be treated with surgical excision, electrocauterization, or laser therapy. Care should be exercised when using electrocauterization and laser therapy on these highly transmissible lesions, due to the potential for aerosolization of viral particles.

Focal Epithelial Hyperplasia (Heck's Disease)

Heck's disease (focal epithelial hyperplasia) is caused by HPV-13 and HPV-32, which are among the low-risk HPVs. Lesions are characterized by pinkish papules that occur diffusely on the mucous membrane of the lips, tongue, or less commonly the buccal mucosa, floor of the mouth, and palate. They are soft, painless, sessile papules about 1 to 4 mm in diameter that occur in clusters (Fig. 3-65) and can be present on more than one intraoral site at a time. Individual lesions are broad based and may appear as a smooth-surfaced plaque rather than a verrucous or papillary lesion (Fig. 3-66).

The condition usually occurs in children and young adults and may have familial predilection. Lesions may last for several months, sometimes years, before running their course. The patient may elect to

Table 3.3   Classification of Intraoral Human Papilloma Virus Lesions

Squamous Papilloma	Verruca Vulgaris	Heck's Disease	Condyloma Acuminatum	Oropharyngeal and Tonsillar Carcinoma
HPV 6, 11	HPV 2, 4, 6, 7, 40	HPV 13, 32	HPV 2, 6, 11, 53, 54	HPV 16, 18, 31, 33
Single	Single	Multiple	Multiple coalesced or low and	Diffuse
Pedunculated[1]	Sessile[2]	Clustered	broad	Not "wart-like", no papillary
Long, cauliflower-like	Short papillary projections or	Sessile[2]	Sessile[2]	projections
projections	rough surface	Pebbly surface	Blunted papillary projections	

[1] Growing on a stalk.
[2] The base is the same size as or larger than the lesion itself.

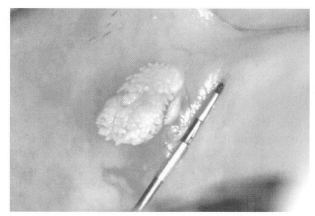

Figure 3–59   Papilloma. Pedunculated mass with prominent cauliflower-like appearance.

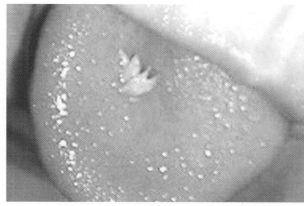

Figure 3–62   Verruca vulgaris. Sessile lesion with prominent finger-like projections.

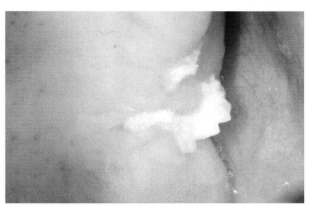

Figure 3–60   Papilloma. White papillary lesions of the alveolar ridge.

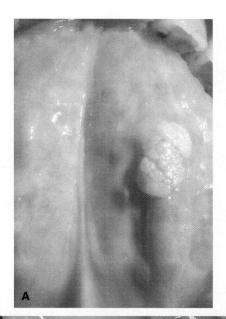

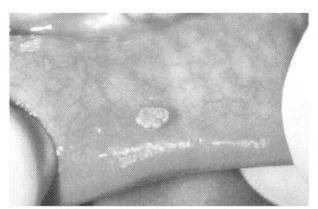

Figure 3–61   Verruca vulgaris. Single sessile exophytic rough-surfaced lesion of the lower lip of a child.

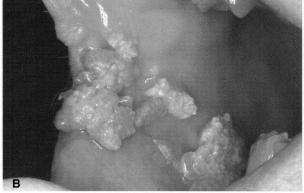

Figure 3–63   Condyloma. A. Small early papilloma-like condyloma on the ventral tongue. **B.** Condyloma of commissure and buccal mucosa.

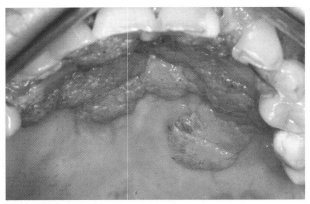

Figure 3–64   Condyloma acuminatum. Confluent lesions of the palate in an immunocompromised patient.

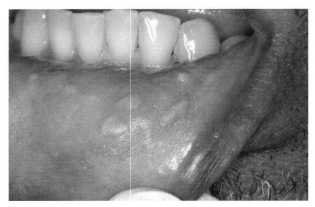

Figure 3–65   Heck's disease. Soft, painless oval sessile papules of the lower lip.

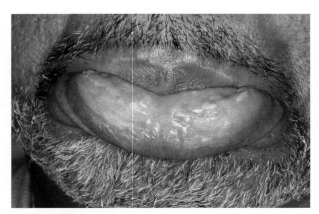

Figure 3–66   Heck's disease. Flat-topped warty lesions, some coalescing.

have lesions removed for cosmetic reasons. The most effective treatment is cryosurgery; however, many cases spontaneously regress once the diagnosis has been established. Heck's disease does not transform into carcinoma.

HPV and Oral Cancer

High-risk HPV types 16, 18, 31, and 33 are capable of causing premalignant epithelial dysplasia and squamous cell carcinoma (SCC) of the genital areas, especially the cervix. HPV infection has also been identified recently as an etiologic factor in oral SCC, particularly of the posterior oropharynx, where HPV can be identified in about 50 percent of cases. HPV-related oropharyngeal SCC appears to be a distinct subset of cancer with a better prognosis compared to other SCCs of the head and neck.

The incidence of oropharyngeal cancer is increasing among a younger, nonsmoking patient population and may be attributed to HPV. In many of these cases, the method of HPV transmission to the oral cavity is uncertain but may be through sexual contact. Prevention of HPV infection is now possible due to the recent development of a vaccine called Gardasil, which is effective against the HPV types that cause most cervical cancers and genital warts. The vaccine is currently recommended for both girls and boys as early as age 9 and up to 26 years of age. Under investigation now is the question of whether HPV vaccines will prevent certain forms of oral cancer.

In conclusion, dental hygienists share an intimate space with their patients and must be aware of methods to prevent potential pathogen transmission. Also, hygienists should be aware of emergence of new infections and resurgences of old infections among their immunocompromised patients and among their immunocompetent patients from developing countries.

Critical Thinking Questions

Case 3-1:   A 65-year-old female presents to your office complaining of a mild burning sensation on the tongue, and sensitivity to spicy foods for the past 2 weeks. The patient's medical history is significant for hypertension, type 2 diabetes, arthritis, and depression. She is taking several medications to manage these problems. Your clinical exam reveals that the patient wears a maxillary removable partial denture. The mucosa underlying the denture is intensely red but nonpainful. A localized portion of the posterior mid-dorsal tongue appears smooth and red. Saliva can be stimulated from the major gland orifices but is viscous and slightly reduced in quantity.

• • •

What is the most likely diagnosis of this patient's acute problem?

What aspect of the local oral environment may be contributing?

Does the partial denture require any attention? If so, what should be done?

Case 3-2:   A 16-year-old male presents with a sore throat, malaise, low-grade fever, and lymphadenopathy that have persisted for the past 10 days. The patient is a healthy, high-school athlete with no known medical conditions or allergies. Your clinical exam is notable for swollen tonsils covered by a yellow-white exudate.

• • •

What is the most likely diagnosis? How can it be confirmed?

What other diseases are associated with this microorganism?

How should this patient be treated?

The patient wants to know if he is contagious. What will you tell him?

Case 3-3:   A 4-year-old girl presents to your office with swollen gingiva and widespread, painful oral ulcers. Cervical lymphadenopathy is identified on your extraoral exam. The patient's mother reports that she has had a fever, irritability, and has been unable to eat.

• • •

What is the most likely diagnosis of this condition?

How should this patient be treated?

Are there future problems that could develop as a result of this process? If so, what signs and symptoms should you tell the mother to look for?

Review Questions

1. **Infections caused by microorganisms that are not normally pathogenic in persons with a healthy immune system are known as**
    A. attenuated.
    B. pathogens.
    C. opportunistic.
    D. compromised.

2. **A type of microorganism that can only cause disease after entering and replicating in a host cell is**
    A. bacteria.
    B. virus.
    C. fungi.
    D. protozoa.

3. **Which of these is NOT one of the three main routes of human disease transmission?**
    A. Sexual
    B. Fecal-oral
    C. Respiratory
    D. Animal vector

4. **Serological testing performed to diagnose a viral infection most often involves the detection of**
    A. antibodies.
    B. toxins.
    C. genetic material (DNA or RNA).
    D. components of the cell wall.

5. A disease control agent that uses live or killed microorganisms or their components to stimulate the immune system and create memory is known as a(n)
    A. antibiotic.
    B. antiseptic.
    C. vaccine.
    D. antibody.

6. Necrotizing ulcerative gingivitis is
    A. usually asymptomatic.
    B. associated with an intense malodor.
    C. treated with systemic antiviral medication.
    D. most often found in elderly patients.

7. Which of the following bacterial infections may be reactivated later in life if a person becomes immunocompromised or debilitated?
    A. Cat-scratch disease
    B. Tuberculosis
    C. Scarlet fever
    D. Actinomycosis

8. Which of the following diseases is NOT caused by a streptococcal infection?
    A. Impetigo
    B. Scarlet fever
    C. Erysipelas
    D. Diphtheria

9. Strawberry tongue and a skin rash resembling "a sunburn with goose bumps" is characteristic of
    A. measles.
    B. herpes zoster.
    C. scarlet fever.
    D. erysipelas.

10. Cervicofacial actinomycosis is most often seen in which of these anatomic locations?
    A. Skin overlying the mandibular angle
    B. Cervical lymph nodes
    C. Maxillary sinus
    D. Hard palate

11. The most common fungal infection seen in the oral cavity is
    A. histoplasmosis.
    B. candidiasis.
    C. actinomycosis.
    D. blastomycosis.

12. Central papillary atrophy and angular cheilitis are both manifestations of
    A. syphilis.
    B. herpes simplex virus.
    C. candidiasis.
    D. human papillomavirus.

13. Which of these therapies is NOT an antifungal agent?
    A. Nystatin
    B. Penicillin
    C. Amphotericin B
    D. Fluconazole

14. A fungal infection that may be acquired by an immunocompromised patient during a hospital stay, particularly in the setting of building renovation, is
    A. aspergillosis.
    B. histoplasmosis.
    C. actinomycosis.
    D. mucormycosis.

15. Among healthy patients, most primary herpes simplex virus infections are
    A. acute herpetic gingivostomatitis.
    B. herpes labialis.
    C. central papillary atrophy.
    D. asymptomatic.

16. Recurrent intraoral herpes simplex virus infections are almost always located on the
    A. attached gingiva or hard palate.
    B. tongue.
    C. buccal or labial mucosa.
    D. soft palate or oropharynx.

17. **Postherpetic neuralgia is a common complication of**

    A. herpes simplex.
    B. herpes zoster.
    C. chickenpox.
    D. herpangina.

18. **Persistent generalized lymphadenopathy raises suspicion for the possibility of**

    A. HIV infection.
    B. measles.
    C. HPV infection.
    D. hand-foot, and mouth disease.

19. **Which of the following infections can cause serious harm to a fetus if the mother is infected during pregnancy?**

    A. Toxoplasmosis
    B. Syphilis
    C. Rubella
    D. All of the above

20. **The etiologic agent responsible for cervical cancer and a growing number of oropharyngeal cancers is**

    A. Epstein-Barr virus.
    B. HIV.
    C. human papillomavirus.
    D. cytomegalovirus.

SUGGESTED READING

Books

Goering, RV, Dockrell, HM, Wakelin, D, Zuckerman, M, et al: Mim's Medical Microbiology, ed. 4. Elsevier Publishing, Philadelphia, 2008.

Marsh, P, Martin, MV: Oral Microbiology, ed. 4. Wright, Oxford, England, 1999.

Neville, BW, Damm, DD, Allen, CM, Bouquot, JE: Oral and Maxillofacial Pathology, ed. 3. Saunders, St. Louis, 2009.

Topazian, RG, Goldberg, MH, Hupp, JR: Oral and Maxillofacial Infections, ed. 4. Saunders, Philadelphia, 2002.

Journal Article

Woo, SB, Challacombe, SJ: Management of recurrent oral herpes simplex infections. Oral Surgery, Oral Medicine, Oral Pathology, Oral Radiology and Endodontology 103(S12):.e1–18.

Online Resources

Coccidioidomycosis. www.cfsph.iastate.edu/Factsheets/pdfs/coccidioidomycosis.pdf Last updated: June 2010. Author unknown.

Centers for Disease Control and Prevention. (2010). Aspergillosis (Aspergillus). Retrieved March 29, 2011 from www.cdc.gov/nczved/divisions/dfbmd/diseases/aspergillosis

Centers for Disease Control and Prevention. (2010). Cytomegalovirus (CMV) and Congenital CMV Infection. Retrieved March 30, 2011 from www.cdc.gov/cmv/index.html

Centers for Disease Control and Prevention. (2011). Diphtheria. Retrieved March 28, 2011 from www.cdc.gov/ncidod/dbmd/diseaseinfo/diptheria_t.htm

Centers for Disease Control and Prevention. (2006). Epstein-Barr Virus and Infectious Mononucleosis. Retrieved March 30, 2011 from www.cdc.gov/ncidod/diseases/ebv.htm

Centers for Disease Control and Prevention. (2010). Histoplasmosis. Retrieved March 28, 2011 from www.cdc.gov/nczved/divisions/dfbmd/diseases/histoplasmosis

Centers for Disease Control and Prevention. (2011). HIV/AIDS. Retrieved March 31, 2011 from www.cdc.gov/hiv/default.htmhttp://www.cdc.gov/hiv/default.htm

Centers for Disease Control and Prevention. (2011). Human Papillomavirus (HPV). Retrieved March 29, 2011 from www.cdc.gov/hpv

Centers for Disease Control and Prevention. (2010). Measles (Rubeola). Retrieved March 30, 2011 from www.cdc.gov/measles/index.html

Centers for Disease Control and Prevention. (2011). Molluscum (Molluscum Contagiosum). Retrieved March 30, 2011 from www.cdc.gov/ncidod/dvrd/molluscum

Centers for Disease Control and Prevention. (2010). Mumps. Retrieved March 31, 2011 from www.cdc.gov/mumps/index.html

Centers for Disease Control and Prevention. (2011). Non-Polio Enterovirus Infections. Retrieved March 31, 2011 from www.cdc.gov/ncidod/dvrd/revb/enterovirus/non-polio_entero.htm

Centers for Disease Control and Prevention. (2010). Rubella (German Measles, Three-Day Measles). Retrieved March 30, 2011 from www.cdc.gov/rubella

Centers for Disease Control and Prevention. (2011). Sexually Transmitted Diseases (STDs): Syphilis. Retrieved March 28, 2011 from www.cdc.gov/std/syphilis/default.htmhttp://www.cdc.gov/std/syphilis/default.htm

Centers for Disease Control and Prevention. (2010). Parasites: Toxoplasmosis (Toxoplasma infection). Retrieved March 29, 2011 from www.cdc.gov/parasites/toxoplasmosis

Centers for Disease Control and Prevention. (2011). Tuberculosis (TB). Retrieved March 28, 2011 from www.cdc.gov/tb

Centers for Disease Control and Prevention. (2011). Varicella-Zoster Virus Infection (VZV Infection, Shingles, Zoster). Retrieved March 30, 2011 from http://www.cdc.gov/ncidod/diseases/list_varicl.htmhttp://www.cdc.gov/ncidod/diseases/list_varicl.htm

Chapter 4

Immunologic Disease

The Immune System
  Self, Nonself, and Antigens
  Structure of the Immune System:
    The Lymphoid Organs
  Immune Cells and Molecules
  Normal Immune Response
Immunopathology
  Hypersensitivity Reactions
  Autoimmune Diseases
  Immunodeficiency Diseases

Clinical Features of Immune and Autoimmune Disorders
  Allergic Disorders
  Ulcerative Conditions
  Lichen Planus
  Lichenoid Mucositis
  Desquamative Gingivitis Associated With Autoimmune
    Vesiculobullous or Vesiculoerosive Disorders
  Orofacial Manifestations of Systemic
    Immunodysregulation

🌑 Learning Outcomes

At the end of this chapter, the student will be able to:

4.1. Distinguish between an antigen and an antibody, differentiate between self and nonself antigens, and define major histocompatibility complex.

4.2. Give examples of the cells of the normal immune system and their functions.

4.3. Differentiate between the humoral and cellular immune responses, and give an example of each.

4.4. Differentiate between active and passive immunity.

4.5. Recognize descriptions of four types of hypersensitivity and give an example of each.

4.6. Explain autoimmunity and list at least two autoimmune diseases.

4.7. Distinguish between primary and secondary immune deficiency disorders.

4.8. Recognize the clinical features of allergic disorders including contact dermatitis, contact stomatitis, plasma cell gingivitis, cinnamon stomatitis, and hypersensitivity to dental restorative materials.

4.9. Differentiate among the key features of minor recurrent aphthous ulcers and herpetiform aphthous ulcers.

4.10. Give examples of systemic disorders associated with major aphthous ulcers.

4.11. Differentiate among the clinical features of the three forms of lichen planus.

Continued

4.12. Differentiate among the diseases that cause desquamative gingivitis.

4.13. Discuss the oral manifestations of systemic immunodysregulation leading to hives and angioedema.

4.14. Recognize the key features of systemic and discoid lupus erythematosus.

4.15. Recognize the oral manifestations of granulomatous disorders of immunity.

4.16. Discuss the key clinical features of Sjögren's syndrome and the long-term outlook for Sjögren's patients.

THE IMMUNE SYSTEM

The main function of the **immune system** is to render the body immune or resistant to disease by protecting it from foreign agents, primarily, but not exclusively, microbes such as bacteria, parasites, fungi, and viruses. The human body is an ideal environment for many microbes to invade and cause infections. The immune system is designed to keep microbes out, or if defenses are breached, to find the invaders and destroy them. The immune defenses are very powerful at maintaining health. However, if the immune defenses are misdirected, they can initiate many disorders that hurt rather than help the individual, including allergic diseases, arthritis, and a form of diabetes. Conversely, when immune defenses are weakened or impaired, other conditions take advantage of decreased defenses, such as AIDS.

The immune system relies on an elaborate and dynamic communications network, which enables it to recognize and remember millions of different enemies, and to produce cells to specifically fight and eliminate nearly all of them.

Self, Nonself, and Antigens

The immune system has the remarkable ability to distinguish between the body's own cells, or "self," and foreign cells, or "nonself." The *major histocompatibility complex* (MHC) molecules are present on almost every cell of the body and act as labels of self. In humans, MHC molecules are also called *human leukocyte antigens* (HLA). Normally, the body's immune defenses react only to foreign cells or organisms that do not carry MHC markers of self.

Any entity that can elicit an immune response is called an **antigen**. An antigen can be a microbe, such as a virus, or a part of a microbe, such as a molecule from the membrane of a bacteria cell, or a toxin produced by the bacteria. MHC markers present on cells that have been "transformed" by cancer or viral infection modify the cells so they are seen as antigenic. They trigger an immune response, which results in the destruction of the transformed cells. MHC markers are highly specific. Tissues or cells from another person, except from an identical twin, are recognized as nonself and act as foreign antigens. This explains why it is so important to match the MHC molecules of transplant recipients and donors to minimize transplant rejection.

In abnormal situations, the immune system can mistake self for nonself and launch an attack against the body's own cells or tissues. The result is **autoimmune disease**, such as some forms of arthritis. In other cases, the immune system may react to a seemingly harmless foreign substance, such as ragweed pollen. This results in **allergy**, and this kind of antigen is called an **allergen**.

Structure of the Immune System: The Lymphoid Organs

The *lymphoid organs* are critical to the functioning of a healthy immune system. They are called lymphoid organs because they house the **lymphocytes**, which are small white blood cells key to the immune response. Lymphoid organs include the following (Fig. 4-1):

- *Bone marrow* represents the soft tissue located in the hollow center of bones. It produces all of the immune cells and blood cells from precursor stem cells.
- The *thymus gland* is located behind the breastbone. The thymus helps render *T lymphocytes* or *T cells* (T stands for thymus) tolerant (acceptant) to self-antigens.
- The lymphatic system is composed of small bean-shaped organs called *lymph nodes* connected to a system of *lymphatic vessels* that run parallel to the arteries and veins. The lymphatic vessels carry a

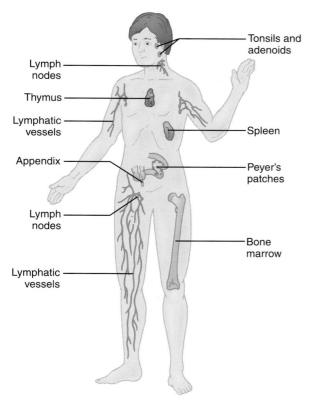

Figure 4–1 Lymphoid organs of the immune system.

Labels: Lymph nodes, Thymus, Lymphatic vessels, Appendix, Lymph nodes, Lymphatic vessels, Tonsils and adenoids, Spleen, Peyer's patches, Bone marrow

clear fluid called *lymph*. Lymph nodes are positioned along the lymphatic vessels, with clusters in the neck, armpits, abdomen, and groin. Each lymph node is highly organized with specialized compartments (Fig. 4-2) as outlined below.

- The germinal centers are located toward the periphery of the cortex layer; this is where another

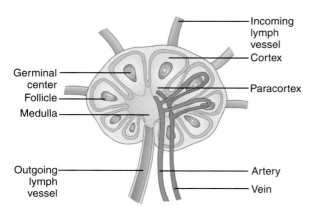

Figure 4–2 Structure of the lymph nodes.

Labels: Germinal center, Follicle, Medulla, Outgoing lymph vessel, Incoming lymph vessel, Cortex, Paracortex, Artery, Vein

type of lymphocyte, *the B lymphocytes or B cells*, develop.

- The intermediary zone, called the paracortex, is where T cells develop.
- The central zone, called the medulla, is the area where a type of mature B cells, called *plasma cells*, reside.
- Immune cells, microbes, and foreign antigens travel throughout the body using lymphatic vessels and blood vessels. With all lymph nodes positioned strategically along the lymphatic vessels, the lymphatic system is specially designed to monitor the body for invading microbes and foreign antigens, initiate an immune response, and eliminate undesirable foreign substances.
- The *spleen* is an organ located in the upper left of the abdomen. It removes old and damaged red blood cells from the general circulation. Because its organization is similar to that of lymph nodes, the spleen can also mount an immune reaction to antigens present in the general circulation.
- *Mucosa-associated lymph tissues (MALT)*, such the lingual, pharyngeal, and palatine **tonsils**, which are located in the oropharyngeal area, as well as *Peyer's patches* and the *appendix*, which are located in the gastrointestinal tract, are also parts of the immune system and function in the same way as the lymph nodes and spleen.

Immune Cells and Molecules

Cells of the immune system include lymphocytes and *phagocytes*, which work together to produce an effective immune response. All immune cells originate from immature stem cells in the bone marrow. They grow into specific immune cell types, such as T cells, B cells, or phagocytes, in response to different chemical signals (Fig. 4-3).

Lymphocytes are long-lived, mobile cells, able to recognize and respond to antigens. B cells and T cells are the main types of lymphocytes, and together represent 20% to 25% of all white blood cells. The other white blood cells present in the circulation include phagocytes and *granulocytes*. In peripheral blood, T cells outnumber B cells with approximately eight T cells for every B cell.

B Lymphocytes and Antibodies, or Immunoglobulins

After maturing in the bone marrow, B cells enter the blood stream and migrate to the germinal centers of the lymph nodes, the spleen, and other lymphoid

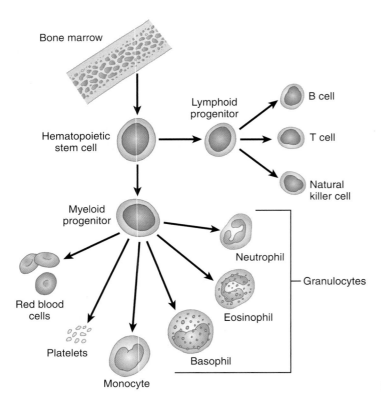

Figure 4–3 Cells of the immune system.

tissues, including the tonsils. Each B cell is programmed to produce one specific **antibody**, a molecule that can bind to one specific antigen. When a B cell encounters the type of antigen that matches the antibody it can produce, the B cell becomes active. It multiplies and creates plasma cells, which are cells that produce antibodies. The activated B cell also produces some B cells that will remain in the body and retain the memory of the encountered antigen.

Antibodies, also called **immunoglobulins (Igs)**, are released into the bloodstream. All Igs have the same basic structure, with two identical *heavy* polypeptide chains and two identical *light* chains arranged in a Y-shaped molecule (Fig. 4-4A). The end of the polypeptides located at the tips of the Y's arms represents the *variable regions* of the antibody, which differ from one antibody to the next and allow one antibody to recognize its matching antigen. The rest of the molecule is the *constant region*, common to antibodies of the same type. Five different types of antibodies exist with different combinations of heavy and light chains, and different structures and functions (Fig. 4-4B).

- *Immunoglobulin G*, or *IgG* (gamma globulin), is a circulating antibody that works by coating microbes and speeding their uptake by phagocytes. IgG accounts for approximately 80 percent of all antibodies in serum.
- *IgM* is the first antibody produced in response to an antigen. It is found on the surface of B cells and can effectively kill bacteria. IgM is the largest-sized antibody and makes up 5% to 10% of the antibodies in serum.
- *IgA* is found in body fluids—tears, saliva, and the secretions of the respiratory and digestive tracts—and guards the entrances to the body. IgA accounts for 10% to 15% of antibodies in serum.
- *IgE* is found in the skin and mucous membranes and triggers the release of **histamine**, an important protein of the inflammatory response. Another function is to naturally protect against parasitic infections. It is also responsible for the symptoms of allergy. IgE antibodies make up only 0.002 percent of total serum antibodies.
- *IgD* remains attached to B cells and participates in regulating B cell responses. IgD antibodies make up only about 0.2 percent of the total serum antibodies.

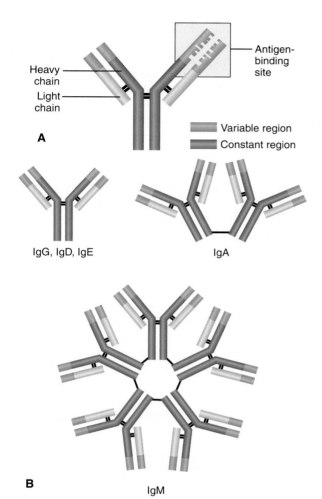

Heavy chain

Light chain

Antigen-binding site

Variable region
Constant region

A

IgG, IgD, IgE

IgA

B

IgM

Figure 4–4   Antibody and immunoglobulin classes.
A. Basic structure of antibodies and variable region that makes antibodies specific. **B.** The five classes of antibodies or immunoglobulins.

T Lymphocytes and T-Cell Receptors

Unlike B cells, T cells do not recognize circulating antigens. Instead, their membranes contain specialized antibody-like receptors, called *T-cell receptors*. These see fragments of foreign antigens bound to MHC molecules (self-markers) on the surface of specialized cells, called antigen-presenting cells (APCs). The most common antigen-presenting cells are macrophages, monocytes, dendritic cells, and B cells. These cells engulf foreign antigens, partially degrade them, and combine digested fragments of antigens to their MHC molecules. The MHC-antigen complex migrates to the cell surface where the self-MHC molecule provides a recognizable scaffolding to "present" the foreign antigen to T cells. As with antibodies, each T-cell receptor is

programmed to recognize and be activated by one specific antigen-MHC complex. Activated T cells divide and produce different types of T cells, depending on the nature of the activating antigen (as will be discussed later). Some activated T cells direct and regulate immune responses, whereas others directly attack infected or cancerous cells. Similar to B cells, some activated T cells will also remain in the body permanently to retain the memory of the activating antigen. Two types of T lymphocytes can be distinguished, based on their functions and some of their surface molecules.

■ *Helper T cells*, or *Th cells*, also designated as *CD4+*, coordinate immune responses by communicating with other cells. Some stimulate nearby B cells to produce antibodies, others mobilize phagocytes, and still others activate other T cells.
■ *Cytotoxic T cells*, or *CTLs*, also designated as *CD8+*, directly attack cells carrying foreign antigens or abnormal molecules on their surfaces, such as virus-infected cells or cancer cells. Cytotoxic T cells act on contact: they bind to their target cells, release granules filled with digestive enzymes, and release toxic chemicals into the target cells to kill and destroy them.

Humans normally have twice as many CD4+ cells than CD8+ cells in their peripheral blood.

A third type of lymphocyte, the *natural killer (NK) cell*, can also attack and destroy virus-infected or cancer cells in a similar way as cytotoxic T cells. However, NK cells differ from T cells in that they do not require activation by antigen-presenting cells or chemical messengers. They can attack their targets immediately and recognize many different types of foreign cells that lack self-MHC molecules. NK cells are not immunologically specific. They are not phagocytic, but must contact the target cell to lyse it.

Phagocytes and Granulocytes

Phagocytes are large white blood cells that can ingest and digest microbes and other foreign particles. *Monocytes* circulate in the blood, then migrate into tissues and become *macrophages*. Specialized types of macrophages can be found in many organs, including the lungs, kidneys, brain, and liver. Macrophages play many roles such as eliminating foreign antigens, dead or damaged cells, and other debris; acting as antigen-presenting cells; and synthesizing and releasing a variety of powerful chemical signals, known as *monokines*. *Dendritic cells*, also derived from monocytes, are found in the parts of lymphoid organs where T cells reside (in the paracortex). Like macrophages, dendritic cells in lymphoid tissues act as antigen-presenting cells and help stimulate T cells.

Granulocytes are named because they contain granules filled with potent chemicals, such as digestive enzymes and reactive oxygen species, which can destroy microorganisms. The predominant granulocyte, the *neutrophil*, is also a phagocyte. The main function of neutrophils is to ingest microorganisms and digest them with the content of their granules. Other granulocytes, *eosinophils* and *basophils*, function by releasing the content of their granules toward harmful cells or microbes that would be too big to be ingested, such as parasites. *Mast cells* are the tissue equivalents of basophils but are found in the lungs, skin, tongue, and linings of the nose and intestinal tract, rather than the bloodstream. Both mast cell and basophil granules contain histamine, which contributes to inflammation and allergy.

Cytokines

Immune cells may communicate by direct physical contact or by releasing and responding to proteins called **cytokines**. Cytokines have various functions, including carrying information to and from immune cells, enhancing cell growth and differentiation, attracting cells to migrate to an area by chemotaxis (in which case the cytokine is called a *chemokine*), and activating immune cells. As mentioned previously, cytokines produced by monocytes and macrophages are called monokines. Conversely, cytokines produced by lymphocytes are called **lymphokines**. Cytokines include a diverse assortment of interleukins, interferons, and growth factors (Table 4-1).

Normal Immune Response

As pathogens attempt to enter our body, the immune response is set in motion in an orchestrated course of events, with different players called to action as time progresses (Fig 4-5). In effect, the immune response can be broken down into two main phases: nonspecific immunity and specific immunity.

Nonspecific Immunity

B and T cells represent a very powerful defense system, but their initial activation when first encountering an antigen requires time. Therefore, the body also has defense mechanisms that are either always in place (acting as preventive measures) or that can act rapidly. These defense mechanisms include physical barriers (such as skin, mucous membranes, nasal hairs, sneezing, coughing); chemical barriers (such as tears, sweat, saliva); the inflammatory response; the clotting system;

Table 4.1	Cytokines and Their Functions		
Cytokine	**Sources**	**Target Cells**	**Activities**
Interleukin 1 (IL-1)	Lymphocytes Antigen-presenting cells	Monocytes Macrophages Neutrophils	Promotes inflammation Induces fever
IL-2 to IL-8	Activated T cells	Macrophages T cells B cells NK cells Mast cells	Stimulate T-cell sensitivity to antigens exposed on antigen-presenting cells Stimulate B-cell activity, plasma cell formation, and antibody production Enhance innate immune defenses Modulate immune response
Tumor necrosis factors	Macrophages Activated T cells	Monocytes Neutrophils Tumor cells	Mimic actions of IL-1 Activate phagocytes Kill or slow the growth of tumor cells
Interferons	Leukocytes Activated T cells	NK cells Macrophages Viruses	Induce NK cell activity Activate macrophages Antiviral activity

Abbreviations: IL = interleukin; NK cell = natural killer cell.

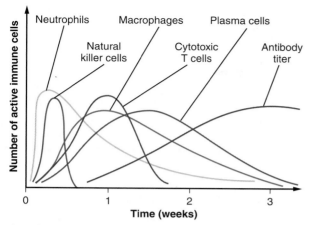

Figure 4–5 Course of immune system response to a bacterial infection over time.

the complement system; and the kinin system. These defense mechanisms of the immune response are *nonspecific*, because they function indiscriminately against any antigen, regardless of prior exposure. They are all examples of *nonspecific immunity*, also called *innate* or *natural immunity*, and share the following properties:

- Immediate and systematic
- Broad-spectrum and directed against any foreign substance
- Based on inborn or inherited defense mechanisms present at birth

Phagocytes, NK cells, and cytotoxic T cells are all participants in the nonspecific immune response. Monocytes and macrophages also contribute to nonspecific immunity, but with their ability to process and present antigens, they also participate in the following line of defenses, called *specific immunity*.

Specific Immunity

Specific immune defenses are also called *adaptive* or *acquired* immunity because they are not present at birth; they develop after exposure to a specific antigen. Once established, specific immune defenses have the ability to remember and respond more quickly to a second exposure to an antigen. Specific immune defenses have the following properties:

- They are *specific*, having developed one type of cells and molecules targeted to one particular antigen and not others.
- They are highly *versatile*, in that they can recognize and react to millions of possible antigens. The immune system stores just a few of each kind of the B

and T cells needed to recognize a multitude of potential antigens. When an antigen first appears, the few matching immune cells that can respond to it multiply intensively to generate the number of cells required to effectively destroy the antigen. They also generate so-called memory cells that will "remember" the antigen.

- They keep a *memory* of the antigens previously encountered and can react to them in a faster, stronger, and longer-lasting way during a second encounter. The concept of vaccination is based on this property.
- They also display *tolerance* towards self-antigens, as previously discussed.

Innate immunity, inflammation, and healing-processes all work together in a concerted way to maintain health.

Antibodies made by plasma cells that arise from B cells and T cells are the two components of the specific immune response and correspond to the **humoral response** and the **cellular response**, respectively.

Humoral Immunity

The surface of each B cell is labeled with the antibody it can produce. When an antigen binds to the antibody present on the surface of a B cell, the B cell processes the antigen and presents it at its surface coupled with its own MHC molecules. A helper T cell with a matching receptor for the complex antigen-MHC molecule can then bind to the B cell and release lymphokines. These lymphokines activate the B cell, which multiplies and matures into antibody-producing plasma cells. Antibodies are then released into the bloodstream, where they bind to the antigens they encounter and form antigen-antibody complexes. These complexes are then eliminated by the complement system or by the spleen and the liver.

Cellular Immunity

Parallel to the humoral response, helper T cells are mobilized when they bind to an APC which displays a complex antigen-MHC molecule that matches with its receptor. The mobilized helper T cell matures and secretes different lymphokines. Some lymphokines will attract phagocytes to the area of infection, including neutrophils and macrophages. Others will stimulate the growth of mature cytotoxic T cells and/or additional mature helper T cells. Together, the phagocytes and cytotoxic T cells will destroy the pathogen and/or the infected cells. Additional mature helper T cells will help recruit more immune cells as needed.

With the integrated efforts of humoral and cellular immunity, the initial response to a new antigen is called *primary response*. The primary response may take up to 2 weeks to fully develop and for the antibody level in the blood (or antibody titer) to reach its peak. During a second exposure to the same antigen, the antigen will trigger a *secondary response* that will be more rapid, extensive, and prolonged than the primary response. Memory B and T cells left behind after the primary response are "primed," which means that they become active more rapidly and can produce a more effective response during a second encounter with the antigen.

Active and Passive Immunity

Depending on the type of antigen (e.g., bacterial or viral), the amount of antigen, and the route of entry into the body, the immune response may be strong or weak, short-lived or long-lasting. The immune response is also influenced by inherited genes, and not all individuals respond to an antigen similarly. Some may easily overcome an infection, others may not. Immunity of a low-responding individual may be boosted in two different ways: active immunity or passive immunity.

In **active immunity**, antibodies are produced in response to an antigen. Active immunity happens naturally when the body fights an infection, such as with the varicella-zoster virus which causes the childhood disease chickenpox. Active immunity may also occur artificially, through vaccination. Vaccines contain either killed or weakened live bacteria or viruses, or chemically altered toxins called toxoids. Memory cells produced in response to the vaccine remain in the body, usually for life. Booster shots can be given to ensure that the memory remains strong. Typical vaccines include polio, tetanus, hepatitis A and B, measles, mumps, and rubella.

In **passive immunity**, the antibodies are not produced by the host but are rather received from another source. Passive immunity occurs naturally in infants who are born with weak immune responses but are protected for the first few months of life by antibodies they receive from their mothers through the placenta. Babies can also receive some antibodies from breast milk that help to protect their digestive tracts. However, passive immunity lasts only a few weeks or months because it is not associated with the production of memory cells in the body. Passive immunity can also occur when someone is given an injection of antiserum or gamma globulins (IgGs). For example, dental health-care workers who incur a needle stick injury may receive an injection of gamma globulins to boost their immune response against potential hepatitis viruses.

IMMUNOPATHOLOGY

Immunopathology represents the study of diseases caused by dysfunctions of the immune system. The diseases can be grouped into three main categories: hypersensitivity reactions, autoimmune diseases, and immune deficiency diseases.

Hypersensitivity Reactions

In **hypersensitivity reactions**, also called *allergic reactions*, the immune system produces an exaggerated response that leads to body tissue destruction. Often the exaggerated response is directed against an antigen that would not be otherwise harmful. This type of antigen is also called an *allergen*. These allergic reactions usually stop when the allergen is removed. These reactions are classified into four main types, based on the nature of the immune reaction that causes them.

Type I Hypersensitivity: Anaphylactic or Atopic Reactions

In type I hypersensitivity, the immune reaction occurs within minutes of an exposure to a previously encountered allergen, such as pollen, latex, penicillin, or cat hair. These antigens are usually not harmful to the general population, only to specific individuals in which plasma cells produce IgE in response to the antigen. IgEs bind to the surface of mast cells, which then release their granules that contain histamine. Histamine increases dilation and permeability of blood vessels, and causes constriction of smooth muscle cells in bronchioles of the lungs.

When the reactions are limited to the skin, such as insect stings or latex allergy, or to upper respiratory manifestations, such as hay fever, they are called **atopic reactions**. Symptoms depend on where the allergen comes into contact with the body and are usually treated with antihistaminic drugs. When the reactions are generalized and systemic, they are called **anaphylactic reactions**. These can be life-threatening if the individual has difficulty breathing. Anaphylactic reactions must be recognized and treated promptly. Treatment options include oral antihistamines, corticosteroids, and epinephrine injections in the most severe cases. Individuals who are aware of their allergies should remain on constant alert and avoid any contact with the allergens.

Type II Hypersensitivity: Cytotoxic Reactions

Type II hypersensitivity reactions, called *cytotoxic reactions*, are also caused by antibodies, usually IgGs or IgMs. In cytotoxic reactions, the antibodies bind to a specific type of cells, either foreign cells that have been introduced to the body, or cells that are wrongly recognized as foreign. As a result, the cells can no longer function well and may even be killed. Examples of cytotoxic reactions include:

■ Reactions to transfusions when a person is given an incompatible blood type.
■ Erythroblastosis fetalis, or Rhesus reaction, during a second pregnancy of an Rh-negative mother with an Rh-positive fetus.
■ Hyperthyroidism, or Graves' disease, in which thyroid cells are damaged but not destroyed by a cytotoxic reaction and end up producing an excess of thyroid hormones.
■ Autoimmune disorders resulting from a change in the MHC molecules of a specific cell type, such as in pemphigus vulgaris, cicatricial pemphigoid, and acute rheumatic fever. In these conditions, the cause of the change in the MHC molecules is usually unknown and irreversible.

Type III Hypersensitivity: Immune Complex-Mediated Reactions

In type III hypersensitivity reactions, immune complexes form between IgM, IgA, or IgG antibodies and circulating antigens such as bacteria, viruses, drugs, chemicals, or endogenous molecules. Normally, immune complexes are rapidly removed from the bloodstream; however, sometimes they continue to circulate and eventually become trapped in the basement membranes of tissues of the kidneys, lungs, skin, joints, or blood vessels. There, they initiate an inflammatory response that leads to localized or systemic tissue destruction. Autoimmune examples of immune complex-mediated reactions include systemic lupus erythematosus, rheumatoid arthritis, and some forms of kidney disease, including glomerulonephritis.

Type IV Hypersensitivity: Cell-Mediated or Delayed Hypersensitivity Reactions

Type IV hypersensitivity reactions are also called *cell-mediated hypersensitivity reactions* because they result from the action of T cells rather than antibodies. Neither B cells nor antibodies are involved in this type of hypersensitivity reaction. In addition, these reactions usually take more time to develop, from 24 to 72 hours or more, which is why they are also called *delayed hypersensitivity reactions*. In these reactions, small antigenic molecules, called *haptens*, combine with the proteins of a specific cell type and trigger a T-cell reaction, resulting in direct tissue destruction by the T cells or by a secondary inflammatory reaction. Examples of cell-mediated hypersensitivity include *contact dermatitis* (skin reaction) and *contact stomatitis* (reaction in the mouth). Examples of substances that may cause a contact allergic reaction include natural rubber latex, poison ivy, metals, cosmetics, and some chemicals used in toothpastes and mouth rinses. The most common dermatologic symptom is the development of an erythematous vesicular rash, which is extremely pruritic (itchy). In the mouth, symptoms include diffuse erythema, ulcers, and vesicles. These symptoms will not stop until the antigen is eliminated or all areas touched by the antigen have been destroyed, which may take several days or weeks. Symptoms may be alleviated with the use of topical corticosteroids.

Allergic contact dermatitis is a type IV hypersensitivity reaction, caused by contact with an allergen such as residues of chemicals used in manufacturing latex gloves. The delayed reaction will occur in a sensitized individual between 24 and 48 hours after exposure to the offensive substances. Symptoms are similar to those observed in *irritant contact dermatitis*, although irritant contact dermatitis is not a hypersensitivity reaction. Irritant contact dermatitis may be caused by chemicals such as surface disinfectants, mechanical rubbing of the gloves against the skin, or by the powder added to some gloves to make them easier to put on. Changing from latex to latex-free gloves may help determine what type of dermatitis is present.

Autoimmune diseases resulting from type IV hypersensitivity include host-versus-graft rejection, type 1 diabetes, and possibly Sjögren's syndrome.

Autoimmune Diseases

In autoimmune diseases, the immune system loses its ability to distinguish self (normal tissues) from nonself (foreign antigens), or a change occurs in the MHC markers of self on some tissues. This triggers activated B cells to produce antibodies against self-antigens, called **autoantibodies**, and/or cytotoxic T cells that attack normal tissues. The result is an immune and inflammatory response that destroys normal body cells, tissues, and/or organs. This response manifests as a type II, III, or IV hypersensitivity reaction similar to that occurring in an allergic reaction. However, in an allergy the immune system reacts to external, normally innocuous substances, whereas in autoimmune disorders, the immune system reacts to normal body tissues. The cause for this abnormal reaction is unknown. Because autoimmune diseases tend to run in families, they are probably associated with predisposing genes. Exposure to specific environmental triggers, such as bacteria or drugs, combined with genetic susceptibility, may be responsible for the necessary changes leading to *autoimmunity*. Women of childbearing age, particularly African American, Hispanic American, and Native American women, have an increased risk of developing autoimmune diseases. Moreover, for unknown reasons, the prevalence of autoimmune diseases is increasing, affecting approximately 5% to 8% of adults in North America and Western Europe.

More than 80 types of autoimmune diseases have been identified (Table 4-2). Some may result in the

Table 4.2 Autoimmune Diseases		
Disease	**Affected Organs**	**Symptoms**
Graves' disease	Thyroid	Tiredness, depression, sensitivity to cold, weight gain, muscle weakness and cramps, dry hair, tough skin, constipation. Sometimes, none.
Rheumatoid arthritis	Joints; also lungs and skin	Inflammation of the joints (hands), muscle pain, deformed joints, weakness, fatigue, loss of appetite, weight loss.
Hashimoto's thyroiditis	Thyroid	Insomnia, irritability, weight loss without dieting, heat sensitivity, sweating, fine brittle hair, weakness in muscles, light menstrual periods, bulging eyes, shaky hands. Sometimes, none.
Vitiligo	Skin melanocytes	White discolored patches appearing in different parts of the skin, mucous membranes, and retina; premature graying of scalp hair, eyelashes, eyebrows, and beard.
Type 1 diabetes	Pancreatic Islets of Langhans	Increased thirst and frequent urination, extreme hunger, weight loss, fatigue, blurred vision.
Pernicious anemia	Stomach	Lack of intrinsic factor production resulting in vitamin B-12 deficiency and anemia. Symptoms of anemia due to vitamin B-12 deficiency, including shortness of breath, fatigue, dizziness, and pale skin; heart murmurs, fast heartbeats, arrhythmias, an enlarged heart (cardiomegaly), or even heart failure. Nervous system symptoms, including feelings of numbness, tingling, weakness, lack of coordination, clumsiness, impaired memory, and personality. Sometimes, none.
Multiple sclerosis	Nervous system	Weakness; trouble with coordination, balance, speaking, and walking; paralysis; tremors; numbness and tingling feeling in arms, legs, hands, and feet.
Glomerulonephritis	Kidneys	Blood in the urine, foamy urine; swelling of the face, eyes, ankles, feet, legs, or abdomen; also abdominal pain, cough, diarrhea, general ill-feeling, fever, joint and muscles aches, loss of appetite, shortness of breath.
Lupus (systemic lupus erythematosus)	Skin, joint, kidneys, heart, brain, red blood cells, others	Swelling and damage to the joints, skin, kidneys, heart, lungs, blood vessels, and brain; "butterfly" rash across the nose and cheeks; rashes on other parts of the body; painful and swollen joints; sensitivity to the sun.
Sjögren's syndrome	Salivary glands, tear glands, joints	Dry mouth (xerostomia), difficulties swallowing, cavities, periodontal disease, mouth sores and swelling, stones and/or infection of parotid glands; eye dryness; joint pain or inflammation.

destruction of one or more types of tissues, others in the abnormal growth or function of an organ. One single organ may be affected, as in type 1 diabetes (pancreas), Graves' disease (thyroid), Hashimoto's thyroiditis (thyroid), celiac disease (gastrointestinal tract), and multiple sclerosis (nervous system), or several organs may be affected, as in rheumatoid arthritis, lupus, scleroderma, and Sjögren's syndrome. Organs and tissues commonly affected by autoimmune disorders include red blood cells, blood vessels, connective tissues, endocrine glands such as thyroid or pancreas, muscles, joints, and skin.

Some symptoms of autoimmune diseases are specific to a disease, but others are more common, including overall ill-feeling, low fever, and muscle aches. Symptoms may suddenly worsen when the autoimmune disease goes through episodes of flare-ups, also called **exacerbations**, and they may disappear when the disease goes through episodes of **remission**. Patients may also have more than one autoimmune disease. All these features make autoimmune diseases difficult to diagnose. Because several autoimmune diseases have oral manifestations, the dental hygienist may be the first health-care professional to observe the signs of these diseases.

These diseases usually cannot be cured and remain chronic, with alternating episodes of exacerbation and remission. The goals of treatment are to reduce symptoms and to control the autoimmune process while maintaining the body's ability to fight disease. The specific treatments used depend on the specific disease and symptoms. Some patients may need supplements to replace a hormone or nutrient the body is lacking. Examples include thyroid supplements, vitamins, or insulin injections. Often, drugs that help control or reduce the immune system response, called **immunosuppressive** medicines, are prescribed. Such medicines may include corticosteroids, such as prednisone, and nonsteroid drugs such as cyclophosphamide, azathioprine, or tacrolimus.

Immunodeficiency Diseases

Although hypersensitivity reactions and autoimmune diseases result from an overactive immune system, *immunodeficiency diseases* arise when one or more components of the immune system are missing or fail to function properly. Patients with immunodeficiency frequently suffer from infections and have an increased risk of developing cancers. When the immune deficit is present at birth, the disease is called primary immunodeficiency; when the deficit is acquired after birth, the disease is called secondary immunodeficiency.

Primary Immunodeficiency

A primary immunodeficiency disease is always due to a **congenital** defect, which means that it is present at birth. In most cases, the immune deficit is inherited and the responsible genetic defect has been identified. However, some cases may result from a spontaneous mutation or a developmental defect, as in DiGeorge syndrome. Primary immunodeficiencies may affect components of either the innate immune response, such as phagocytes or the complement system, or the adaptive immune response, such as B cells, T cells, or both.

More than 70 different types of primary immunodeficiency diseases have been identified and are usually classified by the type of cells involved. Disorders that affect B cells and antibody production range from mild to more severe and include:

- *Selective IgA deficiency* (reduced IgA levels) is the most common and may be asymptomatic or cause recurrent respiratory and genitourinary tract infections.
- *Hypogammaglobulinemia* (reduced IgG levels) usually causes respiratory and gastrointestinal infections.
- *Bruton's (or X-linked) agammaglobulinemia* (very low IgG levels) results in frequent, severe, life-threatening infections early in life.

T-cell disorders can affect both the humoral and cell-mediated responses. Although deficits in the humoral immune response increase the risk for bacterial infections, deficits in the cell-mediated response are associated with increased susceptibility to viral such as cytomegalovirus, protozoan, and fungal infections, such as *Candida albicans*, the agent responsible for common yeast infections.

- *DiGeorge syndrome* is a developmental defect in which the thymus fails to develop normally, resulting in reduction of T-cell numbers and absence of T-cell response, along with characteristic facial abnormalities, reduced parathyroid function, and congenital heart disease.
- *Severe combined immunodeficiency (SCID)* is a rare inherited condition in which T cells, B cells, and NK cells are affected. Patients with SCID have very low numbers of circulating lymphocytes and their thymus fails to develop. They suffer from severe recurrent infections, usually fatal within the first years of life.

Symptoms of primary immunodeficiencies range from very mild to very serious. Many patients with primary immunodeficiency are infants and children who often suffer from multiple infections. These infections may be:

- Mild, but could take longer than usual to treat.
- Caused by microorganisms that would not otherwise cause infections in a child with a normal immune system, in which case they are known as **opportunistic infections**.
- May be *recurrent*, which means that they keep coming back.
- May also be severe and even life-threatening.

Other health problems may develop as complications of the immune deficit, including delayed growth, anemia, arthritis, autoimmunity, or cancer. Some children may have no symptoms at all and the disease may not be discovered until later in life, during adolescence or young adulthood.

Primary immunodeficiency diseases can usually be treated and cured, especially if they are diagnosed early and therapy is started promptly to limit permanent damages and complications. Therefore, discovering these diseases early is very important. The goals of treatment are to clear up the current infection, avoid microbes, prevent exposure to new infections, and correct the immunodeficiency. Current infections may require aggressive treatments, such as long-term use of antibiotics and/or antifungal medications, and preventive measures. When standard medications fail, hospitalization may be required to administer antibiotics and other drugs intravenously. Good hygiene and nutrition practices, as well as avoiding individuals with colds or infections and large crowds, will help avoid and minimize contact with microbes. In severe cases, correcting the immunodeficiency may necessitate a *bone marrow transplant*, a procedure that transfers bone marrow from a healthy individual to the patient. In many cases, *antibody replacement therapy*, consisting of the regular infusion or injection of immunoglobulins taken from healthy blood donors (see passive immunity) will be effective.

Secondary Immunodeficiency

By definition, acquired or secondary immunodeficiencies develop after birth and are not due to a genetic defect. They are more common than primary immunodeficiencies and may be caused by a variety of factors, including therapies that suppress the immune system, such as chemotherapy, radiation, corticosteroid therapy, and any prolonged serious illness, such as diabetes, renal disease, malnutrition, cancer, tuberculosis,

HIV infection, and many more. Critically ill, older, or hospitalized patients are also more susceptible to develop secondary immunodeficiencies. Moreover, common viral infections, including influenza, infectious mononucleosis, and measles, as well as blood transfusions, surgeries, smoking, and stress, may all result in temporary immunodeficiencies. The major manifestations of secondary immunodeficiency are recurrent, opportunistic infections. In the oral cavity, these may manifest as infections with the fungus *Candida albicans* or as aggressive periodontal disease. Usually, the immunodeficiency disappears when the underlying condition is resolved. Therefore, treatment focuses on the underlying disorder.

One common form of secondary immunodeficiency is acquired hypogammaglobulinemia, in which patients have very low but detectable levels of immunoglobulins. The origin of this condition is unknown, and it manifests in young adults in the form of recurrent infections. It can generally be treated with antibody replacement therapy. Another common cause of secondary immunodeficiency is corticosteroid therapy, which is used in the treatment of autoimmune disorders such as rheumatoid arthritis or systemic lupus erythematosus. Currently, the most prominent secondary immunodeficiency is AIDS.

HIV can destroy or disable vital T cells, paving the way for a variety of immunologic shortcomings. The virus can also hide out for long periods (becomes latent) in immune cells. As the immune defenses falter, a person develops AIDS and falls prey to unusual, often life-threatening infections and rare cancers.

CLINICAL FEATURES OF IMMUNE DISORDERS

The central function of the immune system is to distinguish foreign antigens from self-components of body tissues. Sometimes there is failure to discriminate between harmful and harmless antigens. Also, there can be failure to discriminate between self and nonself body proteins. Inappropriate immune responses are responsible for a wide variety of conditions. Depending on the inappropriate reaction, there can be a variety of clinically apparent signs and symptoms, ranging from a skin rash to failure of a major organ system.

Allergic Disorders

An allergy is a disorder acquired by the immune system, also referred to as *hypersensitivity disorder*. This means the body's immune system is overly reactive to a usually harmless antigen, termed an *allergen*, which in another individual may provoke no response at all. Antibodies are produced to the allergen and the subsequent "attack" is experienced as symptoms by the patient. Allergic reactions occur to normally harmless substances in the environment including grasses, pollens, animal dander, and occasionally medications and dental materials.

Allergic Contact Dermatitis

Contact dermatitis is inflammation of the skin (dermatitis) caused by direct contact of an offending agent on the skin. When inflammation is the result of direct contact with an allergen, it is termed *allergic contact dermatitis* and is considered a type IV hypersensitivity reaction. Substances that cause allergic contact dermatitis include such things as poison ivy, base metals, detergents, chemical preservatives, industrial chemicals, or latex rubber. Patients who wear metal watch bands often report tenderness and itching around their wrists (Fig. 4-6). Latex allergy is a common problem among health-care workers who treat patients (Fig. 4-7). Perioral dermatitis may result when a patient uses a new dentifrice or cosmetic

product with an allergen that comes into contact with the skin around the mouth (Fig. 4-8). Initial exposure to the substance does not cause a reaction; it sensitizes the skin. Subsequent exposure causes lesions that are confined to the area of contact. Symptoms include blisters or a pruritic (itchy) red rash that appears within 1 to 2 days post exposure and may take as long as 4 weeks to resolve completely if left untreated (Fig. 4-9). Corticosteroids, such as hydrocortisone, may be applied to small areas of the skin. If the reaction covers a relatively large portion of the skin or is severe, systemic medication, such as the antihistamine diphenhydramine or prednisone, may be prescribed.

Allergic Contact Mucositis

Contact mucositis is inflammation of mucous membranes (*mucositis*) caused by direct contact of an offending allergen. When inflammation is the result of direct exposure to an allergen, it is termed *allergic contact mucositis*. Substances that cause allergic contact mucositis may include dental materials such as denture base acrylic, latex rubber dam material, or orthodontic elastics; oral hygiene products such as flavoring agents; detergent additives; or foods. Often the allergen

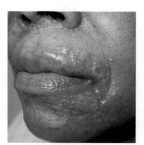

Figure 4–8   Contact dermatitis. Perioral dermatitis from allergy to skin cream. (From Barankin, B: Derm Notes. F.A. Davis, Philadelphia, 2006, p 130.)

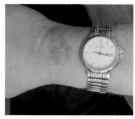

Figure 4–6   Contact dermatitis. Allergy to metals in watch band. (From Barankin, B: Derm Notes. F.A. Davis, Philadelphia, 2006, p 78.)

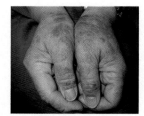

Figure 4–7   Contact dermatitis. Health-care worker with an allergy to latex gloves. (From Barankin, B: Derm Notes. F.A. Davis, Philadelphia, 2006, p 67.)

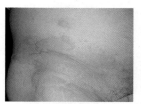

Figure 4–9   Contact dermatitis. Rash of the skin in response to contact with an allergen. (From Barankin, B: Derm Notes. F.A. Davis, Philadelphia, 2006, p 166.)

remains unknown until the patient undergoes allergy testing.

Clinically, contact mucositis appears as an erythematous, edematous, or atrophic zone of mucosa at the point of contact. When the source is toothpaste or mouth rinses, patients will complain of a generalized discomfort and burning sensation, with mild swelling, erythema, and superficial sloughing of the surface epithelium. Deep ulcers or blisters generally do not occur.

Some forms of oral allergic contact mucositis are common enough to warrant their own clinical terminology and are described next.

Plasma Cell Gingivitis

Plasma cell gingivitis has become relatively common since oral health-care products containing essential oils, herbal additives, whitening, and anti-calculus agents are readily available. Although their therapeutic effect is often beneficial to patients, they may cause a hypersensitivity reaction. Plasma cell gingivitis appears as a diffuse enlargement of the free and attached gingiva characterized by erythema and loss of stippling (Fig. 4-10). Other intraoral sites may also demonstrate areas of tenderness and erythema. The name of the condition reflects the presence of a large number of plasma cells present when the tissue is biopsied. Treatment involves discontinuing the use of the allergen. Topical anti-inflammatory agents may be needed to resolve the mucositis.

Cinnamon Stomatitis

Cinnamon stomatitis is an allergic reaction to cinnamon oil (cinnamon aldehyde) used as a flavoring agent in many red-colored cinnamon-flavored gums, candies, and oral health-care products. Patients present with tender or painful "burning" mucosa to which the agent has contact, such as a focal area of buccal mucosa, diffuse gingival lesions, or "chapped" lips. Because patients generally do not associate the pain with the allergen, they continue to use the product. This chronic exposure causes the initial erythematous lesions to transform to thick white plaques that may remain painful (Fig. 4-11). This pain helps to distinguish cinnamon stomatitis from other red and white lesions that occur in the oral cavity. A similar reaction may occur as a result of contact with peppermint, spearmint, or neem oils. Discontinuation of the product brings immediate relief, with resolution within hours or days.

Clinical Implications

Lesions of cinnamon stomatitis may resemble squamous cell carcinoma or an autoimmune mucositis. The key to the diagnosis is sudden onset of pain and tenderness with the use of a product that contains cinnamon aldehyde.

Hypersensitivity Reaction to Dental Restorative Materials

Hypersensitivity reaction to dental amalgam is seen in about 1% to 2% of individuals with amalgam restorations. The word *amalgam* means "several elements merged into a single compound." Dental amalgams are composed of silver, copper, zinc, beryllium,

Figure 4–10 Contact mucositis. Plasma cell gingivitis causes a diffuse enlargement of the free and attached gingiva in response to allergens in oral health-care products.

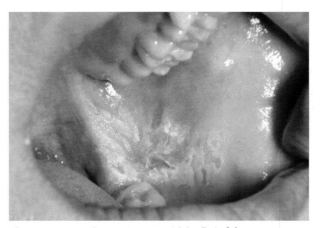

Figure 4–11 Cinnamon stomatitis. Painful erythematous lesion that arose within hours of chewing cinnamon-flavored gum.

nickel, mercury, or other materials in varying quantities depending on the manufacturer's specifications. Patients may be allergic to one or more of these metals. In hypersensitive (allergic) individuals, red and white tender lesions develop wherever the amalgam contacts the mucosa. The buccal mucosa and lateral borders of the tongue are the most common sites (Fig. 4-12). Treatment involves removing the amalgam and replacing it with a composite or other nonmetallic material.

Clinical Implications

When a patient suffers from an allergic reaction to the exposed metal margin of a crown, lesions are typically observed contacting the area on adjacent gingiva, buccal mucosa, or lateral tongue. Enhanced oral hygiene rarely brings improvement. Patients who experience allergic reactions to dental metals may also react to base metals in jewelry. A "quick and dirty" way to help determine this is to ask if they can wear "cheap" jewelry or metal watch bands (refer back to Fig 4-6). If they report developing a rash, they may be allergic to nickel or other metals. Allergy testing should be considered.

Other dental restorations, such as crowns, bridges, and removable partial dentures (RPDs), use metals such as nickel, titanium, gold, chromium cobalt, and palladium. Up to 17 percent of women and 3 percent of men are allergic to nickel and 1% to 3% are allergic to cobalt and chromium. Porcelain-fused-to-metal (PFM) crowns and RPD frameworks contain many of these metals. Contact hypersensitivity reactions to these metals are seen adjacent to the restoration or appliance when it is in place. Intense gingival erythema at the margin of a PFM crown that does not respond to conventional gingival therapy may represent an allergic reaction to one of the metals in the framework of the restoration (Fig. 4-13). Allergy testing for dental materials may be necessary to determine which material causes the reaction. Treatment involves replacing the restorations with non-allergenic materials.

Ulcerative Conditions

An **ulcer** is defined as the loss of epithelial continuity with exposure of the underlying connective tissue (Fig. 4-14 A, B, and C). A crater forms that fills in with fibrin, granulation tissue, and necrotic debris, giving the ulcer the characteristic yellow center with erythematous halo (Fig. 4-15). Although ulcers may be caused by trauma (see Chapter 2) and viruses (see Chapter 3), there are several common immune-related ulcerative conditions. It is clinically important to distinguish among ulcer types because the success of their management and relief of symptoms depends

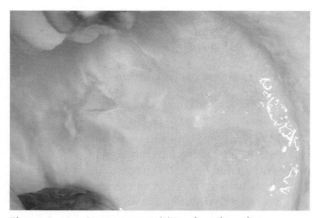

Figure 4–12 Contact mucositis to dental amalgam. Hypersensitivity reaction to dental amalgam. Lesion makes direct contact lower molar restoration when mouth is at rest.

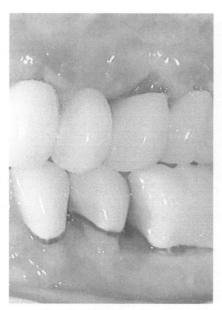

Figure 4–13 Allergy-crown margin. Tender gingival lesions developed within weeks of crown placement. Lesions resolved with removal of restoration.

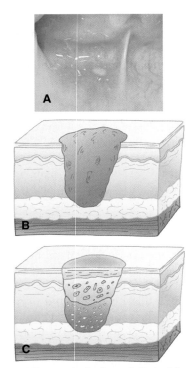

Figure 4–14   Histopathologic and clinical features of a nonspecific ulcer. A. Clinical appearance: Yellow necrotic center with erythematous halo. **B.** Ulcers are craters caused by tissue destruction. **C.** Crater fills with necrotic debris and inflammatory cells, which will be responsible for tissue repair.

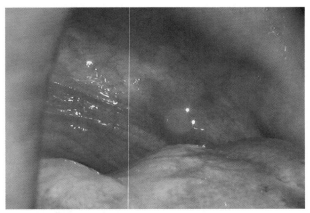

Figure 4–15   Minor RAU. Single painful ulcer of the oral mucosa; note yellow necrotic center and erythematous halo.

on addressing the proper etiology. See Table 4-3 for the primary distinguishing clinical features of he three types of recurrent aphthous ulcers and herpes simplex.

Aphthous Ulcers

The term *aphthous* (pronounced AFF-thus) comes from the Greek word *aphtha*, meaning *ulcer*. So, the term *aphthous ulcer* means "ulcer-ulcer." This fitting term reflects current lack of a precise etiology. The term *recurrent aphthous ulcer (RAU)* is used for several different forms of ulcers that share an immune dysregulation etiology, the presence of painful ulcerations, and a propensity to recur.

Three basic immune defects that may predispose the patient to the development of RAU are: 1) decreased mucosal barrier, 2) increased antigenic exposure and 3) inherited or acquired immunodysregulation. Patients with one or more of these factors may be at increased risk for developing RAU. If these patients have concurrent allergies, blood abnormalities, hormonal imbalance, certain infections, nutritional deficiencies, or experience emotional or physical stress, the risk increases. Any combination of these factors may be responsible for destruction of the epithelium that leads to the development of RAUs. Because no precise etiology exists for RAUs, successful treatment often remains elusive.

Clinical Implications

Traumatic ulcers should clearly be distinguished from RAUs based on the patient's history. The patient will report injuring himself or herself in the area of the ulcer or the clinician might observe a defective restoration or prosthesis contacting the ulcer. Treating a traumatic ulcer with topical anti-inflammatory medication, an acceptable treatment for RAU, may lead to delayed healing and possible infection in a traumatic ulcer.

There are three principal forms of RAUs: minor, herpetiform, and major.

Minor Recurrent Aphthous Ulcers

Minor aphthous ulcers are the most commonly occurring type. They rate second to traumatic ulcers in the oral cavity in number of occurrences. In the immunocompetent patient, they occur as a non-blistering lesion exclusively on nonkeratinized mucosa of the buccal mucosa, labial mucosa, ventral tongue, alveolar mucosa, and less commonly on the soft palate and floor of mouth.

Table 4.3	Clinical Features of Recurrent Aphthous Ulcers Versus Herpes Simplex			
Feature	**Minor RAU**	**Herpetiform RAU**	**Major RAU**	**Herpes**
Etiology	Localized immune defect	Localized immune defect	Systemic immune disorder	Herpes simplex virus
Prodrome	No	No	No	Yes
Intraoral location	Nonkeratinized mucosa*	Nonkeratinized mucosa*	Nonkeratinized mucosa*	Keratinized mucosa*
Preceding vesicle	No	No	No	Yes
Ulcer appearance	Single; less than 5 mm	Cluster less than 5 mm	1 - single, large deep, irregular rolled border 2 - cluster	Cluster that coalesces into large ulcers
Remission period	Yes	Yes	No	Yes
Extraoral sites	No	No	No	Yes
Diagnosis	Clinical features	Clinical features	Systemic disease consultations	Clinical features; cytologic smear
Treatment	Topical anti-inflammatory drugs	Topical anti-inflammatory drugs	Systemic management of underlying disease; systemic immunomodulary drugs for idiopathic etiology	Topical antiviral drugs during prodrome *only;* systemic antiviral drugs for severe recurrent cases

* May occur on any surface in severely immunocompromised patients.

Clinical Implications

Ulcers on the gingiva or hard palate are not recurrent aphthous ulcers. RAUs only occur on nonkeratinized tissue. The gingiva and hard palate are keratinized.

Minor RAUs rarely have a prodrome (warning sign), but the patient may occasionally experience mild burning followed by mild erythema that precedes loss of the surface epithelium. A typical RAU appears as a single shallow ulcer between 3 to 8 mm in diameter with a yellow necrotic center and erythematous halo. The border is not raised or rolled (Fig. 4-16). More than one ulcer may occur simultaneously, but they tend not to cluster together or coalesce, as do herpetic lesions. Once an ulcer forms, the symptoms include pain and burning and the patient reports discomfort eating spicy or acidic foods. In fact, patients often believe these foods cause their ulcer. The mucosa typically returns to normal within 10 to 14 days with no scarring. Patients may experience one to several episodes per year in different anatomic locations.

Herpetiform Aphthous Ulcers

Herpetiform means "herpes-like." This form of RAU occurs as a cluster of small ulcers (Fig. 4-17) that at first glance resemble herpes simplex infection (see Chapter 3). However, on closer investigation, the patient reports no prodrome or cluster of small vesicles. Also, as with other forms of RAU, they occur on loose nonkeratinized squamous epithelium, such as the ventral tongue, soft palate, or buccal mucosa, where herpetic lesions do not occur. The ulcers heal within 7 to 10 days without treatment and leave no scar.

Management of minor and herpetiform RAUs includes identifying the trigger that precipitates the ulcer, keeping in mind that the trigger often remains elusive.

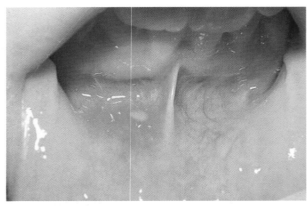

Figure 4–16 Minor aphthous ulcer. Single painful ulcer of the nonkeratinized mucosa. Note yellow necrotic center and erythematous halo.

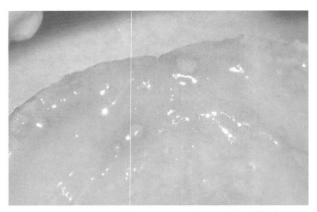

Figure 4–17 Herpetiform RAU. Cluster of small ulcers on nonkeratinized mucosa not preceded by a vesicle.

Once the ulcer develops, there are few medications that can shorten its duration. Because the basic pathology is over-activity of the immune system, medications that suppress the immune and inflammatory responses can be somewhat effective in treating RAUs. However, because they are caused by a variety of immune defects that often cannot be identified in any given patient, not all treatments work for all patients. Many patients experience much trial and error before finding a product that works for them. Analgesic medications may help reduce pain while the ulcer heals. Cauterizing the lesion with chemical agents that "burn" away the diseased tissue and exposed nerve endings may also be used, but must be delivered by a trained oral health professional. Due to significant risk of further tissue damage if used inappropriately, cauterizing agents should never be given to the patient to use at home.

Clinical Implications

Women who suffer from frequent RAUs often report a dramatic remission from the lesions during pregnancy. This is most likely due to increased epithelialization of the oral mucosa in response to pregnancy hormones, thereby increasing the integrity of the mucosal barrier.

Major Aphthous Ulcers

Major aphthous ulcers differ from minor and herpetiform RAUs in several important ways. They are not simply a larger or more severe version of minor RAUs.

Although all aphthous ulcers occur on loose nonkeratinized mucosa, major aphthous ulcers appear in two different clinical patterns:

1. Singly as large, deep ulcers with rolled irregular borders and thick yellow central fibrinopurulent membranes (Fig. 4-18) that heal within 3 to 4 weeks with scarring and are immediately followed by a new similar lesion in a different anatomic location.
2. An outbreak of a cluster of smaller ulcers that develop concurrently, with new small ulcers appearing as older ones resolve.

In both scenarios, patients are rarely without at least one ulcer.

Major RAUs are most common in adolescents and young adults. Some patients suffer for many years and the condition may last into adulthood. Therefore, adults with major RAUs should be questioned about the history of their ulcers because they may have started in childhood or adolescence. The underlying

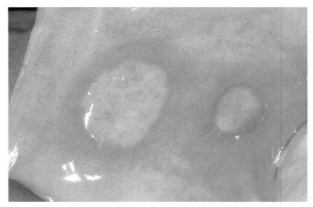

Figure 4–18 Major RAU. Large long-standing ulcers with necrotic center and raised rolled borders.

defect of the immune system that leads to major RAUs is more complex than minor RAUs. Frequently, these indicate underlying systemic disorders that must be investigated. Some examples include Behçet's disease, cyclic neutropenia, HIV/AIDS, and Crohn's disease.

Behçet's Disease

Behçet's disease (pronounced Beh-SET'S) is a multisystem condition that initially affects the oral mucosa and eventually the genitals, skin, joints, eyes, or central nervous system (Fig. 4-19). It is an autoimmune vasculitis, or inflammation of the blood vessels, that, if left untreated, can involve the gastrointestinal tract, pulmonary, musculoskeletal, and neurological systems. To avoid serious life-threatening complications, medical treatment is necessary.

Behçet's disease is considered a rare disease. The cause remains unknown. Persons with a defect of a specific gene in the immune system, called antigen HLA-B51, are predisposed to developing Behçet's disease.

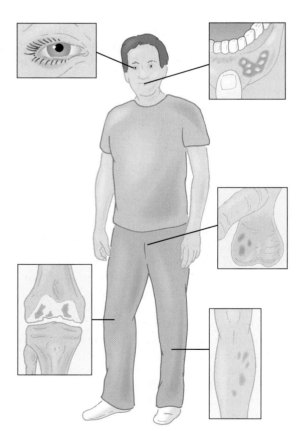

Figure 4–19 Spectrum of systemic involvement in Behçet's disease: Eye lesions, major aphthous ulcers, genital ulcers, arthritis, and skin rashes.

This defect is seen primarily in patients with Turkish, Japanese, or Eastern Mediterranean ancestry, but not limited to these groups. An estimated 15,000 to 20,000 Americans have been diagnosed with Behçet's disease. In the United Kingdom, there are less than 1,000 cases; but in Japan, Behçet's disease is one of the leading causes of blindness due to eye involvement.

The disease first appears in young adults, and often is seen but not recognized before puberty. Onset is marked by the appearance of major RAUs of the oral cavity. Oral lesions are present in 99 percent of cases and are the first sign in nearly 75 percent of cases. Many years may pass before patients develop other Behçet's lesions, so the suspicion may be very low, especially if there is no family history. Patients with oral ulcers of Behçet's disease (Fig. 4-20) without other signs may be misdiagnosed until one of the other signs develops. This lack of multiple features of Behçet's disease may delay the actual diagnosis for years.

Ulcers can vary in size, but patients may have as many as six ulcers at the same time, and are rarely without an ulcer. The diagnosis may be suspected when the ulcers respond to systemic immunosuppressive therapy but not to topical therapy or other palliative measures. When they are misdiagnosed as having an allergy, patients with Behçet's lesions rarely respond to avoidance of the suspected allergen. Biopsy of the oral ulcers rarely leads to the precise diagnosis because the ulcers have nonspecific histopathologic features. Proper testing for Behçet's disease includes blood tests, eye examinations, and skin tests.

Clinical Implications

Patients with major RAUs should be referred to an immunologist or rheumatologist to determine if Behçet's disease is the cause. The diagnosis is not made in a dental office.

Cyclic Neutropenia

Cyclic neutropenia is a rare disease of childhood caused by a mutation of one of the genes called ELA2 that regulates neutrophil growth and development. Neutrophils are the first line of defense in a wide range of infections and other injuries. Although most patients are children, acquired forms of cyclic neutropenia exist in adults. The disease is characterized by reduction or loss of neutrophils in a regular cycle that occurs every 21 days for 3 to 6 days duration. During this time, patients experience infection, including gingivitis and

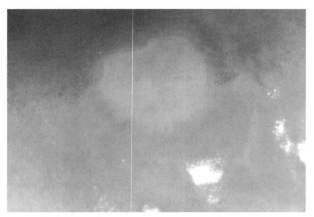

Figure 4-20   Behçet's disease. Typical large long-standing recurrent ulcer seen in Behçet's patient.

severe periodontitis, and a decreased ability to heal after minor trauma. Fever and malaise are characteristic of cyclic neutropenia, as well as recurrent oral ulcerations. Cyclic neutropenia is unusual in that the ulcers occur on keratinized mucosa. This helps distinguish them from RAUs. When neutrophils return to normal, the symptoms regress until the next cycle begins.

Clinical Implications

Cyclic neutropenia is difficult to detect in the dental office due to its cyclical nature. However, when a child presents to the dental office with recurrent severe gingivitis with ulceration, the parent should be asked if the child experiences an unusual number of recurrent infections of the urinary tract, pharynx, or other organ system. This can differentiate cyclic neutropenia from primary herpetic gingivostomatitis (see Chapter 3). Patients must see a physician to have serial blood counts over several weeks or months to determine if their neutrophil counts change over time.

HIV and AIDS

As discussed in Chapter 3, patients with undiagnosed or untreated HIV infection may experience recurrent aphthous-like ulcerations. The ulcers may resemble minor RAU, but herpetiform RAU, the least common of the three types, is common in this population. As immunosuppression becomes more severe, ulcerations become more frequent and also appear on keratinized mucosa. Patients on HAART (**h**ighly **a**ctive **a**nti-**r**etro-viral **t**herapy) tend to have few recurrences of their

ulcerations. However, ulcers that increase in frequency or severity in a patient on HAART may signal treatment failure or noncompliance with the regimen.

Clinical Implications

An underlying systemic disease is not identified in about 50 percent of cases of major aphthous ulcers. These lesions can be treated empirically with topical or locally injected anti-inflammatory agents. Systemic corticosteroids should be reserved for severe outbreaks. Keep in mind that most patients are children or adolescents, so treatment with systemic corticosteroids should be limited due to growth and development considerations. Alternative treatments, including pentoxyphiline and tacrolimus, should be considered.

Erythema Multiforme (EM)

Erythema multiforme (EM) (pronounced multi-FORMEE) is a self-limiting disease that causes a characteristic skin rash and often severe outbreaks of painful ulcerations of the mucous membranes. EM most commonly occurs in young adults and affects males more often than females. EM differs from the three forms of RAU in that EM has a more generalized distribution of ulcerations and erosions accompanied by severe pain. Approximately 50 percent of patients who experience erythema multiforme have had a recent exposure to a known trigger. The exact immunologic mechanism is not fully understood, but it is suspected that once the triggering agent causes production of antibodies, those antibodies are inappropriately identified as foreign by the immune system. The immune system then produces autoantibodies to try to remove them. For example, one of the common triggers for EM is herpes simplex virus. When the patient develops a herpetic lesion, anti-herpes antibodies are produced. After the infection is resolved, the anti-herpes antibodies are seen as foreign instead of normal proteins by the patient's immune system. Autoantibodies against these proteins appear in the blood stream 2 to 3 weeks after the herpes outbreak clears. They erroneously destroy some of the patient's normal tissues, resulting in the lesions of EM.

Besides herpes simplex, triggers include but are not limited to other infectious agents such as *Mycoplasma pneumoniae*, *Bartonella henselae* (which causes cat-scratch disease), *Salmonella spp.*, *Treponema pallidum*, and *Chlamydia*. Some drugs that have been implicated in the development of EM include beta-lactam antibiotics, such as penicillins and cephalosporins, as well as non-beta-lactams, such as clindamycin, tetracycline, and its derivatives. Other triggering drugs include, but are not limited to, phenytoin, barbiturates, aspirin, allopurinol, nonsteroidal anti-inflammatory drugs (NSAIDs), oral antidiabetics, and codeine, furosemide, and protease inhibitors. However, in 50 percent of the cases, a trigger cannot be identified.

As the name *multiforme* implies, a variety of lesions develop in EM. The classic lesions are "target" skin lesions on the arms and legs, occasionally the trunk and face. They appear slightly elevated with concentric erythematous rings less than 3 cm in diameter, often with an ulcer in the center (Fig. 4-21). Target lesions do not occur in the mouth. Oral lesions tend to favor nonkeratinized, non-bound mucosa and begin as erythematous patches that eventually break down to form shallow ulcerations that may involve large areas (Figs. 4-22, 4-23, and 4-24). The lips develop a hemorrhagic-crusted appearance. Some lesions resolve within days, but often lesions take 2 to 5 weeks to fully resolve, during which time the patient experiences severe oral discomfort and risks dehydration due to pain when eating or drinking. Treatment involves supportive and palliative therapy. Discontinuation of the trigger drug is indicated. Avoidance of the trigger helps prevent future outbreaks. A severe form of EM is *Stevens-Johnson syndrome*, also called *erythema multiforme major*. In addition to the skin and oral lesions), patients develop eye and genital lesions (Figs. 4-25 and 4-26). Patients are at risk for blindness if the condition is left untreated. Severe dehydration is also a risk.

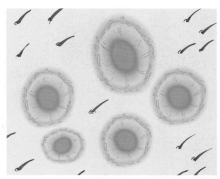

Figure 4–21 **Erythema multiforme.** Cluster of erythematous round "target" lesions on the skin.

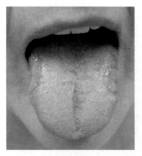

Figure 4–22 **Erythema multiforme.** Painful shallow ulcerations of the lateral tongue. (From Barankin, B: Derm Notes. F.A. Davis, Philadelphia, 2006, p 88.)

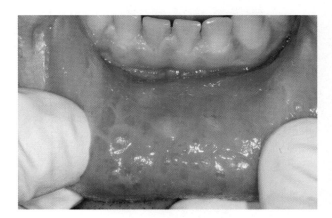

Figure 4–23 **Erythema multiforme.** Painful ulceration of the gingiva and labial mucosa.

Clinical Implications

If a patient with EM reports herpes simplex as their trigger, use of systemic antiviral medication may help prevent herpes outbreaks and hence recurrence of EM.

Lichen Planus

Lichen planus is a common disease of both the skin or mucous membranes or both. Its name is derived from the appearance of the *reticular form* of the disorder that resembles lichens that grow on rocks and trees (Fig. 4-27A and B). Despite its name, it is not related to parasitic or fungal organisms, nor is it infectious or contagious. It is most commonly seen in middle-aged women, but men comprise a large portion of patients.

The etiology of lichen planus is still under investigation. We do know that cytotoxic T-cells (discussed earlier in this chapter) are produced by the host and recognize, as yet undetermined, proteins in the basal layer of stratified squamous epithelium as "foreign."

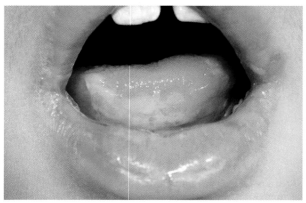

Figure 4–24 Erythema multiforme. Extensive ulceration of lip and tongue.

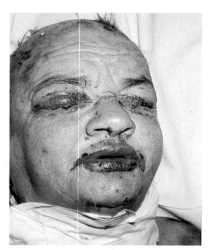

Stevens-Johnson syndrome

Figure 4–25 Stevens-Johnson syndrome. Extensive painful sloughing mucositis following administration of antibiotics. (From Taber's Cyclopedic Medical Dictionary, ed. 21. F.A. Davis, Philadelphia, 2009, p 228.)

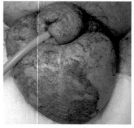

Figure 4–26 Stevens-Johnson syndrome. Genital ulcers. (From Barankin, B: Derm Notes. F.A. Davis, Philadelphia, 2006, p 153.)

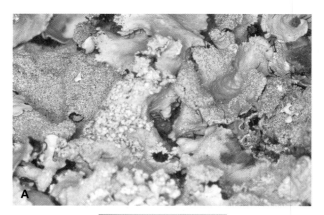

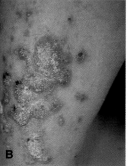

Figure 4–27 Where lichen planus gets its name. **A.** Lichens on rock or tree. **B.** Skin lesions of lichen planus resemble plant lichens. (From Barankin, B: Derm Notes. F.A. Davis, Philadelphia, 2006, p 18.)

These T-cells produce cytokines that are toxic to the basal epithelium and destroy it. Treatment of symptomatic lichen planus involves drugs that suppress T-cells or neutralize their ability to produce these cytokines.

There are three forms of lichen planus that vary in both clinical features and treatment.

Reticular/Papular Lichen Planus

Reticular/papular lichen planus can occur on the skin or mucous membranes. Skin (cutaneous) lesions occur mainly on the extremities as clusters of purple polygonal pruritic papules (called the "4-P's of lichen planus") that may become slightly raised and confluent, forming *plaques* when the patient begins to scratch them (Fig. 4-28). Close observation of oral lesions reveals the hallmark of lichen planus called *Wickham's striae*, which are fine, white, spider-web or lace-like lines on the surface of the plaques. The fingernails also may be involved with a hyperplastic, wrinkled, dry, fragile appearance, called *onconychia*, which may resemble a fungal infection of the nail (Fig. 4-29).

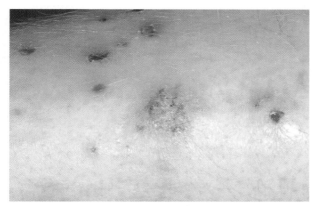

Figure 4–28   Lichen planus. Purple, polygonal, pruritic plaques with overlying Wickham's striae.

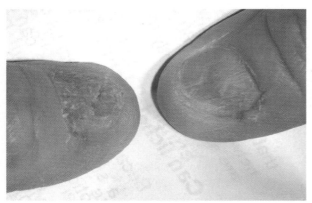

Figure 4–29   Lichen planus. Lichen planus affecting the nails.

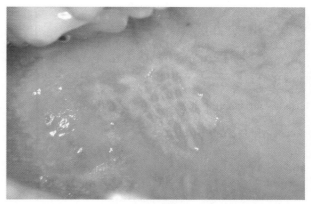

Figure 4–30   Lichen planus. Wickham striae of the buccal mucosa.

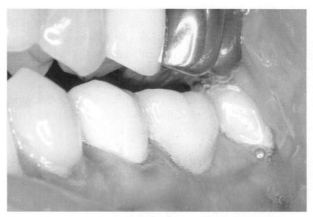

Figure 4–31   Lichen planus. Plaque-like lesions of the attached gingiva.

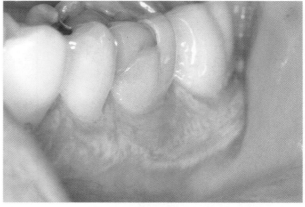

Figure 4–32   Lichen planus. Dried tissue shows Wickham striae in detail.

Intraorally, lesions do not take on the purple color or become pruritic as occurs on the skin. Rather, they appear as Wickham's striae, commonly observed on the buccal mucosa (Fig. 4-30), lateral tongue, and gingiva (Fig. 4-31). Often, small papules appear at the intersection of the white striae. Also, central areas of what appears to be irregular plaque-like hyperkeratosis may occur. Fine striae may be apparent under close observation at the periphery of the lesion. Drying the area with gauze or air often helps in observing striae (Fig. 4-32).

Despite widespread lesions, patients with oral reticular lichen planus remain asymptomatic. A biopsy is necessary to confirm the diagnosis, as other white oral lesions may mimic lichen planus. Biopsy will show an abundance of T-lymphocytes at the junction of the epithelial-connective tissue interface in a linear pattern. Many basal cells show destruction; others appear vacuolated; and some remain normal in appearance. Once the diagnosis is established, the only management is close follow-up for any changes over time. Patients with reticular lichen planus do not tend to progress to the more severe forms, but tend to regress and remit over several years. Treatment with systemic immunosuppressive medications may produce undesirable side effects detrimental to the patient's oral health.

Atrophic Lichen Planus

Atrophic lichen planus is recognized by mucosal thinning and erythema with evidence of Wickham's striae at the periphery of the lesion (Fig. 4-33). Patients complain of pain and tenderness, especially when eating spicy foods or strong mints. Despite the pain, the mucosa remains intact. The gingiva, lateral tongue, and buccal mucosa are the most common areas affected.

Atrophic lichen planus may be confined to the gingiva, where it is often mistaken for recalcitrant gingivitis that does not respond to routine nonsurgical periodontal therapy, including chlorhexidine gluconate rinses. A biopsy is needed to establish the diagnosis because other conditions may mimic atrophic lichen planus and not respond to lichen planus treatment. Because the lesions are symptomatic, treatment with topical immunosuppressive and anti-inflammatory medications may be necessary.

Erosive Lichen Planus

Erosive lichen planus is the least common but most severe form of lichen planus and the most frequent source of complaints by patients who have this disorder. Patients often present to the dental office with painful gingiva, lateral tongue, or buccal mucosa that intensifies when eating even bland foods; eating spicy hot foods is often impossible. Patients often mistakenly believe that spicy foods cause their condition, but avoiding them brings little relief. Lesions of erosive lichen planus present with painful shallow ulcers with red and white borders characterized by peripheral striae (Fig. 4-34A). Details of erosions are seen in Figure 4-34B. Biopsy will identify features similar to other forms of lichen planus, but clinically, large zones of epithelium will be eroded or ulcerated with exposure of underlying connective tissue, a process that is responsible for the intense pain experienced by the patient. Loss of surface epithelium and intense pain may be produced by other conditions, so a biopsy is needed to confirm the diagnosis.

Once a diagnosis of erosive lichen planus is established, the patient may require systemic anti-inflammatory or immunosuppressive medications to relieve the lesions. Topical medications are often not potent enough to lead to re-epithelialization. However, once re-epithelialization has occurred, topical medications may be adequate for maintenance.

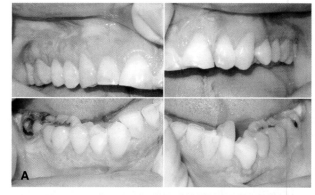

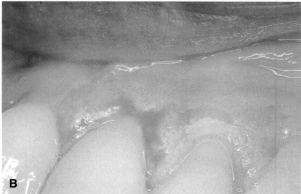

Figure 4–34 **A.** Erosive LP gingiva, tongue, and buccal mucosae. A patient with extensive erosive lichen planus involving most mucosal surfaces. **B.** Close-up of erosive lesion of gingiva.

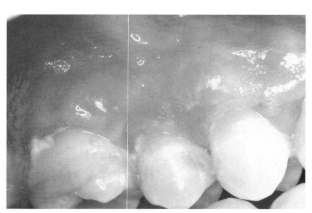

Figure 4–33 **Atrophic lichen planus.** Painful atrophy of gingiva makes brushing difficult.

Lichenoid Mucositis

Many conditions in the oral cavity mimic lichen planus and can fool even an experienced clinician. When a lesion looks like lichen planus, but is caused by something other than an autoimmune disease, it is termed lichenoid mucositis. The suffix **-oid** means "resembles but is not . . ."—in this case, lichen planus. Lichenoid mucositis has several causes, the most common of which is a reaction to a medication or topical agent used in the mouth. Most types of reactions are allergic. Dental amalgams and cinnamon aldehyde previously discussed can develop a lichenoid appearance and therefore fall into the category of lichenoid mucositis.

Lichenoid lesions may resemble any type of lichen planus from reticular to erosive. When a patient presents with a lichenoid lesion, before assuming it is lichen planus, one should:

1. Examine the mouth for dental restorative material in direct contact with the lesion.
2. Obtain an updated medical and drug history. Many drugs have been associated with lichenoid mucositis, including over-the-counter medications and herbal products. Figure 4-35 shows a lichenoid reaction in a patient who had been taking several over-the-counter herbal supplements from the health food store, one of which he was allergic to.
3. If a suspected agent is identified, remove it, if possible. If the lesion regresses, then it most likely was a reaction to the agent. Note that many agents cannot be eliminated, such as essential medications and complex dental restorations.
4. Biopsy the lesion if no suspected agent is found or cannot be removed. If the lesion is allergic, cells

of a hypersensitivity reaction, which differ from the cells seen in lichen planus, will be identified histologically.

These steps help prevent unnecessary treatment for lichen planus in patients who do not actually have the condition.

Desquamative Gingivitis Associated With Autoimmune Vesiculobullous or Vesiculoerosive Disorders

Desquamative gingivitis is a clinical descriptive term rather than a pathologic diagnosis. It describes recalcitrant gingivitis caused by autoantibodies. Patients suffer with erythematous, painful gingiva that appear to slough or "peel" away. This most frequently affects female patients later in life, but males are not excluded. Desquamative gingivitis fails to respond to enhanced oral hygiene or conventional nonsurgical periodontal therapy because it is not caused by periodontal pathogens found in plaque. It is actually a group of separate diseases of altered immunity and autoimmunity referred to as either *vesiculobullous disorders* or *vesiculoerosive disorders*. In each disorder, epithelial cells are destroyed, leaving spaces that fill with tissue fluid, forming small (< 0.5 cm) blisters called *vesicles* or larger (> 0.5 cm) blisters called *bullae* (single = bulla); hence, the term *vesiculobullous*. Clinically, the blisters rupture in a short time, leaving erosions or ulcerations; hence, the term *vesiculoerosive* (Fig. 4-36A, B, C, and D). Each disorder may present with similar signs and symptoms, which makes them difficult to distinguish from each other. A biopsy is essential to determine the correct diagnosis so that proper therapy can be instituted.

In addition to erosive lichen planus, discussed previously, the following autoimmune disorders may produce the clinical presentation of desquamative gingivitis.

Mucous Membrane Pemphigoid

Mucous membrane pemphigoid (MMP) is a type 2 hypersensitivity reaction to specific hemidesmosomal proteins in the basement membrane of the epithelium called *laminins*. Autoantibodies produced by plasma cells destroy this hemidesmosomal "glue" that holds the epithelium to the underlying connective tissue. Biopsy of mucous membrane pemphigoid shows a split between the full thickness of epithelium and the underlying connective tissue. Connective tissue and nerves are exposed to the oral environment, resulting in significant pain for the patient.

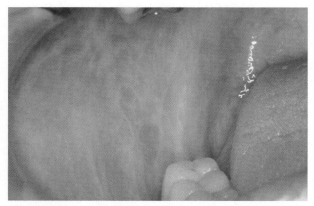

Figure 4–35 Lichenoid mucositis. Patient on over-the-counter herbal medications for memory loss shows reticular lichen planus-like Wickham striae.

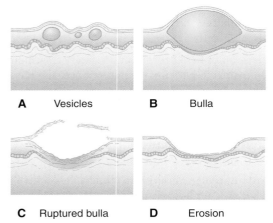

A Vesicles   **B** Bulla

C Ruptured bulla   **D** Erosion

Figure 4–36   Vesiculoerosive disease development. **A**. Tiny vesicles develop on surface of gingiva. **B**. They coalesce to form a bulla filled with fluid. **C**. The bulla ruptures and the epithelium is lost. **D**. Gingiva left behind has little or no protection, which lead to pain.

Clinically, MMP differs from lichen planus in that the MMP lesions are most frequently preceded by the formation of a vesicle or bulla that ruptures and leaves denuded painful mucosa (Fig. 4-37A and B). Sometimes the vesicles are small or occur during sleep so the patient is unaware of them. Mild trauma may induce vesicle and bulla formation, leading to sloughing of the tissue, a phenomenon referred to as **Nikolsky's sign** (Fig. 4-38). A ruptured blister leaves a shallow, mildly tender ulcer bed, which heals in 7 to 10 days. Continuous minor trauma, such as from tooth brushing or eating crispy foods, may dislodge epithelium from the underlying connective tissue. Consequently, patients may modify their diet towards softer foods and decrease oral hygiene home care due to the pain and desquamation. Topical steroid treatment is helpful in the management of mild cases, while systemic corticosteroid therapy may be indicated in more severe cases.

Clinical Implications

MMP does not directly cause periodontitis; however, poor oral hygiene that results from inability to perform proper home care may predispose the patient to periodontal disease.

Other forms of pemphigoid affect the skin and eyes. *Bullous pemphigoid* occurs mainly on the skin, though it can occur intraorally. It is characterized by large bullae that rupture to leave hemorrhagic-crusted lesions that heal

without scarring. *Cicatricial* (pronounced sick-a-TRISH-al) (cicatrix = scar) *pemphigoid* can affect skin or mucous membranes, but is particularly severe when it affects the conjunctiva of the eyes. Severe inflammation resolves with scarring, a condition called *symblepharon* (Fig. 4-39A, B, and C), which eventually leads to blindness. Fortunately, this is a rare occurrence since the advent of improved treatments. Large or secondarily infected intraoral lesions may result in scar formation, but this phenomenon is much less severe in the mouth than the eyes.

Clinical Implications

Patients diagnosed with MMP based on oral biopsy must be referred to an ophthalmologist for an eye exam.

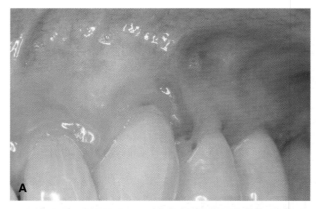

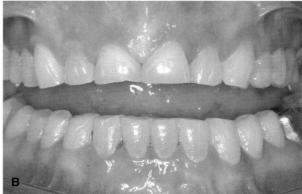

Figure 4–37   Mucous membrane pemphigoid. A. Vesicle formation **B.** Painful sloughing lesions of the oral mucosa.

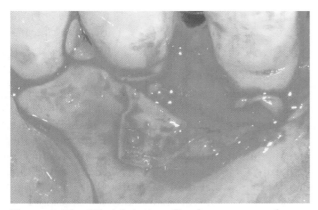

Figure 4–38   Nikolsky's sign. Gentle pressure produces a blister that immediately breaks. This is due to destruction of the basement membrane zone.

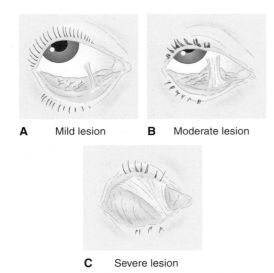

A   Mild lesion   **B**   Moderate lesion

C   Severe lesion

Figure 4–39   Symblepharon. Painful eye lesions that lead to progressive scarring and eventual blindness if left untreated.

Pemphigus Vulgaris

The term *pemphigus* refers to a group of autoimmune blistering diseases of the skin and mucous membranes. The most common form, *pemphigus vulgaris*, is a potentially life-threatening mucocutaneous (both skin and mucous membranes) disorder that often manifests initially in the oral cavity. Pemphigus is derived from the Greek word *pemphix*, meaning bubble or blister. Autoantibodies are produced against proteins called *desmogleins*, which form the desmosomes, the structural units that bind epithelial cells to each other. When the autoantibodies

attack the desmosomes, individual epithelial cells lose the ability to adhere to each other. Hemidesmosomes are not affected. Biopsy of pemphigus vulgaris shows a split in the epithelium above the basal layer. Individual keratinocytes, referred to as *Tzanck cells*, appear to be floating away from each other, providing evidence that the desmosomes have been destroyed. Mild trauma to the area may induce vesicle and bulla formation, leading to tissue sloughing similar to the Nikolsky's sign seen in mucous membrane pemphigoid (Fig. 4-40).

More than 50 percent of patients with pemphigus vulgaris have oral lesions before they develop skin lesions. Oral lesions may affect any anatomic surface, but tend to appear on the buccal mucosa, palate, and gingiva. Patients generally are unaware of the vesicles due to their small size and ease of rupture, but are aware of the ulcerations and erosions (Fig. 4-41). When lesions develop on the gingiva, the term *desquamative gingivitis* is appropriate (Fig. 4-42). However, unlike erosive lichen planus and mucous membrane pemphigoid, pemphigus vulgaris rarely involves the gingiva without involving other oral mucosal surfaces as well. Therefore, examination of the oral cavity often reveals additional erosive, desquamative lesions that follow no consistent pattern. Blistering and erosions secondary to the rupture of blisters may be painful and may limit the patient's daily activities. Patients typically heal without scarring unless the disease is complicated by severe secondary infection

Ocular involvement leads to conjunctivitis, but scarring rarely occurs as in MMP. Skin lesions appear as bullae that rupture to leave large denuded areas that lack epithelium for protection. Before the introduction of effective pemphigus therapy, patients were at risk

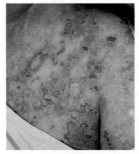

Figure 4–40   Pemphigus vulgaris. Painful blistering lesions of the skin. (From Barankin, B: Derm Notes. F.A. Davis, Philadelphia, 2006, p 128.)

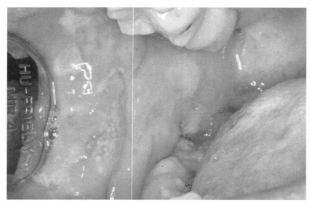

Figure 4-41 Pemphigus vulgaris. Painful blistering lesions of the oral mucosa.

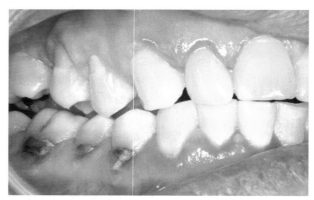

Figure 4-42 Pemphigus vulgaris. Desquamative lesions of the gingiva in a patient with pemphigus.

for sepsis and death due to loss of significant amounts of skin, similar to victims of severe burns.

Linear IgA disease

Linear IgA disease can cause widespread damage to the skin and mucous membranes, similar to that seen in pemphigus. It may affect the eyes and lead to blindness, much like cicatricial pemphigoid, and intraoral lesions heal with scarring. Linear IgA disease, as its name suggests, is characterized by deposits of autoantibodies of the IgA class along the epithelial-connective tissue junction, causing loss of adhesion, which results in vesicle and bullae formation. Like pemphigus vulgaris, patients may develop large areas of skin loss. Unlike others in this group of diseases, there has been some association with administration of medications prior to the onset of the disease. Because linear IgA disease shares several features with other

autoimmune blistering diseases, a biopsy must confirm the diagnosis. Patients are closely followed by a dermatologist with systemic immunomodulary therapy.

Chronic Ulcerative Stomatitis

Chronic ulcerative stomatitis (CUS) occurs when autoantibodies attack the nuclei of oral epithelial cells of the basal and lower spinous layers. Extraoral lesions are rare. Gingiva, buccal mucosa, and the tongue are the most common surfaces affected (Fig. 4-43A and B). Clinically, CUS resembles erosive lichen planus. The first indication that the patient has CUS rather than erosive lichen planus is when lesions fail to respond to standard erosive lichen planus therapy (topical corticosteroids). Therefore, CUS cannot be distinguished without a biopsy. Plaquenil taken systemically has been shown to be an effective treatment.

Clinical Implications

Although specific treatment for autoimmune vesiculobullous disorders will vary depending on the specific diagnosis, most treatment involves use of topical corticosteroids or other immunomodulary agents during some phase of treatment. For patients whose lesions are confined to the gingiva, fabrication of medication carriers, similar to custom fluoride trays, are helpful in delivering the medication directly to the gingiva. These carriers help improve compliance and also reduce the amount of mediation required (Fig. 4-44).

Although topical immunosuppressive therapy is the mainstay for many of these conditions, they have side effects, such as promoting intraoral growth of *Candida albicans*. Patients should be instructed to use topical medications sparingly to help reduce these side effects.

Clinical Implications

If a patient being treated with topical corticosteroids reports that their symptoms have worsened despite compliance to their medication regimen, he or she may be experiencing the symptoms of candidiasis. An oral cytological smear is helpful in making this diagnosis. Individuals who test positive for candida should be placed on antifungal therapy. Dramatic improvement in symptoms often results.

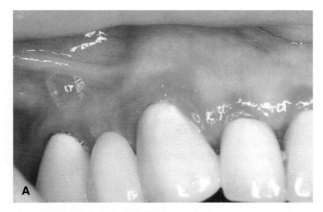

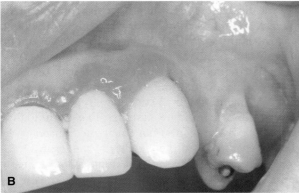

Figure 4–43 **Chronic ulcerative stomatitis**. **A** and **B**. Chronic desquamative lesions of the gingiva that did not respond to nonsurgical treatment or topical corticosteroids.

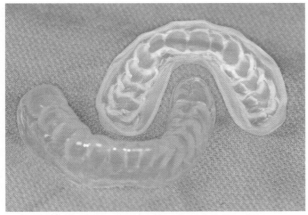

Figure 4–44 **Treatment of desquamative gingivitis**. Custom fabricated medication carriers can be very helpful when vesiculoerosive disease lesions are confined to the gingiva.

Orofacial Manifestations of Systemic Immunodysregulation

Systemic immunodysregulation occurs when the immune system mistakenly attacks and destroys healthy body tissue. Effects can be seen in any organ or organ system in the body. A defect in any arm of the immune system may trigger immunodysregulation. Pathogens, drugs, hormones, and toxins are just a few ways that the environment may trigger dysregulation. Patients suffering from one of the forms of immunodysregulation may have their initial diagnosis missed because signs and symptoms may be vague or overlap with other disorders. Fever, muscle ache, fatigue, joint pain and other constitutional symptoms may be present. Here we will discuss the intraoral and extraoral manifestations seen in some disorders of the immune system.

Hives

Hives, also referred to as *urticaria*, is a type 1 hypersensitivity reaction that is produced by histamine and other compounds released from mast cells. Histamine causes fluid to leak from the local blood vessels, leading to swelling (edema) in the skin. Hives appears as a cluster of circular, red, spongiotic lesions called "wheals," surrounded by areas of erythema called "flares." Hives may appear on any skin surface, but usually spares the palms of the hands and soles of the feet. Hives can vary in size from a few millimeters to involvement of an entire extremity (Fig. 4-45). Lesions tend to change size and move around, disappearing and reappearing in a matter of hours. An outbreak that looks severe may appear during the day and be gone hours later, only to reappear later the same day.

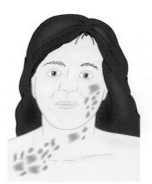
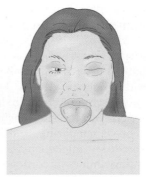

Patient with hives   Patient with angioedema

Figure 4–45 Comparison of clinical features of hives versus angioedema.

There are three classes of hives: 1) idiopathic; 2) immunologic associated with release of histamine in response to an allergen, such as foods and medications; and 3) non-immunologic associated with release of histamine in response to stress or underlying disease with no exposure to an allergen. The most commonly used treatments are oral antihistamines. Oral steroids can help severe cases of hives in the short term but should not be used long term. Topical anti-pruritic and anesthetic agents such as camphor, menthol, and diphenhydramine applied to the skin may provide symptomatic relief.

Clinical Implications

An outbreak of hives in the dental office is more typically associated with the stress of the dental appointment rather than allergy to dental materials.

Angioedema

Angioedema is typically characterized by edema of the facial soft tissues rather than a wheal-and-flare reaction as seen in hives (Fig. 4-45). Edema causes enlargement of the lips and larynx, which leads to hoarseness or shortness of breath. Angioedema can occur as a type I hypersensitivity reaction associated with histamine release or in certain individuals who take angiotensin-converting-enzyme (ACE) inhibitors for control of hypertension. The tendency to develop angioedema may be hereditary or acquired. The hereditary form is associated with lack of or defect in C1 esterase, an important protein in the complement pathway. The acquired form is associated with neoplastic diseases, such as lymphoma, that affect the cells of the immune system. In both forms, anti-C1 esterase antibodies destroy C1 esterase. Without C1 esterase, the resulting complement cascade results in angioedema.

Most patients with mild acute angioedema may be treated similarly to those with an allergic reaction. Mild, limited urticaria is self-limiting, typically disappearing within hours to days, and does not need to be treated. Severe symptoms require immediate medical attention. Emergency measures include use of steroids, subcutaneous epinephrine, and antihistamines. Conversely, hereditary angioedema generally does not respond to antihistamines or corticosteroids, and anabolic steroids may be used for the acute phase of an attack. C1 esterase inhibitor is now available for use in this type of emergency. Transfusions of fresh frozen plasma have been shown to decrease recurring angioedema.

Clinical Implications

The stress of a dental appointment may precipitate angioedema. If the larynx becomes involved, emergency medical attention is essential.

Bone Marrow Transplant Rejection and Graft-Versus-Host Disease

When a patient has a disease of the bone marrow, a bone marrow transplant may be performed in an attempt to save the patient's life. In transplant terminology, the ill recipient of the new bone marrow is referred the *host*, and the healthy donor who supplies the bone marrow is the *graft* (Fig. 4-46A). To receive a bone marrow transplant, the recipient's (host's) own diseased bone marrow is destroyed and replaced with the bone marrow of the donor (graft). The result is that the cells of the recipient's immune system are replaced by cells of the donor's immune system. Two pathological processes may be seen in bone marrow transplant recipients that threaten the viability of the graft. Occasionally, the recipient rejects the donor's bone marrow and the transplant fails. This is referred to as host-versus-graft, or simply *rejection* (Fig. 4-46B).

Another scenario is called graft-versus-host disease (GVHD). It occurs when the recipient's body accepts the new bone marrow, but the donor bone marrow sees the host as foreign. The patient's new immune system may be unable to recognize his or her own tissue. In other words, the new bone marrow cells may "see" the host's own cells and tissues as foreign and attempt to reject and destroy them (Fig. 4-46C).

After a bone marrow transplant, the recipient is given immunosuppressive drugs that attempt to prevent these processes of rejection.

Acute GVHD occurs within approximately 100 days of the transplant and is characterized by a skin rash similar to erythema multiforme, GI symptoms, and liver dysfunction. Chronic GVHD occurs months or years post-transplant and has a more varied presentation. Skin and mucous membrane involvement commonly affects the head, neck, and oral cavity. Symptoms are not unlike those of erosive lichen planus. Patients experience pain and burning of the tongue, buccal mucosa, and labial mucosa accompanied by mucosal atrophy. Tissue may slough, making hydration and proper nutrition challenging. Secondary candidiasis may become a problem, so testing for fungal infection is necessary. If the salivary glands are

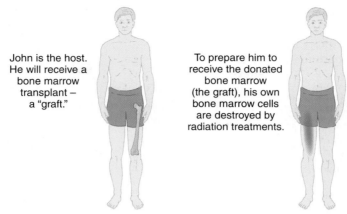

Figure 4–46A **Bone marrow donation**. The host receives the graft.

Rejection of Donated Cells: Host vs. Graft

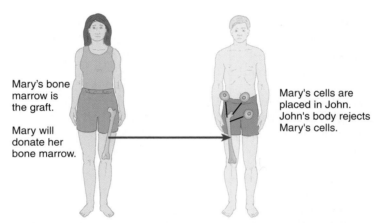

Figure 4–46B **Types of bone marrow transplant rejection**. Host versus graft, or "rejection."

Rejection of New Body: Graft vs. Host Disease

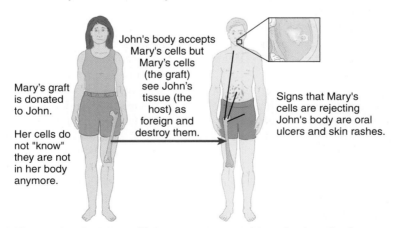

Figure 4–46C **Types of bone marrow transplant rejection**. Graft-versus-host disease.

affected, the patient will develop xerostomia that exacerbates oral discomfort and leads to rampant caries. Most transplant patients experience some degree of GVHD but do well with appropriate treatment.

Clinical Implications

When bone marrow transplant recipients present with oral pain and tenderness, they should be examined for candidiasis. If symptoms persist, referral to the physician for GVHD assessment is essential.

Systemic Lupus Erythematosus

Systemic lupus erythematosus (SLE) is a multisystem disease in which patients develop autoantibodies against proteins within the nucleus of their cells (anti-nuclear antibodies or ANAs). Detection of the *anti-Sm (Smith)* ANA is the most specific test for the diagnosis of SLE. Additional skin and blood tests are used with clinical evaluation of signs and symptoms to confirm the diagnosis.

SLE is a complex disease with many features that may not be present in all patients. A characteristic skin presentation, the "butterfly rash," is often present on the face of a patient with SLE. The "butterfly rash" is a photosensitive erythematous **dermatitis** that covers the bridge of the nose and extends bilaterally onto the cheeks, resembling the shape of a butterfly. The most serious problems associated with SLE involve the kidney and heart. About half of all SLE patients develop *proteinuria*, followed by nephrotic syndrome in which tiny blood vessels in the kidney become leaky, allowing protein to leave the body in large amounts. Patients may go on to develop end-stage renal failure. Other patients develop damage to the heart valves that may predispose the patient to bacterial endocarditis, which can have life-threatening consequences. Most patients suffer from arthritis and myalgia.

Chronic cutaneous lupus (CCL) is a milder form of lupus that presents with no systemic life-threatening symptoms. CCL dermatitis is characterized by multiple scaly patches surrounded by an erythematous halo termed *discoid lupus erythematosus* (Figs. 4-47 and 4-48). Some patients with SLE also develop discoid lupus, but not all patients with discoid lupus develop SLE. In light-skinned individuals, the patches tend to become hyperpigmented. In dark-skinned individuals, the patches tend to become hypopigmented. Sunlight exacerbates the lesions, so the patient should

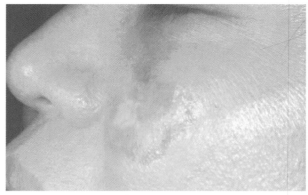

Figure 4–47   Discoid lupus. Skin lesions of patient diagnosed with chronic localized lupus of the skin.

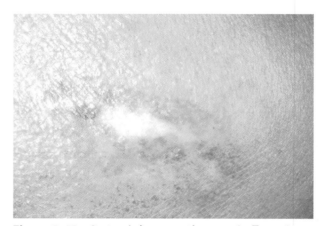

Figure 4–48   Systemic lupus erythematosis. Extensive facial lesions showing loss of pigment with surrounding erythema in a patient with systemic lupus erythematosus.

be advised to use sunscreen and avoid prolonged outdoor exposure.

Oral manifestations of both SLE and discoid lupus develop in less than half of all patients but can be recognized in the dental office. In general, patients with SLE present with signs and symptoms similar to erosive lichen planus (Fig. 4-49). Occasionally, white plaques or erosive areas with a finely speckled keratotic rim rather than Wickham's striae are seen on the buccal mucosa. Desquamative gingivitis may also develop (Table 4-4). Patients with SLE and oral lesions must receive medical attention to resolve their lesions. Patients with discoid lupus in the oral cavity may respond to topical corticosteroids or other immunomodulary drugs, such as tacrolimus.

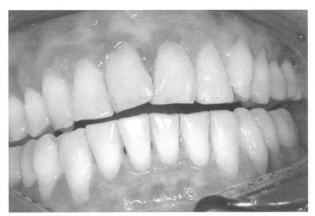

Figure 4–49   Discoid lupus. Painful desquamative lesions of discoid lupus resembling erosive lichen planus.

Granulomatous Diseases

Granulomatous inflammation is a very specific type of inflammation characterized histologically by the presence of granulomas, which are masses of epithelioid histiocytes containing numerous multinucleated giant cells supported by a fibrous matrix. These granulomas replace normal tissues and form irregular firm swellings. Granulomatous inflammation is a response to a number of specific conditions, such as foreign body reactions (see Chapter 2); infections, including tuberculosis, histoplasmosis, and blastomycosis (see Chapter 3); and various autoimmune disorders, as discussed here. Special microscopic techniques and stains can detect foreign bodies, tuberculosis bacilli, and fungal organisms. When these tests are negative, the diagnosis of one of the following immune-based granulomatous disorders should be considered.

Sarcoidosis

Sarcoidosis is a complex multisystem granulomatous disorder of unknown etiology for which the antigenic stimulus has yet to be identified. It is likely that several different antigens are responsible, which affect patients who have a genetic predisposition for development of the disease. Sarcoidosis can be life-threatening if it affects vital organs and is left undiagnosed. The diagnosis of sarcoidosis is often made from a lymph node biopsy. Patients experience an increase in serum or urinary calcium, which can be accompanied by muscle pain and weakness. Sarcoidosis primarily affects two groups of adults: those aged 20-40 and those older than age 60. Because it is a multisystem disease, clinical signs and symptoms are numerous and vary from patient to patient (Fig. 4-50). Signs of sarcoidosis that may be observed in the dental office include *lupus pernio*, a cluster of indurated, violaceous (purple) exophytic lesions of the skin, especially on the skin of the face (Fig. 4-51). Uveitis and conjunctivitis may be seen in the eyes, along with loss of lacrimal gland function, causing *xerophthalmia* (dry eyes).

Table 4.4	Diseases Associated With Desquamative Gingivitis		
Disease	**Classic Intraoral Features**	**Extraoral Signs**	**Target of Autoantibodies***
Erosive lichen planus	Wickham's striae at border of ulcer or erosion	Purple polygonal pruritic plaques on skin of extremities	*Target of T-cells is basal cells
Mucous membrane pemphigoid	Vesicles that rupture; Positive Nikolsky's sign	Symblepharon; Tense bullae on skin	Hemidesmosomes
Pemphigus vulgaris	Additional intraoral sites, rarely gingiva alone; Positive Nikolsky's sign	Flaccid bullae on skin	Desmosomes
Linear IgA disease	Lesions heal with scarring; Occasional "blood" blisters	Erosive skin lesions	Basement membrane zone
Chronic ulcerative stomatitis	Similar to erosive lichen planus but does not respond to steroids; No Nikolsky's sign	Rare	Nuclei of basal and lower spinous cells
Discoid lupus	White plaques with papular rimming	Scaly skin patches; "butterfly rash"; altered pigmentation	Basement membrane zone

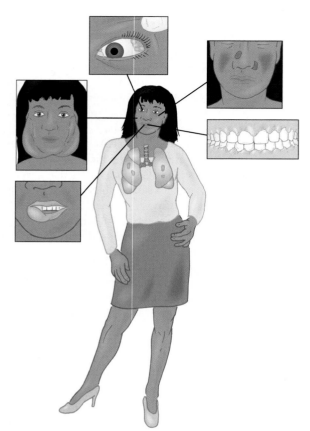

Figure 4–50   Multi-system involvement in sarcoidosis.
Clockwise: Swelling of the lips; swelling of the salivary glands; swelling of the lacrimal glands; violaceous skin lesions of the face; gingival enlargement.

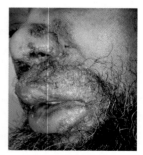

Figure 4–51   Sarcoidosis. Cutaneous red to brown plaques of the face. (From Barankin, B: Derm Notes. F.A. Davis, Philadelphia, 2006, p 141.)

When paratracheal lymph nodes along the trachea in the neck are affected, the patient may present with hoarseness or a change in voice quality.

Intraoral lesions are rare and vary widely in appearance, from discrete papules to hyperkeratotic plaques (Fig. 4-52). If granulomatous inflammation destroys

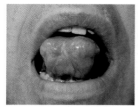

Figure 4–52   Sarcoidosis. Indurated mucosal swelling of the tongue characteristic of granulomatous inflammation of sarcoidosis. (From Barankin, B: Derm Notes. F.A. Davis, Philadelphia, 2006, p 141.)

the salivary glands, the patient will develop xerostomia along with enlargement of the glands as the granulomas increase in size. The combination of sarcoidosis of the salivary glands, uveitis, and facial nerve paralysis is termed *Heerfordt's syndrome*. Lesions may also develop within the bone where they appear as diffuse non-expansile radiolucencies. Treatment includes systemic corticosteroid or other immunomodulary therapy.

Crohn's Disease

Crohn's disease is a chronic autoimmune granulomatous disease of the gastrointestinal (GI) tract, including the mouth, with an uncertain etiology. It primarily affects teenagers and middle-aged adults. Evidence of a hereditary component to Crohn's disease exists, though many patients have no relatives with the disorder. It is also known as *regional enteritis* because it alternately affects and skips some portions of the GI tract, from the mouth to the anus, causing swelling and ulceration that leads to abdominal pain, diarrhea, nausea, and weight loss.

Oral signs and symptoms include diffuse nodular swellings that produce a "cobblestone" appearance (Fig. 4-53) of the buccal mucosa and nonpainful swelling of the lips. Deep ulcers affect the colon and may also be seen intraorally in the form of painful major aphthous ulcers (Fig. 4-54). Some of these ulcerations present with raised rolled borders and develop along linear folds in the buccal and labial vestibules. Crohn's disease has no cure, but symptoms can be controlled using appropriate systemic anti-inflammatory and immunomodulary therapy. Tumor necrosis factor alpha (TNFα) is one crucial mediator involved in this abnormal immune response, and biological therapies targeting TNFα, including infliximab, have significantly improved the management of Crohn's disease.

Clinical Implications

Crohn's disease should be considered when a young patient presents with major aphthous ulcers. Oral ulcers may develop before GI symptoms appear.

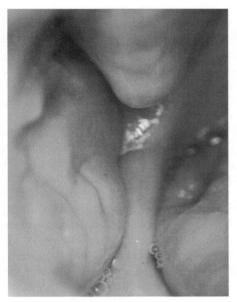

Figure 4–53 Crohn's disease. Cobblestone appearance of the buccal mucosa in a patient with Crohn's disease.

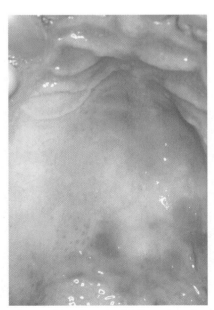

Figure 4–54 Crohn's disease. Diffuse chronic major aphthous ulcers of the palate in a patient with Crohn's disease.

Orofacial Granulomatosis

Orofacial granulomatosis (OFG) can affect any oral tissue, but most frequently involves the lips, which demonstrate sudden onset of unilateral or bilateral nonpainful enlargement called *cheilitis granulomatosum.* (Fig. 4-55). Swelling often remits and recurs, with each episode lasting weeks or months. Eventually, lip enlargement becomes permanent, leaving the lips with a firm or rubbery texture. *Melkerson-Rosenthal syndrome* is an unusual related condition that has as its main features cheilitis granulomatosum, facial nerve paralysis, and fissured tongue.

Linear hyperplastic folds that resemble epulis fissuratum (see Chapter 2) may develop in the buccal and labial vestibules of patients with OFG, despite the fact that the patient does not have dentures. These exophytic, hyperplastic folds of tissue may develop ulcers that are mistaken for RAUs. These are clinically indistinguishable from orofacial Crohn's disease and sarcoidosis, so additional diagnostic testing is necessary. Recent studies have shown that up to 60 percent of children with OFG have subclinical signs of Crohn's disease.

Occasionally, the etiology of OFG can be identified. Cinnamon aldehyde and benzoate preservatives have been implicated as triggers of OFG. Avoidance of suspected triggers often brings relief. When the etiology of OFG cannot readily be identified, cortisone is the most common therapy. Surgery may be required for severe permanent swelling that interferes with esthetics or oral functioning. Spontaneous remission may occur but is rare.

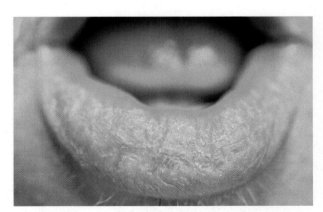

Figure 4–55 Cheilitis granulomatosum. Diffuse firm enlargement of the lips in a patient with no history of Crohn's disease, sarcoidosis, or other chronic granulomatous disease.

Systemic Sclerosis (Scleroderma)

Systemic sclerosis (scleroderma) is a chronic systemic autoimmune disease characterized by autoantibodies that destroy endothelial and smooth muscle cells that line arterioles, replacing them with excess collagen (fibrosis). One of the first signs of scleroderma is *Raynaud's phenomenon*, which features pain of the extremities caused by vasoconstriction that results from fibrosis. Eventually, circumscribed or diffuse areas of hard, smooth, immobile tissue develop.

The disease occurs in diffuse systemic and localized forms. *Diffuse systemic sclerosis/scleroderma* is a rapidly progressive and disabling form that affects a large area of the skin and one or more internal organs, frequently the kidneys, esophagus, heart, and/or lungs. Clinical features include contraction of fingers and hands, ulcerations due to vascular changes, widening of the periodontal ligament space, and inability to open the mouth (Fig. 4-56). In the mandible, pressure exerted by the progressive tightening of overlying skin causes pressure resorption of the underlying bone. Radiographs may show atrophy of the angles of the mandible. Prognosis is guarded for diffuse disease, particularly in older patients. Death occurs most often from pulmonary, heart, and kidney complications.

Localized scleroderma typically affects only isolated areas of skin, causing contraction that resembles large scars, termed "coup de sabre" (cut of the sword). Organ systems are not involved, so the disease is not life-threatening. Patients generally have few complaints other than cosmetic issues. The prognosis is generally good for localized cutaneous scleroderma.

Sjögren's Syndrome

Sjögren's (pronounced SHOW-grins) *syndrome* is a chronic inflammatory autoimmune disorder characterized by replacement of normal salivary and lacrimal gland acini with a progressively increasing number of lymphocytes, resulting in eventual loss of tissue responsible for saliva and tear production. Most patients with Sjögren's syndrome complain of *sicca* (dry) symptoms: xerophthalmia (dry eyes) and xerostomia (dry mouth). Subsequent fibrosis results in salivary, lacrimal, and parotid gland enlargement (Fig. 4-57). Sjögren's syndrome primarily affects women but is not uncommon in men. The pathophysiology of Sjögren's syndrome is not well understood. Inherited susceptibility markers have been identified

Primary Sjögren syndrome occurs in the absence of another underlying autoimmunologic disorder. In other words, Sjögren's syndrome is the patient's primary problem. In addition to xerophthalmia and xerostomia, patients may develop arthralgia, arthritis, Raynaud's phenomenon, myalgia, pulmonary disease, gastrointestinal disease, leukopenia, anemia, lymphadenopathy, neuropathy, and/or vasculitis (see Table 4-5). The diagnosis is based on clinical signs and symptoms, along with laboratory tests that include detection of Sjögren's-specific autoantibodies, called SS-A and SS-B, which are found in some but not all patients. As salivary gland tissue is replaced by lymphocytes and fibrosis, the glands enlarge as firm nontender swellings that may become clinically apparent. A biopsy of salivary gland tissue will demonstrate lymphocytic replacement and fibrosis of normal glandular tissue (Fig. 4-58).

Secondary Sjögren syndrome is seen in patients with another primary underlying autoimmunologic disease,

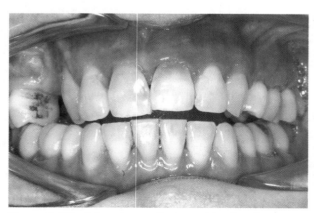

Figure 4–56 **Scleroderma.** Patient with scleroderma unable to open mouth.

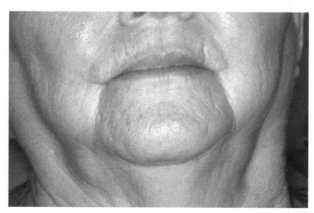

Figure 4–57 **Sjögren's syndrome.** Woman with chronic xerostomia presents with nontender bilateral enlargement of the parotid glands.

Table 4.5	American-European Consensus: Sjögren's Syndrome Classification Criteria

Symptoms	**Ocular** **At Least One**	**Oral** **At Least One**		
	Dry eyes > 3 months	Dry mouth > 3 months		
	Gritty sensation	Swelling of salivary glands		
	Use of artificial tears > 3 x day	Liquids required to swallow dry food		

Signs	**Ocular** **At Least One**	**Oral** **At Least One**	**Histopathology**	**Autoantibodies**
	Schirmer's test < 5 mm/ 5 min	Unstimulated saliva ≤ 1.5 mL /15 mins	Labial salivary gland Focus Score ≥ 1 per 4 mm^2	Anti-SSA(Ro) or Anti-SS-B (La)
	Positive vital dye staining ≥ 4	Abnormal parotid sialography		
		Abnormal salivary scintigraphy		

For a primary Sjögren's syndrome diagnosis:
a. Any 4 of the 6 criteria; must include either Histopathology or Autoantibodies
or
b. Any 3 of the 4 criteria for Signs

For a secondary Sjögren's syndrome diagnosis:
In patients with another well-defined major connective tissue disease, the presence of one symptom plus 2 of the 3 signs are indicative of secondary Sjögren's syndrome.

Exclusion Criteria
• Past head and neck radiation treatment
• Hepatitis C
• HIV/AIDS
• Pre-existing lymphoma
• Sarcoidosis
• Graft-versus-host disease
• Current use of anticholinergic drugs

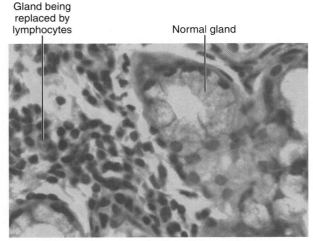

Gland being replaced by lymphocytes

Normal gland

Figure 4–58 Sjögren's syndrome. A biopsy of the minor salivary glands shows destruction of normal gland acini with replacement by lymphocytes.

such as SLE, rheumatoid arthritis (RA), or scleroderma. These patients develop the same features seen in primary Sjögren's syndrome.

The most common symptom of Sjögren's syndrome is xerostomia and its associated problems of dysphagia and dysgeusia. Patients with dentures may be unable to wear them because of lack of moisture necessary to create a seal. Patients may complain of dryness of the eyes accompanied by a sandy or gritty feeling. Depending on the degree of oral dryness, patients may develop rampant dental caries, including Class V lesions that seemingly appear overnight (Fig. 4-59). Fabrication of custom fluoride trays, dietary counseling, and reinforcement of plaque control methods are essential for maintaining optimal oral health. Oral health-care products formulated for patients with xerostomia are available.

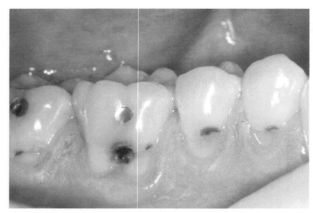

Figure 4–59 Sjögren's syndrome. Patient with recent onset of Sjögren's syndrome and profound xerostomia presents with extensive class V decay.

Clinical Implications

In a patients with residual functioning salivary gland tissue, use of saliva stimulants called sialogogues can help temporarily increase salivary flow. Over-the-counter sialogogues include sugar-free buffered lozenges. Prescription sialogogues, such as pilocarpine, are available. Water-based artificial saliva products are helpful, but they do not have a lasting effect. Vegetable oil-based artificial saliva is longer lasting but is not readily available. Patients can try olive oil as an alternative saliva substitute.

Sjögren's syndrome is a progressively destructive condition that has no effective treatment that will reverse or stop the disease. In both primary and secondary Sjögren's syndrome, the risk of developing lymphoma is increased; therefore, a biopsy of suddenly enlarging glands may be necessary.

Critical Thinking Questions

Case 4-1: Your 49-year-old female patient is diligent about maintaining her home care. She brushes and flosses regularly and has always received positive comments from you on the health of her mouth. On her last visit, you noticed very erythematous gingivitis and bleeding that you have not seen before. You scaled as usual to find no increase in calculus formation. She used chlorhexidine gluconate for 30 days but noticed no improvement. Today she complains that her "gums" hurt whenever she brushes and she cannot floss without bleeding. She also cannot eat Mexican food without having to order something very bland. She says the spicy food "sets her mouth off like it is on fire." She has not changed toothpastes or experienced any new medical problems. She takes no medications.

It is difficult to probe, but you find no pockets greater than 4 mm. Despite her pain, you find little plaque or calculus. Her radiographs appear within normal limits. Lesions are confined to the gingiva in all four quadrants. They appear erythematous and bleed on gentle probing.

• • •

What is a likely explanation for her current complaint?

How can this suspected diagnosis be confirmed?

How will you explain to the patient what is wrong with her mouth?

She wants to know if you can give her a more thorough cleaning and a softer toothbrush. Do you think this will help her?

She wants to know if she is going to lose her teeth. What do you tell her?

Case 4-2: You work for a pediatric dentist. Your otherwise healthy 12-year-old male patient presents with two large ulcers, one on the right lateral border of his tongue and one on the left buccal mucosa. He says the left side has been there for 3 weeks and the tongue lesion has been there for 1 week. He reports that they have occurred off and on since he was 8, but are getting worse. He also states that sometimes they hurt so much that he can only eat soft white bread. Sometimes he misses school because he cannot talk. His mother has taken him to his physician who told her he had herpes simplex and prescribed an antiviral drug. The lesions persisted. Another physician told her he had an allergy and recommended brushing with baking soda instead of toothpaste. His last general dentist said they were aphthous ulcers and there was nothing that could be done about them. He is starting to develop caries and gingivitis because he cannot brush regularly.

• • •

What is the most likely explanation for his problem?

Explain why the antiviral drug did not work.

Explain why brushing with baking soda did not help.

Is there anything that can be done to help him? Who should provide that help?

Case 4-3: Your 54-year-old female patient presents for routine care. During your initial oral inspection, you notice a white lace-like pattern to the left and right buccal mucosae. The patient states that she is unaware of the changes; there is no pain, tenderness, or reaction when she eats hot or spicy foods. The lesions were not present at her last visit 9 months ago. Since that time, she reports she is now taking two new medicines for hypertension. Her history also includes an allergy to several environmental agents, including grasses.

• • •

Name three possible causes for this appearance to her buccal mucosa.

What is the best method to determine the etiology for these lesions?

Should any treatment be instituted today for her lesions?

Case 4-4: Your 27-year-old male patient presents with an asymmetrically enlarged lower lip. The lip is slightly tender to palpation. Upon palpation, the lesion feels "lumpy" but not fluctuant. No exudate is expressed from the lip. It is not warm to the touch. The patient reports no recent history of trauma and states that this anomaly has arisen within the past 3 months.

• • •

List three possible causes for this unusual appearance to his lower lip.

In addition to a biopsy of the lip performed by an oral surgeon, what other specialists should this patient visit?

Case 4-5: You recently enrolled in your dental hygiene program. During preclinical activities, you are asked to wear gloves to get used to the tactile

sensation experienced while wearing them. After several days of preclinical activities, you notice your hands become dry, a little scaly, and somewhat itchy. You apply several different over-the-counter hand lotions, but nothing seems to help. It now appears you are developing a rash.

• • •

What is the most likely cause for this problem? Please be specific in terms of the biological changes associated with this suspected problem.

What two steps should you take to determine the source of the problem?

How do you think this experience will alter the way you practice dental hygiene in the future?

Case 4-6: During Christmas break you travel to a nearby state to visit relatives you have not seen in a while. When your 61-year-old aunt greets you at the door you cannot help but notice that her face has an unusual appearance that you have never noticed before. In front of her ears and along the jaw lines on both sides you notice symmetrical swelling. During Christmas dinner she complains that some of the foods do not taste the way she remembered when she was a girl. You notice that she sips water between each mouthful during the meal. She also complains that her eyes have been bothering her since she cleaned the attic several months ago. She refuses dessert because her dentist recently found three new cavities and had to replace four old fillings.

• • •

What are two possible explanations for your aunt's complaints?

What is causing the swelling of her face?

Why can she not taste food the way she used to?

How does her recent dental history relate to her new complaints?

After dinner, she takes you aside and asks you what you know about why she is getting so many new cavities. What will you say to her?

Review Questions

1. **All of the following are true about the immune response EXCEPT:**
   A. The immune system cannot mistake self for nonself.
   B. If the immune defenses are misdirected they can initiate allergic disease.
   C. Microorganisms are perceived as antigens by the immune system.
   D. Part of a microbe or toxin produced by bacteria can be perceived as antigenic.

2. **Which one of the following is important in minimizing transplant rejection?**
   A. germinal centers
   B. MHC markers
   C. passive antibodies
   D. TCF markers

3. **MHC markers**
   A. act as markers of self.
   B. are not present on cells that have been transformed by cancer or viral infection.
   C. are not highly specific.
   D. play no role in transplant rejection.

4. **Lymphocytes are**
   A. short-lived mobile cells.
   B. represent 20–25% of all white blood cells.
   C. are a specialized form of B granulocytes.
   D. are also known in tissue as histiocytes.

5. **B cells**
   A. become inactive when they encounter antigens.
   B. remain in the bone marrow for the life of the individual.
   C. are mature neutrophils.
   D. become plasma cells and produce one specific antibody.

6. **Which one of the following is the first antibody produced in response to an antigen?**
   A. IgG
   B. IgM
   C. IgA
   D. IgE

7. **Which one of the following is found in body fluids, including tears and saliva?**
   A. IgG
   B. IgM
   C. IgA
   D. IgE

8. **All of the following are true about activated T cells EXCEPT:**
   A. They can remain in the body permanently to retain the memory of an antigen.
   B. They can directly attack infected or cancerous cells
   C. They may direct and regulate the immune response.
   D. Activated T cells release histamine, responsible for the symptoms of allergy.

9. **Macrophages**
   A. circulate in the blood.
   B. play a role in eliminating foreign antigens in tissue.
   C. release powerful chemical signals called antibodies.
   D. are rare in the lungs, kidneys, brain, and liver.

10. **Which one of the following is not a function of cytokines?**
    A. Carrying information to and from immune cells
    B. Enhancing cell growth and differentiation
    C. Releasing histamine to kill parasites
    D. Attracting cells to migrate to an area by chemotaxis

11. **All of the following are true about the primary immune response EXCEPT:**
    A. It involves the integrated efforts of both humoral and cellular immunity.
    B. The primary response may take up to a year to fully develop.
    C. During a second exposure to the same antigen, there will be a secondary response.
    D. Memory B cells left behind after a primary response are "primed."

12. **In active immunity**
    A. antibodies are not produced by the host.
    B. antibodies are transmitted from mother to infant.
    C. the protection normally lasts only a few weeks.
    D. antibodies are produced in response to an allergen.

13. **Allergic reactions in which exaggerated response leads to body tissue destruction are known as**
    A. hypersensitivity reactions.
    B. passive immunity.
    C. immunodeficiency reaction.
    D. hyposensitivity reactions.

14. **Reactions to transfusions and erythroblastosis fetalis are examples of which type of hypersensitivity reaction?**
    A. Type I
    B. Type II
    C. Type III
    D. Type IV

15. **What type of hypersensitivity reaction is involved in autoimmune diseases such as rheumatoid arthritis?**
    A. Type I
    B. Type II
    C. Type III
    D. Type IV

16. **In autoimmune diseases**
    A. the immune system is activated to distinguish self from nonself.
    B. activated B cells produce antibodies against self-antigens called autoantibodies.
    C. immunity occurs when cytotoxic T cells attack abnormal tissues.
    D. symptoms usually manifests as a type I hypersensitivity.

17. **All of the following are examples of primary immunodeficiency diseases EXCEPT**
    A. selective IgA deficiency.
    B. hypergammaglobulinemia.
    C. DiGeorge syndrome.
    D. erythroblastosis fetalis.

18. **Contact dermatitis**
    A. requires direct contact with an allergen.
    B. results in lifelong immunity when re-exposed.
    C. has no known treatment.
    D. is considered a type I hypersensitivity reaction.

19. **All of the following immune defects predispose patients to developing recurrent aphthous stomatitis EXCEPT**
    A. decreased mucosal barrier.
    B. hormonal changes during pregnancy.
    C. increased antigenic exposure.
    D. inherited immune dysregulation.

20. **Major aphthous ulcers**
    A. occur on keratinized mucosa, such as the hard palate.
    B. frequently occur in the elderly.
    C. are contagious and easily transmitted.
    D. are most common in adolescents and young adults.

21. **Children with cyclic neutropenia may demonstrate all of the following EXCEPT**
    A. recurrent severe gingivitis with ulceration.
    B. frequent systemic infections.
    C. decreased ability to heal after minor trauma.
    D. ulcerations only on the non-keratinized mucosa.

22. **Your patient has an acute extensive blistering, erosive disease of the oral mucosa that erupted suddenly. There are large pruritic, red, concentric circular macules on his arms and neck. He is in pain and cannot eat. Which one of the following most likely precipitated your patient's current condition?**
    A. A recent episode of recurrent herpes labialis
    B. Recent exposure to a child with chickenpox
    C. A hereditary vascular disorder
    D. An HIV infection

23. **The clinical hallmark of reticular oral lichen planus is**

    A. pruritic purple papules.
    B. Wickham's striae.
    C. target lesions.
    D. major aphthous ulcerations.

24. **Which one of the following does not produce the clinical presentation of desquamative gingivitis?**

    A. Erosive lichen planus
    B. Mucous membrane pemphigoid
    C. Sjögren's syndrome
    D. Pemphigus vulgaris

25. **A chronic blistering disease of the skin and mucous membranes that features erosive gingivitis, blisters of mucous membranes and other skin surfaces, and symblepharon is**

    A. erosive lichen planus.
    B. chronic ulcerative stomatitis.
    C. pemphigoid.
    D. erythema multiforme.

26. **Butterfly rash on the face is most characteristic of which one of the following?**

    A. Linear IgA disease
    B. Cutaneous lupus erythematosus
    C. Lichen planus
    D. Erythema multiforme

27. **Which of the following is FALSE regarding Crohn's disease?**

    A. It is an autoimmune granulomatous disease.
    B. Painful major aphthous ulcers can occur.
    C. In the oral cavity nodular swellings can produce a cobblestone appearance.
    D. One of the first signs of this disease is development of Raynaud's phenomenon.

28. **Your 45-year-old patient presents with dry eyes and dry mouth and you suspect Sjögren's syndrome. Which of the following steps should be in the plan to manage this patient?**

    A. Daily home fluoride therapy and intensive oral health-care instructions.
    B. Dietary analysis for excessive sugar intake.
    C. Use of artificial saliva and possible prescription for a sialogogue.
    D. All of the above

SUGGESTED READINGS

Books

Abbas, AK, Lichtman, AH: Basic Immunology: Functions and Disorders of the Immune System, ed. 3. Saunders Elsevier, Philadelphia, 2008.

Eisen, D, Lynch, D: The Mouth, ed. 1. Mosby, St. Louis, 1998.

Martini, FH, Nath, JL: The lymphoid system and immunity. In: Fundamentals of Anatomy and Physiology, ed. 8. Pearson/Benjamin Cummings, San Francisco, 2009.

National Institute of Allergy and Infectious Diseases: Understanding the Immune System. How it Works. Bethesda, MD: NIH Publication No. 07-5423; 2007.

Neville, BW, Damm, DD, Allen, CM, Bouquot, J: Oral and Maxillofacial Pathology, ed. 3. Saunders Elsevier, St. Louis, 2009.

Neville, BW, Damm, DD, White, DH: Color Atlas of Clinical Oral Pathology, ed. 2. Williams and Wilkins, Baltimore, 1999.

Regezi, JA, Scuibba, JJ, Jordan, RC: Oral Pathology: Clinical Pathologic Correlations, ed. 4. Saunders Elsevier, St. Louis, 2003.

Journal Articles

Al Johani, KA, Moles, DR, Hodgson, TA, Porter, SR, Fedele, S: Orofacial granulomatosis: Clinical features and long-term outcome of therapy. Journal of the American Academy of Dermatology 62(4):611–620, April 2010. Epub 2010 Feb 4.

Altiner, A, Mandal, R: Behçet syndrome. Dermatology Online Journal 16(11):18, Nov 15, 2010.

Dale, DC, Bolyard, AA, Aprikyan, A: Cyclic neutropenia. Seminars in Hematology 39(2):89–94, April 2002.

Endo, H, Rees, TD: Clinical features of cinnamon-induced contact stomatitis. Compendium of Continuing Education in Dentistry 27(7):403–409, quiz 410, 421, July 2006.

Fabbri, P, Cardinali, C, Giomi, B, Caproni, M: Cutaneous lupus erythematosus: Diagnosis and management. American Journal of Clinical Dermatology 4(7):449–465, 2003.

Fatahzadeh, M, Rinaggio, J: Diagnosis of systemic sarcoidosis prompted by orofacial manifestations: A review of the literature. Journal of the American Dental Association 137(1):54–60, January 2006.

Graves, B, McCullough, M, Wiesenfeld, D: Orofacial granulomatosis - A 20 year review. Oral Diseases 15:46–51, 2009.

Haztmut, F, Hildebrand, CV, Maxtin, P: Nickel, chromium, cobalt dental alloys and allergic reactions: An overview. Biomaterials 10, October 1989.

Hernández-Molina, G, Avila-Casado, C, Cárdenas-Velázquez, F, Hernández-Hernández, C, Calderillo, ML, Marroquín, V, Soto-Abraham, V, Recillas-Gispert, C, Sánchez-Guerrero, J: Similarities and differences between primary and secondary Sjögren's syndrome. Journal of Rheumatology 37(4):800–808, April 2010. Epub 2010 Mar 1.

Jadwat, Y, Meyerov, R, Lemmer, J, Raubenheimer, EJ, Feller, L: Plasma cell gingivitis: Does it exist? Report of a case and review of the literature. Journal of the South African Dental Association 63(7):394–395, August 2008.

Lee, SJ, Flowers, ME: Recognizing and managing chronic graft-versus-host disease. American Society of Hematology Education Program 134–141, 2008.

Messadi, DV, Younai, F: Aphthous ulcers. Dermatologic Therapy 23(3):281–290, May–June 2010.

Porter, SR, Bain, SE, Scully, CM: Linear IgA disease manifesting as recalcitrant desquamative gingivitis. Oral Surgery, Oral Medicine, Oral Pathology, Oral Radiology and Endodontology 74(2): 179–182, August 1992.

Porter, S, Scully, C: Connective tissue disorders and the mouth. Dental Update 35(5):294–296, 298–300, 302, June 2008.

Pullen, RL Jr, Hall, DA: Sjögren's syndrome: More than dry eyes. Nursing 40(8):36–41, August 2010.

Rowland, M, Fleming, P, Bourke, B: Looking in the mouth for Crohn's disease. Inflammatory Bowel Diseases 16(2):332–337, February 2010.

Saalman, R, Mattsson, U, Jontell, M: Orofacial granulomatosis in childhood - A clinical entity that may indicate Crohn's disease as well as food allergy. Acta Paediatrica 98(7):1162–1167, July 2009. Epub 2009 Apr 17.

Sciubba, JJ: Autoimmune oral mucosal diseases: Clinical, etiologic, diagnostic, and treatment considerations. Dental Clinics of North America 55(1):89–103, January 2011.

Sciubba, JJ: Oral mucosal diseases in the office setting - Part II: Oral lichen planus, pemphigus vulgaris, and mucosal pemphigoid. General Dentistry 55(5):464–476; quiz 477–478, 488, Sept–Oct 2007.

Thyssen, JP, Menné, T: Metal allergy - A review on exposures, penetration, genetics, prevalence, and clinical implications. Chemical Research in Toxicology 23(2):309–318, February 15, 2010.

Vitali, C, Bombardieri, S, Jonsson, R, Moutsopoulos, HM: European Study Group on Classification Criteria for Sjögren's Syndrome. Classification criteria for Sjögren's syndrome: A revised version of the European criteria proposed by the American-European Consensus Group. Annals of the Rheumatic Diseases 61(6):554–558, June 2002.

Wetter, DA, Davis, MD: Recurrent erythema multiforme: Clinical characteristics, etiologic associations, and treatment in a series of 48 patients at Mayo Clinic, 2000 to 2007. Journal of the American Academy of Dermatology 62(1):45–53, January 2010. Epub 2009 Aug 7.

Online Resource

Shy, BD, Schwartz, DT: Contact dermatitis. Updated: March 19, 2014. Retrieved from http://emedicine.medscape.com/article/762139-overview.

Developmental Disorders of the Orofacial Complex

Learning Outcomes

At the end of this chapter, the student will be able to:

5.1. Discuss how disturbances during orofacial embryological development contribute to abnormalities of the head, neck and oral cavity.

5.2. Explain the etiology of developmental abnormalities of the teeth.

5.3. Explain how disturbances in tooth development affect oral health.

Continued

5.4. Discuss the origins of the most common odontogenic cysts.

5.5. Explain the difference between an inflammatory odontogenic cyst (see Chapter 2) and a developmental odontogenic cyst.

5.6. Discuss the origins of nonodontogenic cysts of the head and neck.

5.7. Recognize and describe the clinical and/or radiographic characteristics of developmental cysts.

5.8. Explain the difference between "true cysts" and nonepithelial cyst-like entities.

FUNDAMENTALS OF OROFACIAL EMBRYOLOGY AND DEVELOPMENT

An understanding of embryological development is useful in explaining developmental disorders. **Developmental disorders** are defined as those that occur during development of a part or organ. Interference with development may occur that causes the organ or part to be too small, too large, malformed, or absent. The cause of interference is referred to as the **etiologic agent**. Etiologic agents in the environment that cause abnormalities are known as **teratogens**. This chapter focuses on disorders resulting from environmental disturbances during development. It is important to note that the precise cause of many developmental disorders is not clear. Inherited developmental disorders are discussed in Chapter 6.

Facial Development

Embryology is fundamental in understanding developmental anomalies of the face and oral cavity. The origins of tissues, formation of organs and body parts, and the timeline of their development are precise. A primitive head is observed in utero in the fourth week of gestation, as the embryo begins to lengthen and bend (Fig. 5-1). The developing embryo is covered with a layer of tissue called *ectoderm*. Externally, ectoderm forms the skin, its appendages (hair, sweat glands), fingernails, and toenails. Ectoderm also gives rise to the neural tube and covers the interior of the forming primitive mouth, or stomodeum. Inside the primitive mouth, ectoderm becomes the oral mucosa and eventually contributes to the formation of teeth. In the early stages, the mouth is separated from the intestinal tube (primitive gut) by the buccopharyngeal (oropharyngeal) membrane, which consists of two layers: ectoderm on the mouth side and endoderm on the gut side. Normally, this membrane ruptures around the fourth week to allow communication between the mouth, throat, and gastrointestinal tract. The tonsillar pillars mark the point where this membrane existed.

Development of Neural Crest Cells

The frontal prominence contains the developing brain. The brain, along with the rest of the central nervous system, arises in the neural tube that extends from the developing head toward the tail of the embryo (Fig. 5-2). The neural tube is formed by infoldings called neural folds, which arise from ectoderm during the third week *in utero*. Special cells, called **neural crest cells,** develop along the lateral margins (crests) of the neural tube. In the head and neck region, these cells undergo extensive migration and form tissue known as *ectomesenchyme*. Ectomesenchyme contributes to the formation of craniofacial connective tissues, including bone and cartilage, dermis, and tissues making up the tooth, except enamel (Fig. 5-3).

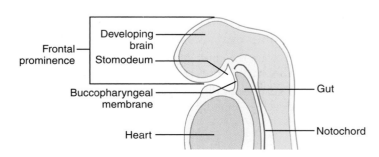

Figure 5–1 Human embryo, 4 weeks. Primitive head at 4 weeks, covered by ectoderm. Oropharyngeal membrane separates primitive mouth from gut.

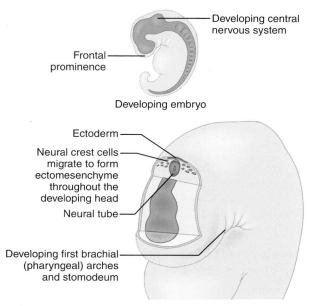

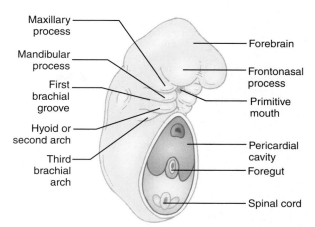

Figure 5–4 **Pharyngeal arches.** Developing pharyngeal arches.

Figure 5–2 Developing nervous system, neural tube, and migration of neural crest cells to craniofacial areas.

mandible, muscles of mastication, trigeminal nerve, and maxillary artery. If there is a disturbance in the first arch during development, the result may appear as a defect in any or all of the associated tissues.

Pharyngeal or Branchial Arches

Six paired bars of tissue in the head and neck region, known as pharyngeal (branchial) arches, form structures with pouches and grooves. They are the organizational units of development and each gives rise to specific body parts. Each arch has specific bones, muscles, nerves, and blood vessels that arise from it. These tissues remain "related" throughout life. They give rise to adult craniofacial structures, including the facial processes above and below the primitive mouth (Fig. 5-4). For example, the first arch, called the *mandibular arch*, gives rise to the maxilla and

Development of the Nose, Lips, and Palate

The maxillary processes grow forward to eventually fuse with medial and lateral nasal processes that have grown downward from the frontal process. The contribution of each of these to the formation of the face is depicted in Figure 5-5. Bilateral, medial, and lateral nasal processes contribute to the formation of the nasal placodes and pits, which eventually form the nose. By the sixth week in utero, the medial nasal processes form the philtrum of the lip, while the right and left maxillary processes form the sides of the upper lip. A disturbance at this time may result in a cleft lip.

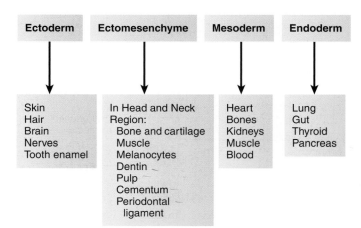

Figure 5–3 **Derivatives of embryonic germ layers.**

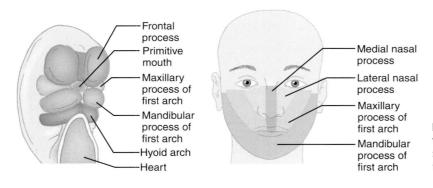

Figure 5–5 Formation of the face. Contributions of the frontal, mandibular, and maxillary processes to the development of the face.

Growth of the medial nasal processes produces a wedge of tissue known as the **intermaxillary segment**. Contact and fusion of this segment with the medial aspect of the maxillary processes forms what is known as the primary palate, or premaxilla (Fig. 5-6). The primary palate eventually contains the lateral and central incisors. Outgrowths from the surfaces of the maxillary processes form two lateral palatine processes, or shelves. At the eighth week in utero, these elevate over the forming tongue and, at weeks 9 to 12, fuse to form the secondary palate. Fusion of these processes with the primary palate completes palate formation. The mid-palatal suture marks the line of fusion of the lateral palatine processes. A disturbance at this time may result in a cleft palate.

Development of the Tongue and Thyroid Gland

The tongue develops from contributions of the first, second, and third pharyngeal arches, which form the floor of the primitive mouth. At the fourth and fifth weeks in utero, tissue swellings from these arches appear (Fig. 5-7). A central swelling in the floor of the mouth, the tuberculum impar, arises along with two lateral (lingual) swellings. The lateral swellings grow rapidly and merge with the tuberculum impar

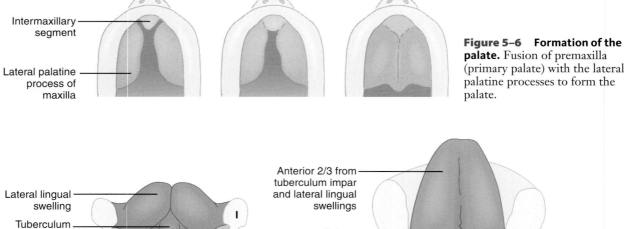

Figure 5–6 Formation of the palate. Fusion of premaxilla (primary palate) with the lateral palatine processes to form the palate.

Figure 5–7 Development of the tongue. A. Pharyngeal arches that contribute to development of the tongue. **B.** Mature tongue with pharyngeal arch contributions to the anterior and posterior tongue.

to form the anterior two-thirds of the tongue. Another midline swelling from the third arch, the hypobranchial eminence, rapidly forms and fuses to form the posterior third of the tongue. The complex contributions of more than one pharyngeal arch to tongue development explain its innervation by multiple cranial nerves. Failure of one or more of these arches to develop properly may result in a tongue that is too small or absent.

A V-shaped groove on the dorsum of the tongue, called the terminal sulcus, marks the boundary between the posterior and anterior tongue. This sulcus terminates posteriorly in a depression called the *foramen cecum*.

The thyroid gland begins its formation at the foramen cecum. Thyroid-forming cells develop in this area and migrate along the thyroglossal tract (duct) to the site of the future thyroid gland in the neck. Failure of the cells to migrate may result in ectopic thyroid gland development or formation of cysts along the tract.

ABNORMALITIES OF THE FACE AND ORAL CAVITY

Defects present at birth or shortly after birth are referred to as **congenital** abnormalities. Some congenital abnormalities are not observed until the development of a body part is complete. **Teratology** can be broadly defined as the study of developmental abnormalities, both congenital and developing after birth. Inherited mechanisms and/or agents called teratogens interfere with embryonic development, resulting in developmental malfunctions or defects. The precise etiology of many developmental defects is unknown; however, some well-known examples of environmental teratogens include drugs (thalidomide, alcohol), radiation (x-rays), and microorganisms (rubella, syphilis). Teratogens often affect forming tissues only at specific stages of development.

Cleft Lip and Cleft Palate

Clefts are considered the most common developmental facial abnormality. They represent failure of fusion of adjacent embryological processes that normally fuse to form one continuous structure. Cleft lip and cleft palate occurrence differs between genders and among ethnic groups. Cleft lip and cleft lip with cleft palate are more common in males, while cleft palate alone is more common in females. Cleft lip and cleft palate occur more frequently in some ethnic groups when compared to others. For example, when observing 700 births per group, clefts occur in one birth among Caucasians, almost four births among Native Americans, and about two births among the Japanese. African Americans have a low rate of 0.3 clefts per 700 births.

In general, clefts of the face, lip, and/or palate are thought to be multifactorial in terms of etiology. Both inheritance and environmental factors are important. Environmental factors linked to development of clefts include drug and alcohol abuse, cigarette smoke, chemicals such as insecticides, and microorganisms such as treponema pallidum and cytomegalovirus. Cleft lip and cleft palate may occur alone or together.

Cleft lip results from impaired fusion of the median nasal process with the maxillary process. Clefting of the lip is depicted in Fig. 5-8. It may be partial or complete (Fig. 5-8 B and C), unilateral or bilateral (Fig. 5-8 D). It almost always involves the upper lip. Clefts of the lower lip are rare. Cleft lip occurs early in embryonic life, between the sixth and ninth weeks during lip formation. After birth, it appears as either a small gap or an indentation in the lip at the philtrum. A partial cleft lip involves only the lip, but a complete cleft will involve the lower portion of the nose. In decades past, the condition was sometimes referred to as *harelip*, but that term is no longer used.

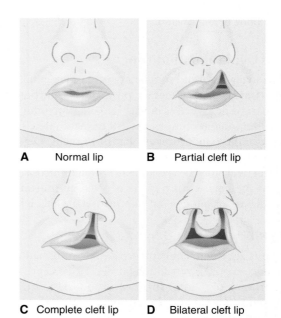

A   Normal lip   **B**   Partial cleft lip

C   Complete cleft lip   **D**   Bilateral cleft lip

Figure 5–8   **Cleft lip.** Cleft lip can be unilateral or bilateral, partial or complete. Complete cleft lip involves the lower portion of the nose.

Cleft palate represents failure of fusion of any of the palatal processes. Failure of fusion can be bilateral (Fig. 5-10A) or unilateral (Fig. 5-10B). The palate begins to fuse at the eighth week in the anterior segment. If failure of fusion occurs at this time, none of the palate will fuse (Fig. 5-10C). Fig. 5-10D is a radiograph showing failure of fusion in bilateral cleft palate. Fig. 5-10E is a CT-generated image showing a unilateral cleft of the maxilla. If failure of fusion occurs in the ninth to tenth week, the lateral palatal processes fail to fuse. If failure occurs at the eleventh week, then only clefting of the soft palate will be seen. Bifid uvula is considered a mild form of cleft palate.

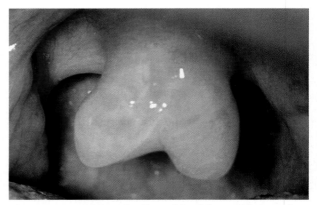

Figure 5–9   Bifid uvula. Caused by failure of fusion of palatal processes at around 11 weeks in utero.

Clinical Implications

Clefts may present as openings between the oral cavity and nasal passages, resulting in feeding and speech problems. In untreated cleft lip and/or palate, facial growth results in increased separation of the involved processes. This creates disordered dental development and malpositioned teeth, requiring surgical and orthodontic interventions. Facial clefts most often are treated with surgery. In some cases, the process of distraction osteogenesis is employed. This uses a bone-lengthening procedure in which a mechanical device applies tension over time to induce new bone formation, promoting closure of the bone defect or cleft.

Bifid Uvula and Bifid Tongue

Bifid uvula and bifid tongue are often incidental findings. A uvula or tongue that appears to be splitting into two parts is described as bifid (Fig. 5-9). Both bifid uvula and bifid tongue occur as a result of incomplete fusion of the embryonic processes that form them. Defective or incomplete fusion of the palatal processes that result in bifid uvula may be accompanied by submucosal clefting of the palate. Bifid uvula is often an indicator to investigate for undetected submucosal palatal clefts.

Lip Pits

Lip pits are small, congenital, sac-like invaginations of lip mucosa on the vermillion border with a depth ranging from 1 to 4 mm. In most instances, lip pits are not symptomatic and are an incidental finding. Depending on their location, size, and depth, there may be cosmetic considerations. They may occur singly or in pairs and are commonly located at the corners of the mouth, where they are called *commissural*. Commissural lip pits result from defective embryonic development of the lip and are unrelated to cleft lip and/or palate. Lip pits may also occur near the midline, where they are called *paramedian*. Paramedian lip pits may be associated with cleft lip and/or cleft palate and are seen in van der Woude syndrome (see Chapter 6).

Double Lip

Double lip is characterized by the presence of a fold of redundant lip mucosa. Double lip varies in severity and may be an incidental finding, only noticeable upon smiling (Fig. 5-11). It most often affects the upper lip and may be related to altered lip formation during embryonic development. Alternately, double lip may be acquired later in life from injury, such as chronic lip sucking. It can be an inherited component of Ascher syndrome, which is characterized by double lip, edema, sagging of eyelid tissue (blepharochalasis), and benign, nontoxic thyroid enlargement.

Aglossia and Ankyloglossia

Aglossia is characterized by partial formation or complete absence of the tongue. It may occur congenitally as the result of failure of fusion of the components of the branchial arches responsible for tongue formation. It may also result from the surgical treatment of disease. *Ankyloglossia* describes attachment or tethering of the anterior tongue to the floor of the mouth, usually by a tight cord of tissue or frenum (Fig. 5-12). This may be partial or complete and is referred to as "tongue tie." Significant speech and swallowing problems may result, depending on the severity of restricted tongue movements. Treatment options

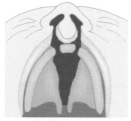

A Bilateral cleft palate with lip involvement

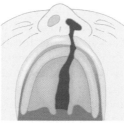

B Unilateral cleft palate with lip involvement

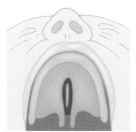

C Late failure of fusion with partial cleft palate; lip is not affected

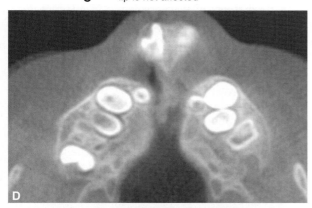

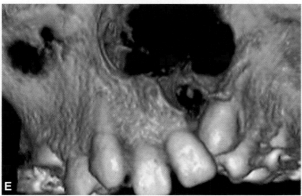

Figure 5–10   Cleft palate. A. Bilateral cleft palate often involves the lip. **B.** Unilateral cleft palate with lip involvement. **C.** Partial cleft palate with no lip involvement. **D.** Radiograph of bilateral cleft palate. **E.** CT-generated image showing unilateral cleft of maxilla.

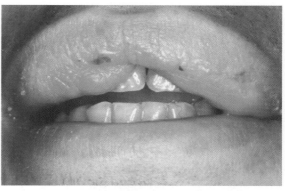

Figure 5–11   Double lip. Extra fold of tissue in a patient with Ascher syndrome.

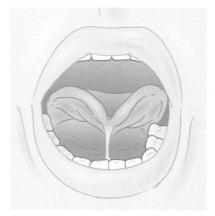

Figure 5–12   Ankyloglossia. Abnormally short attachment of the lingual frenum.

include frenotomy (frenectomy) to release the tongue from the mouth floor.

Macroglossia and Microglossia

Macroglossia is defined as abnormal increase in size of the tongue. It may be congenital, as in Down syndrome (Fig. 5-13), or occur as a result of neoplasia, such as lymphangioma (see Chapter 7). *Microglossia* is a rare, congenital disorder in which the tongue is abnormally small due to lack of development of the tuberculum impar and other structures involved in tongue development. An excessively large or small tongue can significantly affect speech and impact feeding or swallowing. Normal growth and development of the mandibular alveolar processes may be altered by lack of tongue forces, resulting in malocclusion.

Fissured Tongue

Fissured tongue is a condition in which one or more deep grooves are present on the dorsum of the tongue

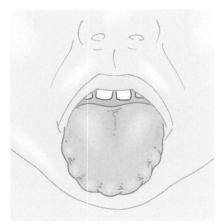

Figure 5–13 Macroglossia. Large tongue that overfills the mouth with scalloping of borders from pressure on teeth.

(Fig. 5-14). Fissured tongue may be seen in both children and adults, and its prevalence in the general population has been estimated at around 5 percent. Fissured tongue has been associated with geographic tongue (see Chapter 2), with many patients having both conditions. Fissured tongue is a component of Melkersson-Rosenthal syndrome (see Chapter 4). Food particles and oral debris may become trapped in the deep crevices of a fissured tongue, creating an oral hygiene problem. Oral health-care procedures that address this issue include cleaning the tongue by brushing and rinsing.

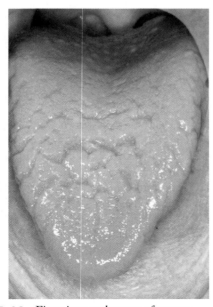

Figure 5–14 Fissuring on dorsum of tongue.

Lingual Thyroid (Ectopic Thyroid)

Lingual thyroid occurs when normal thyroid tissue remains at the **foramen caecum**, the initial site of thyroid gland formation on the dorsum of the tongue. It is referred to as **ectopic**, meaning out of normal position. Appearance of lingual thyroid is most commonly a mucosal-colored round nodule, reaching up to 4 cm in diameter, located at or near the terminal sulcus (Fig. 5-15). Ectopic thyroid tissue can remain anywhere along the thyroglossal tract, the route of thyroid gland migration to its final site in the neck.

Clinical Implications

Lingual thyroid is most often asymptomatic, an incidental finding, and requires no treatment. In unusual cases, it can interfere with normal swallowing and breathing, which necessitates removal. However, because removal of a lingual thyroid may result in hypothyroidism (see Chapter 9), the presence of adequate thyroid gland tissue in the neck must be carefully evaluated.

Lingual Varicosities

Varicosities (varicose veins) are swollen, twisted, and sometimes painful veins that have filled with an abnormal collection of blood. They are seen most commonly on the legs. Lingual varicosities are similar in appearance to varicose veins in the legs. They present as nonpainful, large, dilated, blue masses on the ventral surface of the tongue (Fig. 5-16) and are more common in older individuals, with few if any seen in children and adolescents. Most

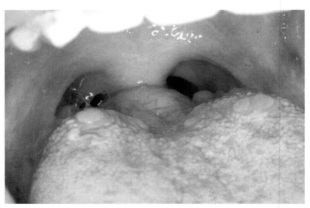

Figure 5–15 Lingual thyroid. Nodule at foramen caecum.

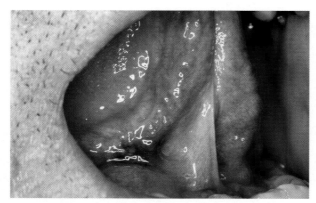

Figure 5–16   Lingual varicosities. Tortuous veins on ventral tongue.

lingual varicosities are asymptomatic and require no treatment.

Hemifacial Microsomia

Hemifacial microsomia is a congenital condition in which one-half of the face is underdeveloped (Fig. 5-17). Also called Goldenhar syndrome, or Oral-Mandibular-Auricular syndrome, it is the second most common birth defect after facial clefting. The affected structures include the mouth, mandible, and ears. The condition is believed to arise around the fourth embryonic week due to a decreased vascular supply to the affected region that compromises growth.

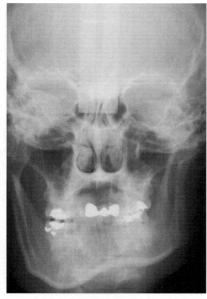

Figure 5–17   Hemifacial microsomia. Underdevelopment of the left jaw, compared to normal development of the right jaw.

In addition to cosmetic problems, individuals with hemifacial microsomia may experience varying degrees of difficulty with hearing, breathing, eating, and facial movements. Surgery to correct defects and improve aesthetics may be warranted, depending on the severity of the condition.

FUNDAMENTALS OF TOOTH DEVELOPMENT

Tooth development begins at approximately the sixth week in utero and ends with the eruption of the third molars. Teeth are vulnerable to deleterious environmental influences during this time. Ectoderm covering the external surface of the embryo and lining the primitive mouth as oral mucosa, is vital for tooth development. Around the sixth week in utero, two horseshoe bands of thickened epithelium called dental lamina appear over the upper and lower alveolar ridges (Fig. 5-18A). Ten localized epithelial buds in the maxilla and ten in the mandible extend downward into the underlying connective tissue to form germs of the primary (deciduous) teeth (Fig. 5-18B). They are tethered to the overlying epithelium by the *dental lamina*. Lingual outgrowths from these epithelial buds will form 20 successor (succedaneous) or permanent teeth. Twelve additional permanent tooth buds develop from continued distal growth of the dental lamina.

Enamel Organ

Bud, cap, and bell stages comprise the earliest tooth development. Epithelial *buds* grow down into the underlying ectomesenchyme to form a *cap* shape which further proliferates into the shape of a *bell* (Fig. 5-18C). This structure is called the *enamel organ*. Each enamel organ is composed of inner and outer enamel epithelium, with intervening stellate reticulum and stratum intermedium. The inner enamel epithelium later differentiates into ameloblasts that will form enamel.

Rests of Serres

At the end of the bell stage, the dental lamina is no longer needed, so it degenerates. Small fragments of epithelium, referred to as **rests of Serres** (Fig. 5-18D), are left behind. Later in life, these residual fragments of epithelium may develop into cysts.

Reduced Enamel Epithelium

Enamel formation continues until crown formation is complete. When enamel formation is finished, the inner and outer enamel epithelium meet and fuse to form the

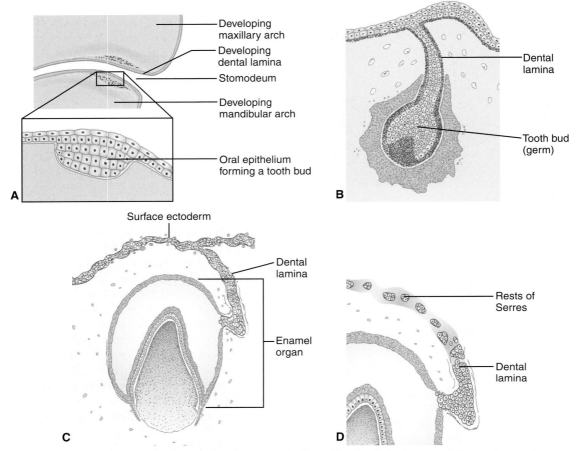

Figure 5–18   Fundamentals of tooth development. A. Dental lamina in bud stage. **B.** Formation of the dental lamina's umbilicord-like structure. **C.** Bell stage. **D.** Breakdown of the dental lamina and formation of the Rests of Serres.

reduced enamel epithelium. This forms a covering that protects the enamel surface during tooth eruption.

Dental Papilla and Dental Sac

The concave inner surface of enamel organ surrounds a connective tissue core of ectomesenchyme referred to as the *dental papillae.* Eventually, dentin and pulp form from the dental papilla. Tissues surrounding the enamel organ and dental papilla are known as *dental follicle* or *dental sac.* Odontoblasts differentiate from cells of the dental papilla adjacent to the ameloblast layer. They secrete a layer of predentin, which signals ameloblasts to begin enamel production. At the future cemento-enamel junction (CEJ), the inner and outer enamel epithelia meet, fuse to form the cervical loop, and continue to develop apically, forming *Hertwig's epithelial root sheath* (Fig. 5-19A). The epithelial root sheath forms the outline of the developing root.

Eventually, the root sheath breaks apart, allowing cementum formation to proceed along the root surface.

Rests of Malassez

Remnants of Hertwig's epithelial root sheath are known as **rests of Malassez** (Fig. 5-19B). In the developed jaw, these epithelial rests are located within the periodontal ligament space. Later in life, these small fragments of epithelium may develop into a cyst or tumor that appears to be arising within or from the periodontal ligament space.

DEVELOPMENTAL ABNORMALITIES OF THE DENTITION

Developing teeth are vulnerable to deleterious environmental influences during their years of development. While heredity may influence some aspects of tooth

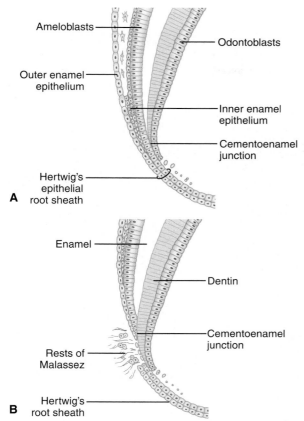

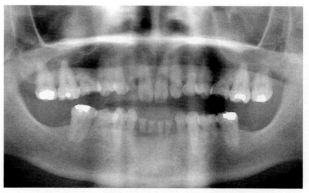

Figure 5–20 **Hypodontia.** Congenitally missing premolars and molars.

Figure 5–19 **Hertwig's epithelial root sheath. A.** Hertwig's root sheath is made up of cells of the inner enamel and outer enamel epithelium. **B.** Rests of Malassez are remnants of Hertwig's root sheath when it breaks down during root formation.

associated with abnormalities of ectoderm. Because teeth arise from ectoderm, their formation is affected in these syndromes.

> **Clinical Implications**
>
> Congenitally missing teeth may not be apparent until radiographic evaluation reveals the failure of tooth formation. Depending on the number and location of missing teeth, clinical implications may include aesthetics, speech, and mastication of food. Interdisciplinary management of anodontia or hypodontia often incorporates the specialties of pediatric dentistry, orthodontics, and prosthodontics.

development, most common tooth anomalies are the result of local or systemic factors that affect the developing teeth.

Congenitally Missing Teeth

Variations in the number of teeth may occur. Failure of all teeth to form is known as *anodontia*. Failure of some teeth to form, leaving a fewer than normal number, is termed *hypodontia* or *oligodontia*. Hypodontia can range from one to multiple missing teeth (Fig. 5-20). It may affect either the permanent or primary dentitions, but is more common in the permanent dentition. The most common congenitally missing permanent teeth are the third molars, maxillary lateral incisors, and mandibular second premolars. Anodontia or hypodontia may be familial or inherited as a part of a syndrome. Ectodermal dysplasia (see Chapter 6) describes a group of inherited syndromes that are

Hyperdontia (Supernumerary Teeth)

Extra teeth are called *supernumerary teeth*. They occur when extra tooth buds develop from dental lamina, or when tooth buds erroneously divide. There may be one or many supernumerary teeth present in the dentition (Fig. 5-21). The most common supernumerary tooth is the *mesiodens*, which occurs in the midline between the maxillary central incisors and often has a conical or peg shape. A *paramolar* is a supernumerary tooth lying lingual to, or buccal to, maxillary or mandibular molars (Fig. 5-22). Supernumerary teeth may block other teeth from erupting successfully. Crowding of developing teeth may impinge on the tooth germ or Hertwig's epithelial root sheath and result in altered crown and root shapes. Supernumerary teeth are commonly impacted. They may be seen in inherited disorders, such as cleidocranial dysplasia or Gardner's syndrome (see Chapter 6).

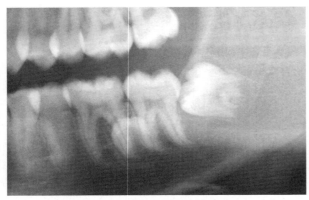

Figure 5–21 Supernumerary tooth. Premolar-shaped supernumerary tooth developing between tooth #18 and tooth #19.

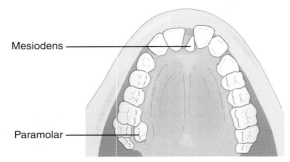

Figure 5–22 Common examples of microdontia. Mesiodens and paramolar.

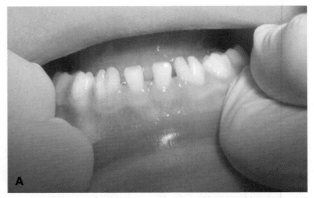

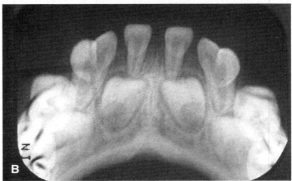

Figure 5–23 Fusion. A. Clinical photo of child with fusion of laterals and canines bilaterally. **B.** Radiograph of same child.

Fusion and Gemination

Fusion occurs when the dentin of two adjacent tooth buds fuses together to become a single mass (Fig. 5-23A and B). Fusion may occur between two normal tooth buds or between normal and supernumerary tooth buds. Both deciduous and permanent anterior teeth are commonly affected.

Gemination, or twinning, occurs when a single tooth bud attempts to divide into two teeth. It is distinguished from fusion by counting tooth crowns. In fusion, less than the normal number of crowns/teeth appear to be present. In gemination, more than the normal number of crowns/teeth appear to be present (Fig. 5-24).

Concrescence

Concrescence occurs during cementum formation and deposition. Teeth in close approximation become bound together by cementum. It is seen most frequently in maxillary molars (Fig. 5-25) and may be an incidental finding on radiographic examination.

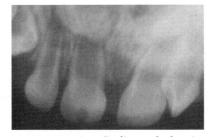

Figure 5–24 Gemination. Radiograph showing attempted twinning of central incisor.

Extraction of teeth with undetected concrescence may result in fracture and loss of facial- or lingual-supporting alveolar bone. With maxillary molars, fracture or loss of the entire tuberosity is possible. Discerning concrescence on radiographs is often problematic due to the similar radiodensities of cementum and adjacent alveolar bone.

Abnormalities of Tooth Shape

Shapes of teeth are determined during the *morphodifferentiation stage* of tooth development. Final shapes

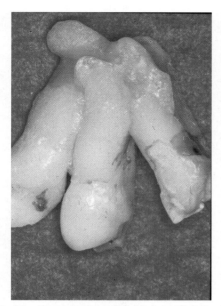

Figure 5–25 **Concrescence.** Multiple teeth joined by cementum.

may be affected and altered by injury or space constraints during development.

Microdontia and Macrodontia

Microdontia and *macrodontia* refer to teeth that are smaller (micro-) or larger (macro-) relative to the other teeth in the dentition. A single tooth or multiple teeth may be affected. True microdontia most often affects a single tooth, such as a maxillary third molar (Fig. 5-26), or supernumerary teeth. Generalized macrodontia has been associated with gigantism and generalized microdontia has been associated with certain types of dwarfism (see Chapter 9).

Peg Lateral

Peg lateral describes an alteration in the shape of maxillary lateral incisors that causes the lateral incisor to have a conical shape. Peg laterals are smaller than normal laterals and are considered microdonts. One or both laterals may be affected (Fig. 5-27). Peg laterals may require restoration to improve aesthetics.

Talon Cusp

An extra cusp on the lingual or palatal surface of an anterior tooth in the cingulum area is known as *talon cusp* (Fig. 5-28). This occurs as an extra outgrowth of the enamel organ during crown formation. The cusp is often triangular-shaped and thought to resemble the talon of an eagle. Talon cusps are susceptible to wear and fracture and contain an extension of pulp. Noncarious or restorative pulp exposures may occur, resulting in pulpal necrosis and apical pathology. Endodontic treatment may be necessary.

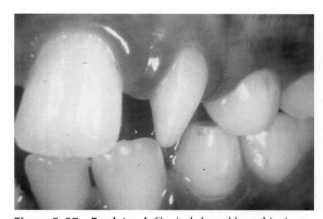

Figure 5–27 **Peg lateral.** Conical shaped lateral incisor.

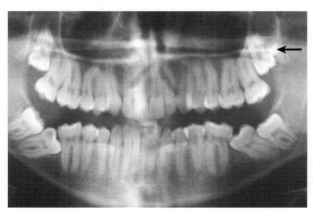

Figure 5–26 Microdont fourth molar.

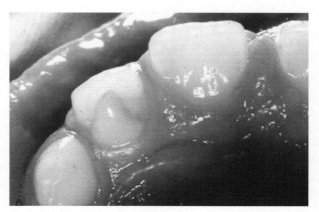

Figure 5–28 **Talon cusp.** Extra cusp on the cingulum of maxillary lateral incisor.

Dens Evaginatus

Dens evaginatus is formation of a supernumerary cusp, most often on a posterior tooth. It may occur unilaterally or bilaterally on any tooth, most frequently on the occlusal surface of premolars (Fig. 5-29). An extension of pulp is usually present within the extra cusp. There is increased risk of pulp exposure with cusp wear or fracture. This can result in pulpitis, pulpal necrosis, and apical pathology. Endodontic treatment may be required.

Dens Invaginatus (Dens-in-Dente)

Dens invaginatus (dens-in-dente) results from an infolding of the enamel organ during crown formation. This produces a bulb- or pear-shaped defect that projects from the crown downward to varying depths in the root canal space and gives the appearance of a "tooth within a tooth" (Fig. 5-30). Dens invaginatus occurs most frequently in the anterior teeth, especially the maxillary lateral incisors. Direct communication with the pulp in the cingulum area is a common complication. This can result in pulpal necrosis and apical pathology soon after tooth eruption. In some cases, early intervention may consist of preventive restorations to seal any pulpal communication in the cingulum area. Endodontic treatment is most often employed, either preemptively to prevent pathology or to treat existing apical pathology.

Enamel Pearl

Enamel pearl most commonly occurs as a round concretion, resembling a small pearl, in or adjacent to the furcation area of the maxillary molars (Fig. 5-31). These are often first detected on radiographic examination as

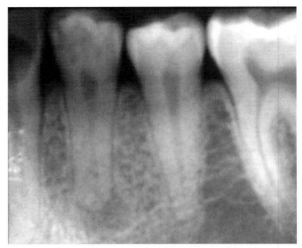

Figure 5–30 Dens-in-dente. Note the periapical radiolucency indicating nonvitality of the first premolar.

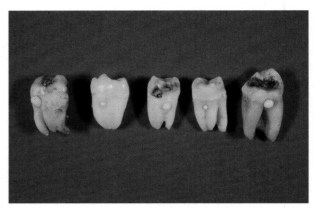

Figure 5–31 Enamel pearl. Group of molars showing enamel pearls.

small, radiopaque spheres and may be mistaken for calculus. The concretion is covered with enamel and may contain dentin and sometimes an extension of pulp. Enamel pearls are thought to result from displacement of ameloblasts during dental hard tissue formation. Depending on their precise location, they may alter the gingival epithelial attachment, contributing to plaque and calculus accumulation and periodontal pocket formation. Enamel pearls are not routinely removed unless they cause periodontal problems.

Dilaceration

Dilaceration is a condition in which a tooth root exhibits abnormal curvature (Fig. 5-32). This may occur anywhere along the root, from the cemento-enamel junction to the apex. Dilaceration is thought to result

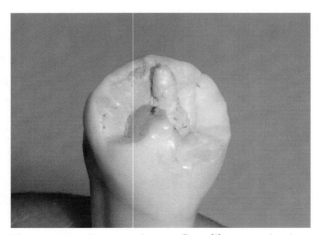

Figure 5–29 Dens evaginatus. Cusp-like protrusion in central groove of mandibular premolar.

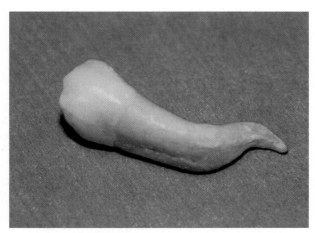

Figure 5–32 Dilaceration. Abnormal curvature of the apical one-third of the root.

from trauma to Hertwig's root sheath, causing displacement of forming tissues. Dilacerated teeth are not usually a significant finding, unless they pose problems during tooth extraction or endodontic treatment.

Taurodontism

Taurodontism is an anomaly of molar teeth caused by alteration of Hertwig's root sheath. Clinically, it may not be apparent and is often an incidental finding on radiographic examination. Taurodontism is characterized by an increase vertically in the size of the body (crown) of the tooth at the expense of the roots. Pulp chambers appear elongated, with short, pointed roots located in the apical one-third of the tooth (Fig. 5-33). The prefix *tauro-* means "bull." The teeth are named after their similarity to bovine teeth, which typically have large crowns and short roots. Taurodontism is

seen in both primary and permanent dentitions and may occur in one or more teeth either unilaterally or bilaterally. Taurodontism has been reported in such syndromes as Klinefelter's syndrome and can be a component of one form of amelogenesis imperfecta (see Chapter 6). Clinical findings of taurodontism may necessitate the evaluation of the patient for a syndrome.

Supernumerary Roots

Supernumerary or extra tooth roots arise from additional extensions of Hertwig's root sheath. The exact cause is unknown. They are most often an incidental finding on radiographic examination, but may be difficult to detect. Supernumerary roots may occur on any tooth, but tend to be more common in the mandibular and maxillary third molars (Fig. 5-34). They may complicate endodontic therapy or tooth extraction, but otherwise cause no problems.

Abnormalities of Tooth Color

Coloration of teeth may be inherited as well as influenced by environmental factors. **Extrinsic stain** or **exogenous stain** on external surfaces of the teeth may be due to exposure to foods such as tea and coffee; vitamins, such as iron; and habits, such as smoking or chewing tobacco. Extrinsic stain can usually be removed. Over time, stains may become incorporated within cracks, crevices, and defects of enamel. **Intrinsic** (internal) staining, also known as **endogenous** staining, is incorporated during tooth development. Endogenous stains may result from ingested medications or systemically produced pigments.

Tetracycline Stain

Tetracycline is a broad-spectrum antibiotic that chelates calcium ions and becomes incorporated within any

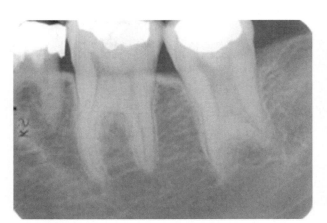

Figure 5–33 Taurodont. Mandibular molars showing increase in size of pulp chamber with small roots.

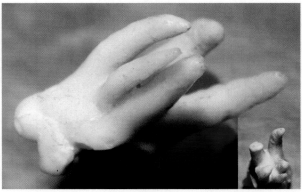

Figure 5–34 Supernumerary root. Maxillary molar with five roots.

mineralizing tissues, including bone, cartilage, enamel, and dentin. When ingested during tooth formation, it can be incorporated into the developing enamel and dentin. This may result in yellow to gray-brown intrinsic discolorations of the teeth (Fig. 5-35). The degree of staining is related to the patient's age at the time of administration, dosage, and duration of use. Staining is most often of concern in the permanent dentition, especially the anterior teeth, because it cannot be removed by conventional means. In addition to staining, tetracycline may also affect ameloblast metabolism, which results in defective enamel formation. (enamel hypoplasia). Tetracycline use should be avoided during the years of tooth formation. This includes use in pregnant and nursing mothers, because the drug can cross the placenta and enter breast milk.

Hemoglobin Pigment (Erythroblastosis Fetalis)

Erythroblastosis fetalis (Rh disease) develops in utero when the mother and fetus have different blood types. This commonly occurs as a result of a red blood cell surface antigen known as Rh. Antibodies produced by an Rh-negative mother cross the placenta and attack red blood cells in an Rh-positive fetus. This, in turn, produces anemia in the fetus and initiates the release of increased numbers of immature red blood cells into the fetal circulation. Destruction of the red blood cells, called **hemolysis,** produces elevated levels of hemoglobin and its breakdown product bilirubin. The yellow-brown pigments are deposited and incorporated in developing teeth, most often the primary dentition (Fig. 5-36), which eventually exfoliates; therefore, no treatment is needed. The permanent dentition is normal in coloration.

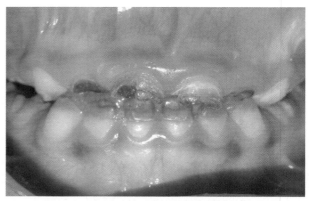

Figure 5–36   Bilirubin staining of teeth. Green discoloration of primary teeth in a child with congenital liver disease.

Enamel Hypoplasia

Enamel hypoplasia refers to incomplete or defective development of enamel as a result of disruption of ameloblast metabolism during enamel production. This can result from environmental factors, such as fluoride ingestion, nutrition, infection, and trauma. Inherited disorders of enamel formation are covered in more detail in Chapter 6.

Turner Tooth

Turner tooth describes enamel hypoplasia of one or two permanent teeth caused by localized disturbance of amelogenesis. The most common cause is infection or trauma associated with a primary tooth. Contact of the disturbance with the underlying developing permanent tooth may interfere with enamel formation by destroying or injuring the ameloblasts. Upon eruption, the tooth or teeth may appear misshapen and/or discolored (Fig. 5-37). Treatment is cosmetic restoration.

Contemporaneous Enamel Hypoplasia

Contemporaneous enamel hypoplasia is enamel hypoplasia that affects all teeth that are developing at the time of exposure to a harmful environmental agent. It affects multiple permanent teeth in a band-like pattern, reflecting the times of tooth development at which amelogenesis was disrupted. Contemporaneous enamel hypoplasia has usually been associated with systemic infections in young children, which produce a high fever affecting amelogenesis. Areas of enamel hypoplasia are prone to discoloration and staining. Cosmetic considerations are the main clinical concern, and treatment often consists of tooth-colored restorations or veneers.

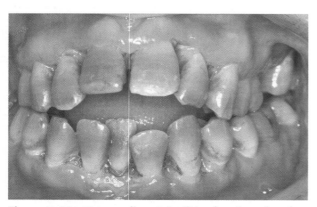

Figure 5–35   Tetracycline stain. Discoloration of teeth due to tetracycline use during childhood.

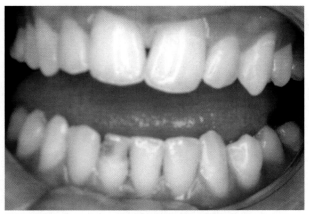

Figure 5–37 Turner tooth. Enamel hypoplasia and discoloration of tooth #25; deciduous tooth fractured, leading to pulpal necrosis.

Dental Fluorosis

Dental fluorosis is a condition in which amelogenesis is affected by ingestion of high levels of fluoride during tooth development. This can occur by drinking water with levels of fluoride exceeding 1 ppm, or ingestion of excess fluoride in vitamins. Fluorosis occurs during crown formation. Tooth eruption does not occur until crown formation is complete, so fluorosis only becomes apparent after eruption. The condition is characterized by generalized spotty defective enamel that ranges in severity from small, white, chalky spots and pitted defects to teeth that are extensively affected and described as "mottled." Defective areas are prone to staining and discoloration (Fig. 5-38). The main clinical concern with dental fluorosis is cosmetic. Treatment consists of surface restoration.

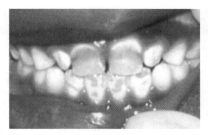

Figure 5–38 Fluorosis. Mottled enamel and hypocalcification in child who ingested excessive fluoride during tooth development.

DEVELOPMENTAL CYSTS OF THE HEAD AND NECK

A **cyst** is defined as a cavity or space within tissue that is lined by epithelium, and contains semisolid or fluid material. Cysts grow or increase in size by osmotic attraction of fluids into an interior space. They are called **intraosseous** when they occur within bone, and **extraosseous** when they occur outside of bone. Cysts that arise from remnants of epithelial tissue left over from tooth development are called **odontogenic cysts.** These only occur in the jaws or on the gingiva, as shown in Table 5-1. **Nonodontogenic cysts** arise from epithelial tissues unrelated to tooth development, as shown in Table 5-2.

Combination of both clinical and microscopic features is necessary to precisely identify a cyst. All true cysts have an epithelial lining, which can only be seen under the microscope. Microscopically, the majority of cysts have similar linings, composed of unremarkable nonkeratinizing simple or stratified squamous epithelium. Therefore, the location of the cyst is an important piece of information in formulating the diagnosis.

Table 5.1	Classification of Developmental Odontogenic[a] Cysts and Their Origins	
Intraosseous Cysts[b]	**Origin**	**Clinical Features**
Dentigerous cyst	Tooth follicle and reduced enamel epithelium	Pericoronal radiolucency
Primordial cyst	Failure of tooth germ to develop	Unilocular radiolucency where tooth did not form
Lateral periodontal cyst	Rests of Malassez	Unilocular radiolucency in periodontal ligament space
Odontogenic keratocyst	Any odontogenic epithelial tissue	Unilocular or multilocular radiolucency anywhere in jaws
Calcifying odontogenic cyst	Any odontogenic epithelial tissue	Well-defined mixed radiolucent/radiopaque; wide variety of locations
Buccal bifurcation cyst	Crevicular epithelium	Radiolucency in furcation of molars; swelling

Continued

Table 5.1	Classification of Developmental Odontogenic[a] Cysts and Their Origins—cont'd	

Extraosseous Cysts[c]

| Eruption cyst | Tooth follicle and reduced enamel epithelium | Bluish swelling in gingiva over erupting tooth; no radiographic features |
| Gingival cyst (also called dental lamina cyst) | Rests of Serres | Bluish swelling of gingiva over root surface; no radiographic features |

[a]Odontogenic cysts arise from remnants of tooth tissues.
[b]Intraosseous lesions develop inside bone and have radiographic features.
[c]Extraosseous lesions develop outside bone and will not have radiographic features.

Table 5.2	Classification of Nonodontogenic[a] Cysts of the Jaws	
Intraosseous Cysts[b]	**Origin**	**Clinical Features**
Nasopalatine duct cyst (also called incisive canal cyst)	Nasopalatine duct of the incisive canal	Heart-shaped radiolucency between maxillary central incisors; often intraoral swelling
Median palatine cyst	Remnants of fusion of palatine processes	Radiolucency along midline of palate; often intraoral swelling
"Globulomaxillary" cyst	Remnants of fusion between pre-maxilla and lateral palatine process[b] vs. odontogenic epithelium	Unilocular radiolucency between maxillary lateral and canine
Extraosseous		
Nasolabial cyst	Remnants of fusion of lateral nasal and maxillary processes during lip formation	Soft tissue swelling along nasolabial fold
Thyroglossal duct cyst	Remnants of the thyroglossal duct or tract, route of migration of thyroid gland	Soft tissue swelling in midline of neck above thyroid cartilage; may move upon swallowing
Cervical lymphoepithelial cyst	Unknown; remnants of developing lymphoid tissue within developing salivary gland within the upper neck	Soft tissue swelling of the lateral neck
Oral lymphoepithelial cyst	Remnants of developing lymphoid tissue entrapping surface epithelium	Small white or yellow nodules of oral epithelium in Waldeyer's ring
Epidermal inclusion cyst	Surface epithelial remnants inadvertently implanted within the submucosa	Small white or yellow nodules of oral epithelium in any oral location
Epidermoid cyst	Hair follicle epithelium	Dome-shaped soft tissue swelling of facial skin
Dermoid cyst	Surface skin entrapped in submucosal tissues	Soft tissue swelling of the midline floor of the mouth

[a]Nonodontogenic cysts arise from tissue in the orofacial region, not including tooth tissues.
[b]Source is disputed. Most globulomaxillary cysts are other odontogenic cysts (Table 5-1).

Other non-epithelial-lined spaces and anatomical defects that mimic cysts are found in the jaws; however, these are not true cysts because they lack an epithelial lining. They are best called **pseudocysts**. Table 5-3 lists several common pseudocysts encountered in the jaws.

Odontogenic Cysts

Odontogenic cysts arise from epithelial remnants of the developing tooth germ, called "rests." Rests of Serres are epithelial remnants of dental lamina that are found in the gingiva. Rests of Malassez are remnants of Hertwig's epithelial root sheath that are found in the periodontal ligament space. Epithelial cells in these rests multiply when they are stimulated, most often by the inflammatory response. They multiply to form small clusters of epithelium around a center that attracts fluid from adjacent connective tissues. This results in a cystic sac that gradually expands as fluid accumulates. For rests of Serres, the pressure from the growing cyst will cause a visible soft tissue swelling of the gingiva. For rests of Malassez, the pressure from the growing cyst will cause resorption of adjacent bone that appears radiographically as a well-defined radiolucency. This section includes a brief discussion of the commonly encountered odontogenic cysts in the oral cavity.

Follicular Cysts: Dentigerous Cyst and Eruption Cyst

There are two types of *follicular cysts*. Both occur when the reduced enamel epithelium surrounding the crown of an unerupted tooth (the *follicle*) becomes separated from the enamel surface and fluid accumulates within the newly formed space (Fig. 5-39). If the tooth is

embedded within alveolar bone, the cyst is referred to as a *dentigerous cyst*. Radiographically, a well-defined unilocular radiolucency is present around the crown of an unerupted tooth, attached at the cemento-enamel junction (Fig. 5-40A and B). These occur most frequently around impacted third molars, maxillary canines, and mandibular second premolars. Treatment is

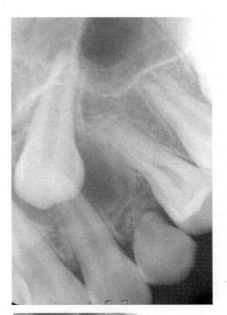

A

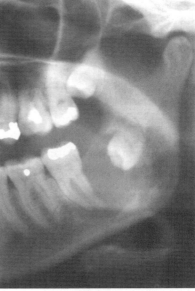

B

Figure 5–40 **A.** Dentigerous cyst: Canine; pericoronal radiolucency appears attached at CEJ. **B.** Dentigerous cyst: Third molar; pressure from developing dentigerous cyst is causing resorption of root of tooth #18.

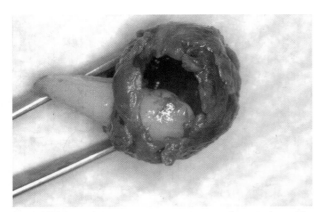

Figure 5–39 **Dentigerous cyst.** Extracted premolar with dentigerous cyst attached at cemento-enamel junction.

enucleation or removal of the entire cyst lining and contents.

Eruption cysts have the same origin as dentigerous cysts, but occur later in tooth development. They are located around the crown of an erupting tooth, in overlying soft tissue after the tooth has emerged through bone. Clinically, they appear as firm, pink or bluish swellings over an erupting tooth (Fig. 5-41). Radiographic examination reveals an erupting tooth attempting to penetrate surface soft tissues. Eruption cysts with a bluish coloration have been confused with mucoceles (see Chapter 2). However, mucoceles do not occur on gingiva, because gingiva does not contain minor salivary glands.

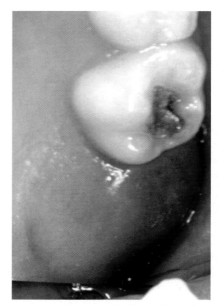

Figure 5–41   Eruption cyst. Molar under soft tissue has failed to erupt. Note the bluish appearance to the soft tissue.

Clinical Implications

Dentigerous cysts may become very large in size due to continued expansion. They are capable of resorbing surrounding bone and/or adjacent tooth roots. The diagnosis of dentigerous cyst cannot be made until the cyst is removed and examined microscopically. Other pathological conditions, such as odontogenic tumors, may mimic dentigerous cysts radiographically. Removal of the affected tooth and/or cystic tissue is the usual treatment.

In most cases of eruption cysts, the tooth eventually breaks through the overlying tissue and no treatment is necessary. If the cyst and/or dense tissue continue to hinder eruption, an opening may be created surgically to allow the tooth to erupt.

Primordial Cyst

Primordial cysts are believed to arise from degeneration of tooth germs during embryological development. Remnants of the enamel organ are thought to be the source of the epithelial lining. Primordial cysts are located in the space where a tooth should have formed. Clinical history is most often that of a missing tooth that never developed. The posterior mandible, especially the third molar region, is the most common site. Radiographic appearance is that of a unilocular, well-defined radiolucency in place of a tooth. Primordial cysts most frequently turn out to be odontogenic keratocysts, discussed next.

Odontogenic Keratocyst

Odontogenic keratocysts (OKCs) occur anywhere in the jaws, but are most commonly found in the posterior mandible. They only occur within bone. OKCs are well-defined unilocular (Fig. 5-42) or multilocular radiolucencies that may displace teeth or resorb tooth roots. Radiographically, their location may suggest dentigerous, primordial, or other odontogenic cysts or tumors. Microscopically, the epithelial lining of OKCs is uniquely parakeratinized (Fig. 5-43). Tiny *satellite cysts* arising away from the main cyst lining make OKCs difficult to eradicate. These cysts have a much higher recurrence rate than any other cyst. Their aggressive behavior and propensity for recurrence

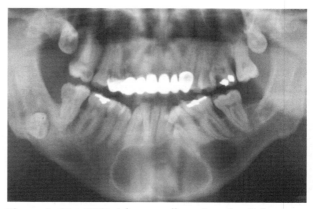

Figure 5–42   OKC. A large, well-corticated radiolucent lesion.

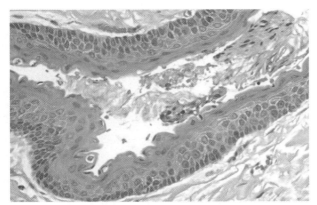

Figure 5–43 Lining of OKC showing keratin in the lumen. Parakeratotic stratified squamous epithelium with dark-staining basal cells lining lumen of odontogenic keratocyst.

have lead pathologists to suggest that this lesion actually is a cystic neoplasm, called **keratinizing cystic odontogenic tumor (KCOT)**. This tumor is discussed further in Chapter 7.

Clinical Implications

Multiple OKCs have been associated with the genetically linked nevoid basal cell carcinoma syndrome. Individuals with this syndrome have been reported to develop an initial OKC at an early age and then multiple cysts throughout their lifetime. See Chapter 6 for more details on identifying this syndrome.

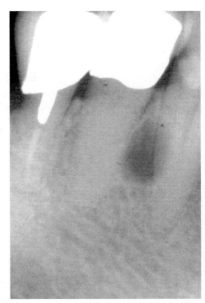

Figure 5–44 Lateral periodontal cyst. Unilocular radiolucency arising in periodontal ligament space of premolar; teeth are vital.

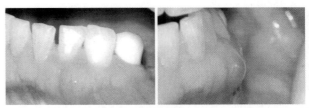

Figure 5–45 Gingival cyst. Soft fluctuant mass on facial surface at mucogingival junction. Note bluish coloration.

Lateral Periodontal Cyst

Lateral periodontal cysts arise in the periodontal ligament space from the rests of Malassez, most frequently in the mandibular premolar area. Pressure causes resorption of alveolar bone lateral to the tooth (Fig. 5-44). Radiographically, they appear as small unilocular radiolucencies between premolars. Lateral periodontal cysts are treated surgically and rarely recur.

Gingival Cyst

Gingival cysts are located in soft tissues surrounding the teeth, most often on the facial gingiva (Fig. 5-45). Believed to arise from the Rests of Serres, they are often referred to as *dental lamina cysts*. Gingival cysts may be seen in newborns at or shortly after birth, or in adults. They are typically small, fluctuant, and may have a bluish tint. Because they do not involve bone, they do not appear on radiographs. Gingival

cysts are treated surgically and are not known to recur.

Calcifying Odontogenic Cyst

Calcifying odontogenic cysts, also known as *Gorlin cysts*, are most common in the second to third decades of life, but can be seen at almost any age. Radiographically, this cyst differs from other odontogenic cysts in that it has a mixed radiolucent/radiopaque appearance caused by irregular calcifications within the cyst lining. Other odontogenic tumors and cysts may need to be ruled out depending on the location and appearance. Surgical excision is curative and recurrence is not expected. This cyst is not found as a part of a syndrome.

Buccal Bifurcation Cyst

Buccal bifurcation cysts are most commonly associated with the mandibular first molar. They are most likely to occur when the tooth has a defect referred to as cervical enamel extension. In this defect, enamel develops along the root surface and extends into the bifurcation area, preventing periodontal ligament attachment. The defect creates a "gap" where bacteria can accumulate and symptomatic infection can occur. Swelling that occurs is enclosed by crevicular epithelium. While the cyst itself is not "developmental," it is the result of an unusual developmental defect of enamel formation.

Nonodontogenic Cysts

During embryonic and fetal development, numerous processes must meet and fuse. Small fragments of residual ectoderm at these points of fusion may remain trapped within the underlying connective tissues. These embryonic rests can be stimulated in the same fashion as the rests of Malassez and Serres to form cysts. The resulting developmental cysts are unrelated to tooth development and are referred to as **nonodontogenic cysts.** Below are some of the more common nonodontogenic cysts that occur in the head and neck.

Nasopalatine Duct Cyst (Incisive Canal Cyst)

Nasopalatine duct cysts are the most common nonodontogenic cysts in the jaws. They originate in the nasopalatine duct located within the incisive canals. The terminal branch of the descending palatine artery and nasopalatine nerve are also located here. The duct and canals are so intimately related that it is often difficult to determine the source of the cyst, hence the two names. Cystic changes within the epithelial lining of the duct may lead to soft tissue swelling behind the maxillary central incisors. Radiographically, there is an intraosseous, well-defined, unilocular radiolucency between or adjacent to the roots of the central incisors (Fig. 5-46). This may give the cyst a heart-shaped appearance. Drainage from the cyst via the canal can occur, and patients may complain of a salty or metallic taste.

Median Palatine Cyst

Median palatine cysts are located in the midline of the hard palate in a more posterior location than the nasopalatine duct cyst (Fig. 5-47). The origin is believed to be from remnants of embryonic epithelium trapped during fusion of the lateral palatine shelves. Another theory is that the median palatine cyst represents a nasopalatine duct cyst that develops in the posterior-most portion of the incisive canal.

Clinical Implications

Nasopalatine duct cysts, nasolabial cysts, and median palatine cysts are treated with surgical excision and do not recur. Although these cysts are not associated with pulpal pathology, pulp testing of adjacent teeth prior to treatment is necessary to rule out chronic apical periodontitis (granuloma) or apical cyst formation.

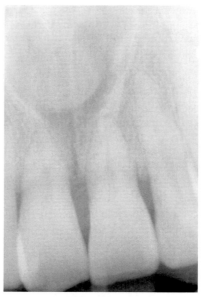

Figure 5–46   Nasopalatine duct cyst. Well-defined unilocular radiolucency originating between the maxillary central incisors, which are vital.

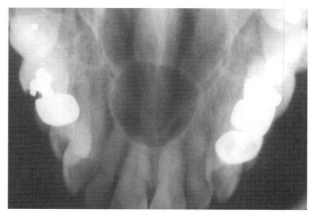

Figure 5–47   Median palatal cyst. Anteriorly positioned median palatal cyst.

Nasolabial Cyst

Nasolabial cysts are found within soft tissues of the lip and below the ala of the nose (Fig. 5-48A). This cyst is thought to arise from embryonic remnants of epithelium trapped during fusion of the lateral, medial, and maxillary processes during formation of the upper lip. The cyst presents as a facial swelling that expands the gingivolabial sulcus and nasolabial fold (Fig. 5-48B). Because this represents a remnant of soft tissue fusion, there is no bone component and radiographs are negative.

Epidermal Inclusion Cyst

Epidermal inclusion cysts most commonly occur within the soft tissues of the skin, but may occur within the oral cavity. They are the result of implantation of epidermal elements into the dermis of skin or submucosa of the oral cavity as a result of minor trauma, surgery, or other unknown cause. These cysts are usually small, white, and asymptomatic. They may be somewhat movable beneath the surface, except when located on masticatory mucosa.

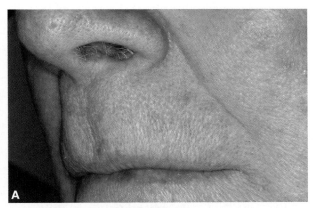

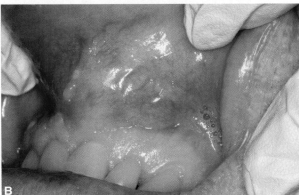

Figure 5–48 **Nasolabial cyst. A.** Soft tissue swelling in nasolabial fold. **B.** Intraoral swelling fills maxillary vestibule.

Epidermoid Cyst of the Skin (Sebaceous Cysts)

Epidermoid cysts are slow-growing, painless, freely movable lumps beneath the skin. They originate from a hair follicle that has become inflamed, known as *folliculitis*. Hair follicles contain several layers of epithelium, some of which become involved in formation of the cyst. Because hair follicles have an associated sebaceous gland, these cysts are often referred to as *sebaceous cysts*. Clinically, they have a nodular or pimple-shaped appearance and contain keratinaceous material made up of desquamated keratin and sebum.

Clinical Implications

Epidermal inclusion cysts and epidermoid cysts are treated with surgical excision and do not recur. Epidermoid cysts may be seen as a clinical feature in Gardner's syndrome (see Chapter 6).

Dermoid Cyst

Dermoid cysts appear to arise from entrapped surface epithelial tissue remnants during embryonic development. Unlike epidermoid cysts, skin structures such as sebaceous glands, sweat glands, and hair follicles are found within the epithelium that lines the central cavity of dermoid cysts. Dermoid cysts range from several millimeters to centimeters and are commonly located in the floor of the mouth at the midline. Dermoid cysts most commonly occur above the mylohyoid muscle, although an occasional dumbbell-shaped cyst extends into the submental area, giving the patient a "double chin" appearance. Cysts that occur above the mylohyoid muscle may displace the tongue back and upwards toward the roof of the mouth. Large dermoid cysts that cause significant displacement of the tongue may interfere with eating, swallowing, and speaking. Surgical removal is indicated.

Cervical Lymphoepithelial Cyst (Branchial Cleft Cyst)

Cervical lymphoepithelial cysts present as unilateral, soft-tissue, fluctuant swellings that arise in the lateral aspect of the neck anterior to the sternocleidomastoid muscle. They most commonly occur late in childhood or in early adulthood. The origin was once thought to be from remnants of the second branchial arch, hence the older name of *branchial cleft cyst*. Other theories of development include an origin from entrapped salivary duct epithelium in the lymph nodes of the lateral neck. Clinically, the cysts are well circumscribed and can reach 2 to 5 cm in diameter. They may begin after a respiratory infection and gradually increase in size. Treatment consists of surgical excision.

Oral Lymphoepithelial Cyst

Oral lymphoepithelial cysts are much smaller than cervical lymphoepithelial cysts. They develop within benign lymphoid aggregates in the oral or pharyngeal mucosa, wherever lymphoid tissue is located. The most common location is the floor of the mouth, lateral and ventral tongue, and soft palate, especially the mucosa above the pharyngeal tonsils. This zone of the oral cavity is referred to as Waldeyer's ring. Oral lymphoepithelial cysts present as movable, painless, submucosal nodules with yellow or yellow-white coloration. They are most often less than 0.5 cm in diameter and can occur at any age, but are more common during the teen years, after which they may regress. Treatment consists of conservative surgical excision.

Thyroglossal Duct Cyst

The *thyroglossal duct* (tract) is the route that the thyroid gland follows from foramen caecum on the posterior tongue to its permanent location in the anterior neck. Remnants of the duct may form cysts anywhere from the foramen cecum to just above the suprasternal notch (Fig. 5-49). Thyroglossal duct cysts are soft, fluctuant, and range in size from small (1 cm) to large (10 to 12 cm) (Fig. 5-50). Because of their origin, they are almost always observed in the midline of the neck. If they adhere to the hyoid bone, the mass appears to move as the patient swallows. Surgical excision is required to relieve the mass.

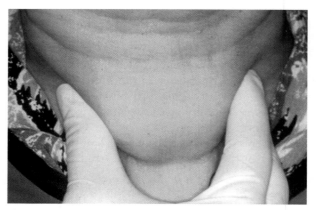

Figure 5–50 **Thyroglossal duct cyst.** Adult female with midline swelling of the neck that moves when she swallows.

Globulomaxillary Cyst

Globulomaxillary is a term used to describe an anatomical area between the roots of the maxillary lateral incisors and cuspids. This area represents the junction of the "globular" portion of the medial nasal and the maxillary processes during embryonic development. The origin of this cyst was thought to be from remnants of embryonic epithelium trapped along the fusion line of the primary and secondary palate; however, recent evidence suggests that cysts in this location are of odontogenic origin because the majority exhibit odontogenic features when examined under the microscope. Radiographically, cysts in this area appear as a well-defined, unilocular radiolucency with an oval or inverted pear shape (Fig. 5-51). Vitality testing is required to rule out chronic apical periodontitis (granuloma) or an apical cyst (Chapter 2). The final diagnosis is dependent

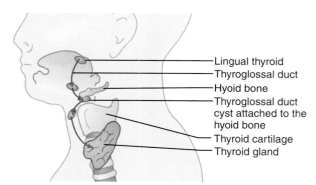

Lingual thyroid
Thyroglossal duct
Hyoid bone
Thyroglossal duct cyst attached to the hyoid bone
Thyroid cartilage
Thyroid gland

Figure 5–49 Path of thyroglossal duct and associated pathology.

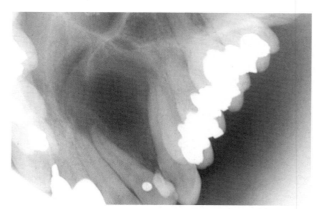

Figure 5–51 **Globulomaxillary cyst.** Radiolucent lesion of the globulomaxillary area between maxillary lateral and canine.

Table 5.3	Pseudocysts of the Jaws*	
Interosseous	**Origin**	**Clinical Features**
Static bone cavity	Depression on lingual surface of mandible due to presence of sub-mandibular gland during development	Well-defined radiolucency of posterior mandible below the mylohyoid line
Simple bone cavity / traumatic bone cavity	Degeneration of blood clot during healing of bone injury	Well-defined radiolucency that may "scallop" between roots; at surgery, cavity empty
Hyperplastic dental follicle	Degeneration of reduced enamel epithelium of enamel organ	Pericoronal radiolucency

*Intrabony lesions with no epithelial lining.

on microscopic features. Most pathologists do not consider the globulomaxillary cyst to be a distinct pathologic entity because they are typically diagnosed as odontogenic keratocysts, radicular cysts, or other odontogenic cysts.

Developmental Anomalies That Mimic Cysts of the Jaws (Pseudocysts)

Static bone cavity, also known as *Stafne defect*, is an anatomical defect of the mandible that forms during jaw development. When a large submandibular gland is present along the lingual surface of the mandible, forming bone may accommodate the gland, resulting in a concavity where the gland was located. This appears radiographically as a well-circumscribed, oval to round radiolucency near the angle of the mandible below the mylohyoid line (Fig. 5-52). Static bone cavities are not symptomatic nor can they be palpated intraorally. Most static bone cavities are an incidental finding observed in adults, predominantly males. Because they have no epithelial lining, they are not true cysts. Depending on their location, they may mimic odontogenic cysts. An occlusal radiograph or a CT scan may reveal the true nature of the defect. No treatment is indicated.

Simple bone cavity, formerly known as *simple bone cyst*, is also known as *traumatic bone cavity*. These do not have an epithelial lining and so are not true cysts. Simple bone cavities consist of an empty air-filled space. They are found most frequently in the mandible in young adult males. Radiographically, a unilocular, well-defined radiolucency may appear to scallop between the roots of existing vital teeth (Fig. 5-53). The exact cause is unknown. It is believed that trauma to the mandible is followed by formation of a blood clot. For reasons unknown, the clot is destroyed or resorbed, leaving behind an empty cavity. Surgical exploration reveals an

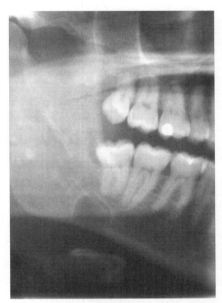

Figure 5–52   Static bone cavity also known as Stafne defect. Well-defined radiolucency in posterior mandible below the mylohyoid line.

air-filled empty space. Curettage of the cavity walls stimulates new clot formation, followed by new bone formation, which eventually fills the empty space.

Hyperplastic dental follicle is seen around the crowns of unerupted teeth. The exact cause is unknown. Most likely it occurs as the tooth attempts to erupt, causing pressure and tension in surrounding soft tissues. This provokes a reactive response, resulting in soft tissue hyperplasia, which appears radiolucent on radiographs. This creates the impression of a cystic cavity (Fig. 5-54) and may mimic a dentigerous cyst. The treatment is excision of the hyperplastic follicle and/or extraction of the tooth.

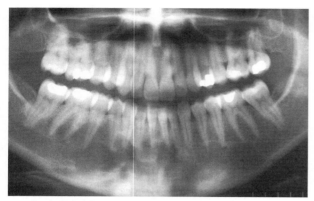

Figure 5–53 Simple bone cavity. Simple bone cavity extends from right first molar to left first molar; note scalloping between teeth.

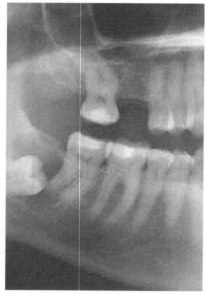

Figure 5–54 Hyperplastic dental follicle. Well-defined radiolucent lesion around crown of tooth #32; no cyst cavity was found at surgery, only dense connective tissue.

Critical Thinking Questions

Case 5-1: A female infant was born with a cleft lip. She is the only child born to this family who has this congenital defect. Her mother is concerned that she "did something wrong" by drinking champagne at her sister's wedding while she was 6 months pregnant.

• • •

Describe when and how the cleft developed during embryonic life.

Explain to the mother whether or not the glass of champagne influenced the formation of her daughter's lip.

Discuss the role of teratogens in cleft development.

Discuss future dental considerations and problems for this patient.

Case 5-2: A mother brings her 10-year-old son to the dental office with a chief complaint that "his tooth came in with a cavity." You observe an otherwise healthy dentition. Tooth #20 has a malformed crown and appears discolored (brown). The enamel is not "soft"; the explorer does not penetrate the enamel. The mother wants to know how it got this way, as her understanding of caries includes exposure to sugars and poor oral hygiene. She wants to know if it is possible he was eating candy at school.

• • •

Describe when and how this developed during development of the tooth.

What questions can you ask the mother to help you explain to her what happened?

What possible etiologic factors could have contributed to the development of this defect?

Is there anything the child or the mother did to cause this problem?

What steps can be taken to address the concerns with this tooth?

Case 5-3: A 24-year-old man presents with the chief complaint that his lower right jaw is sore. A panoramic radiograph shows that tooth #32 is impacted. You detect a 4-mm radiolucent space around the crown. Bone expansion is not detected intraorally. The patient wants to know how he got "a cavity" in this tooth.

• • •

What are some possible diagnoses for this pericoronal radiolucency?

Explain to the patient why this occurred.

Explain to the patient how this is different from a cavity.

The patient says he is reluctant to have the tooth removed, he simply wants pain medication. What information can you give him to help with his decision-making process?

What steps should be taken to address the patient's chief complaint?

Case 5-4: Your 32-year-old new female patient presents with a bluish fluctuant swelling on the facial gingiva over tooth #20. She says her previous dentist told her she has a "blocked saliva gland." He said it does not have to be removed right away.

• • •

Explain to the patient why this is not likely a mucocele.

Describe to her what the most likely diagnosis is.

She wants to know how it happened. What can you tell her?

Review Questions

1. **Clefts are considered the most common developmental facial abnormality. They occur during embryonic life between weeks**
   A. one to three.
   B. three to five.
   C. six to eleven.
   D. twelve to twenty-four.

2. **Tethering of the anterior tongue to the floor of the mouth is called**
   A. ankyloglossia.
   B. aglossia.
   C. microsomia.
   D. macroglossia.

3. **Which one of the following is often associated with Down syndrome?**
   A. Commissural lip pits
   B. Hemifacial microsomia
   C. Lingual thyroid
   D. Macroglossia

4. **Lingual thyroid is most frequently observed**
   A. near the foramen cecum.
   B. in the floor of the mouth.
   C. on the ventral tongue.
   D. at the junction of the hard and soft palates.

5. **Hemifacial microsomia**
   A. rarely develops before embryonic week 16.
   B. is the most common birth defect in the head and neck.
   C. commonly presents as underdevelopment of one-half of the face.
   D. has few cosmetic implications for the patient.

6. **Which one of the following is the most common supernumerary tooth?**
   A. Maxillary lateral incisor
   B. Mesiodens
   C. Maxillary third molar
   D. Mandibular central incisor

7. **In which one of the following is less than the normal number of teeth present?**
   A. Fusion
   B. Gemination
   C. Peg lateral
   D. Mesiodens

8. **Talon cusp is an example of**
   A. dens-in-dente.
   B. dens invaginatus.
   C. dens evaginatus.
   D. gemination.

9. **The most important dental complication of both dens invaginatus and evaginatus is**
   A. pulp exposure and subsequent apical pathology.
   B. aesthetics and malocclusion.
   C. increased incidence of gingivitis and periodontal disease.
   D. calculus and dental plaque retention.

10. **Radiographically, enamel pearls may be mistaken for**
    A. caries.
    B. internal resorption.
    C. tori.
    D. calculus.

11. **Which one of the following conditions is characterized by an elongated pulp chamber and short, pointed roots?**
    A. Dens-in-dente
    B. Macrodontia
    C. Taurodontism
    D. Dens invaginatus

12. **The union of one or more teeth by cementum is**
    A. fusion.
    B. concrescence.
    C. gemination.
    D. ankylosis.

13. **Which one of the following conditions develops *in utero* and results in intrinsic staining of the primary dentition?**
    A. Contemporaneous enamel hypoplasia
    B. Fluorosis
    C. Turner tooth
    D. Erythroblastosis fetalis

14. **Enamel hypoplasia affecting the facial surface of multiple, anterior permanent teeth in a band-like pattern is known as**
    A. contemporaneous enamel hypoplasia.
    B. fluorosis.
    C. Turner tooth.
    D. erythroblastic enamel hypoplasia.

15. **The most useful clinical feature for determining the type of cyst is**
    A. size.
    B. location.
    C. duration.
    D. degree of discomfort or pain.

16. **Cysts with an origin related to tooth development are termed?**
    A. Intraosseous
    B. Extraosseous
    C. Odontogenic
    D. Pseudocysts

17. **Which cyst is always located around the crown of an unerupted tooth?**
    A. Dentigerous
    B. Primordial
    C. Odontogenic keratocyst
    D. Lateral periodontal

18. **A firm, pink or bluish swelling over an erupting tooth best describes which cyst?**
    A. Dentigerous
    B. Primordial
    C. Odontogenic keratocyst
    D. Eruption

19. **A patient with multiple odontogenic keratocysts should be evaluated for**
    A. cleidocranial dysplasia.
    B. Gardner's syndrome.
    C. nevoid basal cell carcinoma syndrome.
    D. contemporaneous enamel hypoplasia.

20. **Which one of the following cysts may occur anywhere from the foramen cecum to the suprasternal notch?**
    A. Static bone
    B. Simple bone
    C. Thyroglossal tract
    D. Oral lymphoepithelial

REFERENCES

Avery, J, Chiego, D: Essentials of Oral Histology and Embryology: A Clinical Approach, ed 3. Elsevier Mosby, St. Louis, 2006.

Cawson, RA, Odell, E: Cawson's Essentials of Oral Pathology and Oral Medicine, ed. 8. Churchill Livingstone, London, 2008.

Kumar, GS: Orban's Oral Histology and Embryology, ed. 12. Elsevier, St. Louis, 2008.

Nanci, A: Ten Cate's Oral Histology: Development, Structure, and Function, ed. 7. Elsevier Health Sciences, St. Louis, 2007.

Neville, B, Damm, DD, Allen, CM, Bouquot, J: Oral and Maxillofacial Pathology, ed. 3. Saunders, Philadelphia, 2009.

Regezi, JA, Sciubba, JJ, Jordan, RCK: Oral Pathology, ed. 5. Saunders, Philadelphia, 2008.

Scully, C, de Almeida, OP, Bagan, J, Dios, PD, Taylor, AM: Oral Medicine and Pathology at a Glance. Blackwell, London, 2010.

Shear, M, Speight, P: Cysts of the Oral and Maxillofacial Regions, ed. 4. Wiley-Blackwell, Oxford, 2007.

Disorders of Genetics and Inheritance

● Learning Outcomes

At the end of this chapter, the student will be able to:

6.1. Define DNA, chromosome, genes, and alleles.

6.2. Compare autosomal versus x-linked modes of genetic disease transmission.

6.3. Differentiate between dominant and recessive modes of transmission.

6.4. Define genetic mutations and chromosomal damage.

6.5. Discuss carrier state, incomplete penetrance, and variable expressivity.

6.6. Define the term *syndrome*; recognize the major features of Papillon-Lefèvre syndrome and describe its effects on the periodontium.

6.7. Recognize the principal features of hereditary gingival enlargement.

6.8. Recognize and describe the principal features of the craniosynostosis syndromes and Treacher-Collins syndrome.

6.9. Explain why early detection in the dental office may be crucial in hereditary hemorrhagic telangiectasia, Gardner's syndrome, Cowden syndrome, and Peutz-Jegher's syndrome.

6.10. Recognize and describe the principal features, including mode of transmission, for the bone disorders osteogenesis imperfecta, osteopetrosis,

Continued

fibrous dysplasia, cherubism, and cleidocranial dysplasia.

6.11. Describe the principal features of nevoid basal cell carcinoma syndrome.

6.12. Recognize and describe the principal features of disorders of the oral soft tissues, including white sponge nevus and hereditary benign intraepithelial dyskeratosis.

6.13. Recognize and describe the principal features of the three forms of amelogenesis imperfecta.

6.14. Recognize and describe the two inherited disorders of dentin, dentinogenesis imperfecta and dentin dysplasia.

6.15. Describe the dental problems experienced by children with odontohypophosphatasia.

BASIC PRINCIPLES OF GENETIC AND INHERITED DISORDERS

Currently, the study of **genetics** is a major focus in scientific investigation of disease, seeking to solve the mysteries of causation and develop new treatments. Although it is beyond the scope of this book to explain all aspects of genetics, an understanding of the basic principles of genetic and inherited diseases is essential. Patients may present with inherited syndromes and disorders that directly impact dental practice. This chapter seeks to familiarize dental hygienists in recognizing inherited abnormalities that result in alteration in form or function of the head and neck, and directly or indirectly impact dental care.

Basics of Genetics

Deoxyribonucleic acid (DNA) is the material in most organisms that transmits inheritance. All cells of a given individual have the same DNA, which is located in the cell nucleus. DNA can replicate, or make copies of itself. Strands of DNA are arranged in a double-helix formation that serves as a pattern for duplication, so inherited characteristics can be passed on to new generations of cells (Fig. 6-1). Newly formed cells should contain an exact copy of DNA from the parent cell.

Chromosomes

DNA molecules are packaged into tiny units of organization called **chromosomes** (see Fig. 6-1). Chromosomes are only visible in the cell's nucleus when it is dividing. Each chromosome has a tight central point called the *centromere*, which separates the chromosome into two sections or arms. The short arm of the chromosome is called the *p arm*. The long arm of the chromosome is called the *q arm*. The location of the centromere on each chromosome gives the chromosome its characteristic shape, as can be seen in Figure 6-1. The letters *p* and *q* are also used to designate the location of specific genes on the chromosome. If the gene is located on the short arm, it is designated *p* for *petit* (French); on the long arm it is indicated as *q*. The combination of numbers and letters provide a gene's "address" on a chromosome. An example would be the gene *BRCA2*, which is associated with breast cancer. It is located on 13q12, which means it is seen on the long arm of chromosome 13 in the twelfth position. These designations help geneticists develop a genetic map that identifies where on a chromosome a particular trait is located.

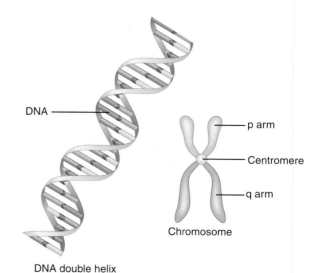

DNA double helix

Figure 6–1 **DNA and chromosomes**. Each chromosome has a centromere that gives the chromosome its characteristic shape. The "p" and "q" designate the location of specific genes on the chromosome.

Genes

Genes are segments or sequences of the DNA that determine specific traits or characteristics of a person. They determine the traits of individual cells and tissues. A *gene* is a unit of nucleoprotein (protein found in the nucleus of a cell) that carries the basic instructions for a characteristic capable of being passed on to offspring. Genes determine eye color, hair color, tooth shape, etc. The precise part of a gene that actually determines specific color or shape is called an **allele** (Fig. 6-2).

Chromosomal Abnormalities

Karyotype is the term used to describe the number and appearance of chromosomes in the nucleus. The study of karyotypes is part of *cytogenetics*. A *karyogram*, seen in Figure 6-3, depicts pairs of chromosomes taken from the nucleus of a cell. The normal human karyotypes contain 22 pairs of autosomal chromosomes and one pair of sex chromosomes. Any variation from the standard karyotype may indicate the patient is at risk for developmental abnormalities.

Euploid refers to the correct or normal number of chromosomes. In humans, each cell normally contains 23 pairs of chromosomes, for a total of 46. The majority of human cells are *diploid*, having the normal two sets of chromosomes. Reproductive or sex cells (spermatozoon or an ovum) have half the number of chromosomes and are termed *haploid*. Diseases can result if the number or structure of the chromosomes is altered. *Aneuploid* cells are missing one or more chromosomes. *Trisomy* is the term used when there are three rather than the normal two chromosomes. *Monosomy* refers to a cell with one chromosome, a condition that does not support life.

Even if the correct number of chromosomes is present, structural defects may occur when the cell is actively dividing. **Deletion** occurs when a portion of the chromosome goes missing during cell division. **Translocation** occurs when two chromosomes exchange parts. **Inversion** occurs when the chromosome breaks and is reinserted in the wrong location.

Modes and Patterns of Gene Transmission

Inheritance patterns trace the transmission of genetically encoded traits, conditions, or diseases to offspring. The mode of transmission refers to the way the

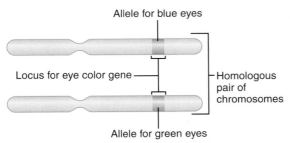

Allele for blue eyes

Locus for eye color gene

Homologous pair of chromosomes

Allele for green eyes

Figure 6–2   Two chromosomes showing the location of the eye color gene. One parent donates a green eye allele and the other donates a blue eye allele.

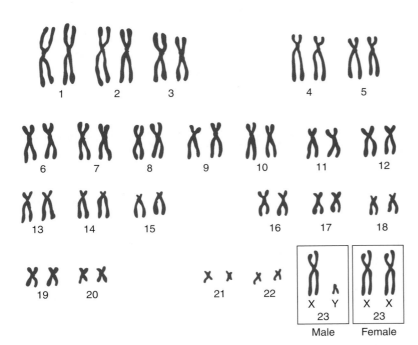

Figure 6–3   Cytogenetics uses a karyotype of an individual's chromosome to help identify any abnormalities. (From Taber's Cyclopedic Medical Dictionary, ed. 21. F.A. Davis, Philadelphia, 2009, p 1258.)

gene is expressed, or becomes operational. Several modes of inheritance are discussed here.

Autosomal Versus X-Linked Disorders

Twenty-two pairs of chromosomes, out of the normal 23 pairs, are called **autosomes**. They appear the same in both males and females. The twenty-third pair, the **sex chromosomes**, differs between males and females. Females have a pair of X chromosomes, whereas males have one X and one Y chromosome. When an allele for a disorder is carried on an autosomal chromosome, it is referred to as an *autosomal disorder*. If the allele is carried on a sex chromosome, it is referred to as an *X-linked* or *Y-linked disorder*. Y-linked disorders are exceptionally rare, whereas X-linked are more common.

Dominant Versus Recessive

Genes come in pairs. A pair of genes from each parent participates in determining a trait such as eye color. There are two alleles for each inherited trait. These may be the same (homozygous) or different (heterozygous). If one parent has blue eyes and the other has green eyes, and the child's eyes are blue, then the allele on the gene from the parent with the blue eyes was expressed. Another term for this is **dominant**. The allele that was not expressed, the green eye allele, was **recessive**. When both parents pass on a recessive allele, then the offspring has that allele. For example, if both of your parents have green eyes, then most likely your eyes are also green because there is no blue allele to dominate the green allele and block it from expressing itself. The term **express** in genetics indicates a process that takes inherited information in genes to make a specific functional product. Alleles rather than genes are the main reason each of us is unique.

In disease, only one copy of a gene is required for a person to be affected by an *autosomal dominant disorder*. Each affected person usually has one affected parent; therefore, there is a 50 percent chance that a child will inherit the mutated gene (Fig. 6-4).

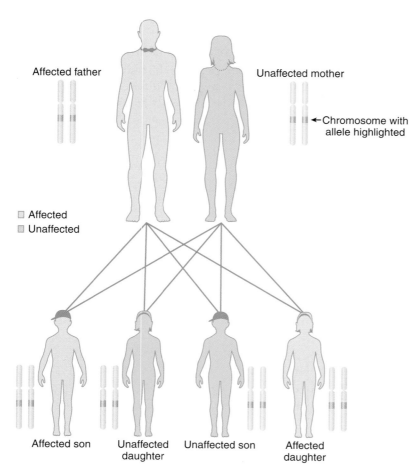

Autosomal dominant

Affected father

Unaffected mother

←Chromosome with allele highlighted

☐ Affected
☐ Unaffected

Affected son

Unaffected daughter

Unaffected son

Affected daughter

Figure 6–4 Pattern of autosomal dominant inheritance. The "affected" allele represents a genetic defect that may be passed on to offspring.

Autosomal recessive disorders require two copies of the disease allele for a person to be affected. Affected individuals usually have unaffected parents who each carry a single copy of the disease allele. The parents are referred to as *carriers*. Two unaffected people who each carry one copy of the disease (mutated) allele have a 25 percent chance with each pregnancy of having a child affected by the disorder. At conception, each sibling of an affected individual has a 25 percent chance of being affected, a 50 percent chance of being an asymptomatic carrier, and a 25 percent chance of being unaffected and not a carrier (Fig. 6-5).

X-linked recessive disorders are caused by mutations in genes on the X chromosome. Males are more frequently affected than females. The sons of a man with an X-linked recessive disorder will not be affected because their X chromosome comes from their mother. All daughters will carry one copy of the mutated allele. A woman who is a carrier of an X-linked recessive disorder has a 50 percent chance of having sons who are affected and a 50 percent chance of having daughters who carry one copy of the mutated allele, and are therefore carriers (Fig. 6-6).

Carriers are seen mainly in recessive disorders. These individuals have inherited a genetic trait or mutation but do not show symptoms of the disorder. They are able to pass the gene on to their offspring, who may then express the gene (have the disorder). The disease appears only when two carriers have children. Each child has a 25 percent chance of having the disease. Examples of disorders involving carriers are hemophilia and sickle cell disease.

X-linked dominant disorders are very rare and are caused by mutations in genes on the X chromosome. Males and females are both affected in these disorders, with males typically being more severely affected than females. Some X-linked dominant conditions are fatal in males either *in utero* or shortly after birth, and are therefore predominantly seen in females.

Autosomal recessive

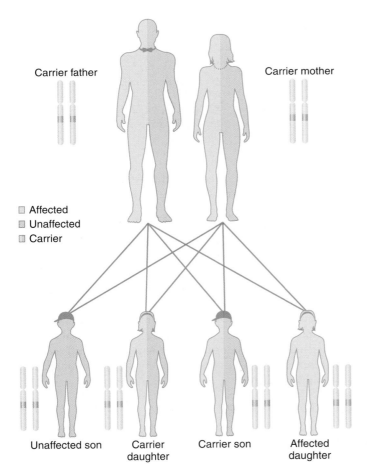

Carrier father

Carrier mother

☐ Affected
☐ Unaffected
☐ Carrier

Unaffected son
Carrier daughter
Carrier son
Affected daughter

Figure 6–5 Pattern of autosomal recessive inheritance with identification of carriers.

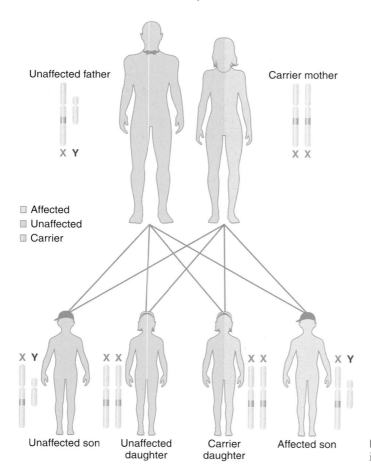

X-linked recessive, carrier mother

Unaffected father

X Y

Carrier mother

X X

☐ Affected
☐ Unaffected
☐ Carrier

X Y   X X   X X   X Y

Unaffected son   Unaffected daughter   Carrier daughter   Affected son

Figure 6–6 X-linked recessive disorder pattern of inheritance with identification of carrier.

Penetrance and Expressivity

Reduced penetrance and *variable expressivity* are factors that influence the effects of particular genetic changes. These factors usually affect disorders that have an autosomal dominant pattern of inheritance.

Penetrance is the proportion of individuals carrying a particular variation of a gene or allele that also express an associated trait. Not all individuals who possess a defective gene or allele actually have the disease. Penetrance is said to be *reduced* or *incomplete* when some individuals fail to express the trait, even though they carry the allele. For example, if a gene responsible for a particular disorder has 95 percent penetrance, then 95 percent of those with the mutation will develop the disease, whereas 5 percent will not. "Lack of penetrance" means that the individual carries a gene with a dominant effect without presenting any clinical manifestations of the gene.

Reduced penetrance probably results from a combination of unknown genetic, environmental, and lifestyle factors.

Variable expressivity refers to the range of signs and symptoms that may occur in different people with the same genetic condition. It is the degree of clinical manifestations of a trait or characteristic. Many genetic disorders can demonstrate signs and symptoms that differ among affected individuals. For example, some Down syndrome patients have a lower than normal IQ, while others present with normal intelligence. Variable expressivity is probably caused by a combination of unknown genetic, environmental, and lifestyle factors.

Genotype Versus Phenotype

An individual's **genotype** is the set of genes that it carries—its full hereditary information. In other words, genotype is an individual's genetic composition. An individual's **phenotype** is all of its visibly observable characteristics that are created by the genes' codes. In other words, phenotype is the observable appearance. For example, when the genotype melanocortin-1 receptor (MC1R) is found on chromosome 16, the phenotype is red hair.

Mutations

A **mutation** is a permanent change in the DNA sequence that makes up a gene. Mutations may occur before birth or after birth. Before birth, there are two ways mutations can occur. They may be inherited from a parent at the time of fertilization of egg and sperm. These are called *germline mutations* and are present throughout a person's life in all cells. Mutations may occur just after fertilization, often as a result of exposure to a teratogen. Teratogens are agents that may disturb the development of an embryo or fetus. Examples of teratogens include radiation, maternal infections, chemicals, and drugs. These may produce what are called *new (de novo) mutations*. De novo mutations may explain genetic disorders in which an affected child has a mutation but has no family history of the disorder because it was not carried in either the sperm or the ovum.

Another type of mutation that occurs after birth is called *acquired* or *somatic*. Environmental factors, such as ultraviolet radiation from the sun, chemical exposure, or radiation exposure, cause damage to the DNA that is then carried on in each subsequent cell division. Also, if a mistake is made as DNA copies itself during cell division, an acquired mutation may occur. Cells carry a "toolkit" of DNA repair enzymes, but if the damage overwhelms the cell's ability to repair itself, the mutation results. Acquired mutations cannot be passed on to offspring.

Syndromes

A **syndrome** is a collection of signs and symptoms that occur together and characterize a particular abnormality or condition. A syndrome includes a number of *essential* characteristics, which, when concurrent, lead to the diagnosis of the condition. The signs and symptoms may appear completely unrelated. An example is Down syndrome. This disease is caused by trisomy on chromosome 21. The signs include cardiac abnormalities; intussusceptions; gastric reflux; hypothyroidism; excess skin at the nape of the neck; flattened nose; single crease in the palm of the hand; small ears; small mouth; upward slanting eyes; wide, short hands

with short fingers; white spots on the colored part of the eye (Brushfield spots); impulsive behavior; short attention span; and slow learning. One must wonder how such a widely varied and seemingly unrelated group of symptoms all arise together from one altered chromosome.

There are hundreds of syndromes, only some of which will be discussed here. Many syndromes are **eponymous**, which means they were named after the person who first described them. For example, Gorlin syndrome is named after Dr. Robert Gorlin, who helped describe this and many syndromes involving the head and orofacial structures.

Genetic disorders rarely have effective treatments, though gene therapy is being tested as a possible treatment. Gene therapy is a technique for correcting defective genes responsible for disease development. Researchers may use one of several approaches for correcting faulty genes, such as inserting a normal gene to replace a nonfunctional gene, swapping the abnormal gene for a normal gene, repairing the abnormal gene, or turning the abnormal gene off. Gene therapy is currently not standard of care, but is still in experimental stages.

GENETIC AND INHERITED DISORDERS OF THE HEAD AND NECK

Genetic and inherited malformations of the head and neck are common, with approximately 2 percent of infants being born with abnormalities that usually arise during fetal life. Many of these malformations can be attributed to defects in genes that regulate the formation of the head, neck, and oral structures. Several hundred of these conditions exist. In this section, the focus will be on some disorders of periodontium, jaws, facial structures, and oral soft tissues.

Disorders of the Periodontium/Gingiva

Inherited disorders of the periodontium and the gingiva are rare but are of interest to the dental hygienist because of their impact on oral health.

Papillon-Lefèvre Syndrome

Papillon-Lefèvre syndrome is inherited in an autosomal recessive manner and is characterized by both dermatological and oral manifestations. It affects approximately 1 to 4 per million people and an additional 2 to 4 per 1,000 people are carriers. It is caused by a mutation in the cathepsin C gene that leads to loss of cathepsin C function. Cathepsin

C is an enzyme that assists in proper development of the skin. It also is important in the inflammatory response (Chapter 2) because it aids in chemotaxis of neutrophils and allows for phagocytosis, two important steps in fighting infections. Therefore, in this disease patients have abnormal skin and a decreased ability to fight infection because of their defective gene.

The most prominent clinical features that result from loss of cathepsin C are palmoplantar keratosis and advanced periodontitis. *Keratosis* is a buildup of keratin on the skin that is the result of the loss of the ability of the epithelium to desquamate at its regular rate. Keratosis begins within the first 3 years of life on the palms of the hands and soles of the feet and is called *palmoplantar keratosis*. Lesions are white-to-yellowish-to-brown plaques that undergo crusting and cracking. Some patients report a worsening of the condition during winter. Other less common manifestations of Papillon-Lefèvre syndrome include dystrophic lesions of the nails, increased sweating, and keratosis of elbows and knees. Every region of the skin may be involved in some cases.

Intraoral manifestations include severe periodontitis, affecting both primary and permanent dentitions (Fig. 6-7A). Loss of chemotaxis and phagocytosis leads to uncontrolled inflammation in response to periodontal pathogens. The inflammatory process appears immediately after eruption of teeth. Gingivitis is followed by rapid loss of attachment and bone support, at which stage the teeth appear to be "floating in space" on radiographs (Fig. 6-7B) with eventual loss of teeth in the order in which they erupted. Once the teeth are lost or extracted, the gingival soft tissues return to normal health.

Studies have suggested that the pathogenesis of Papillon-Lefèvre syndrome includes an infectious etiology and is not merely a manifestation of immune dysfunction. Most of the common periodontal pathogens have been isolated, including *Actinobacillus actinomycetemcomitans* and *Porphyromonas gingivalis*.

Skin lesions are usually treated by topical *keratinolytic* (keratin destroying) agents, such as retinoids, a class of chemical compounds related to vitamin A that regulate epithelial cell growth. Once removed, keratosis will eventually recur due to the genetic foundation of the disease. There is no effective treatment for the periodontitis and patients generally require dentures at a young age. Antibiotic therapy has been unsuccessful in the long term.

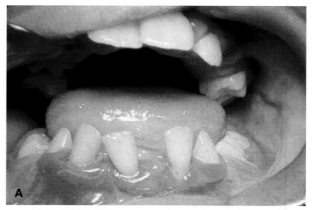

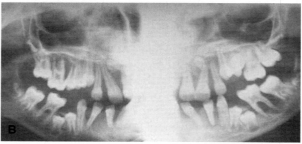

Figure 6–7 Papillon-Lefèvre syndrome. A. Intraoral manifestations include severe periodontitis, affecting both primary and permanent dentitions. **B.** Teeth appear to be "floating in space" on radiographs.

Hereditary Gingival Enlargement

Hereditary gingival enlargement, formerly termed *hereditary gingival fibromatosis*, presents as localized or generalized enlargement of the attached gingiva. Recent findings report a defect in the Son of sevenless-1 gene on chromosome 2p21-p22 as a possible cause. It is transmitted through both autosomal dominant and recessive modes, depending on its association with a syndrome (see below). Onset usually begins with eruption of the permanent teeth. In either isolated or syndromic forms, the gingiva is characteristically pink, firm, and very fibrous, with little tendency to bleed. The gingiva is markedly enlarged, asymptomatic, nonexudative, and appears as either focal nodules or generalized enlargement. The gingiva may even cover the crowns of the teeth. Pressure caused by the overgrowth of very dense collagen predisposes malpositioning of the teeth and retention of deciduous teeth that leads to aesthetic and functional problems (Fig. 6-8A and B).

Hereditary gingival enlargement may present as an isolated feature or as part of a syndrome. See Table 6-1 for a list of some of the syndromes associated with

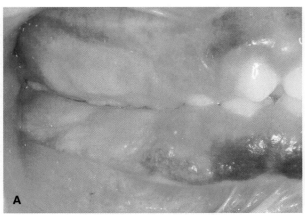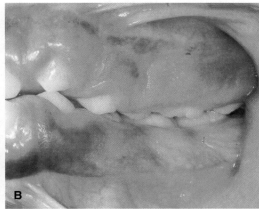

Figure 6–8 Hereditary gingival overgrowth. A. Child with massive overgrowth of the gingiva. **B.** The tissue regrew following gingivectomy.

Table 6.1	Syndromes Associated With Hereditary Gingival Overgrowth	
Syndrome	**Orofacial Characteristics**	**Other Features**
Rutherford	Delayed eruption; dentigerous cysts	Mental retardation; corneal opacities
Zimmerman-Laband	Defects of ears, nose	Hepatosplenomegaly; defects of fingers
Cowden	Papillomatosis of gingival, oral mucosa, and face	Hamartomas; neoplasms
Goltz-Gorlin	Gingival, oral papillomatosis; lip and tooth defects	Poikiloderma; adactyly; syndactyly; 90% female
Murray-Puretic- Dresher	Fibromas of head, trunk, and extremities	Suppuration of skin and mucosa; intellectual disabilities; flexion contractures
Cross	Microphthalmia; hypopigmentation	White hair; intellectual disabilities; athetosis; corneal clouding
Ramon	Hypertrichosis; cherubism	Juvenile rheumatoid arthritis; intellectual disabilities; epilepsy

hereditary gingival enlargement. The clinical condition generally requires repeated periodontal surgical procedures throughout the patient's lifetime to manage continued gingival enlargement.

Acatalasia

Acatalasia is a rare hereditary metabolic autosomal recessive disorder caused by the lack of an enzyme called catalase. This enzyme's job is to assist in the decomposition of hydrogen peroxide, a harmful byproduct of many normal metabolic processes. Catalase converts hydrogen peroxide into harmless water and oxygen. Without this enzyme, hydrogen peroxide builds up and destroys tissues. Though usually mild and asymptomatic, about half of the affected persons have recurrent infections of the gingiva that may lead to gangrenous lesions.

It is postulated that the gingival lesions result from damage to tissue from hydrogen peroxide generated by organisms in gingival plaque. The hydrogen peroxide produced by plaque microorganisms cannot be degraded by leukocytes genetically lacking the enzyme catalase. Early tooth loss results from periodontal destruction.

 Clinical Implications

Patients with acatalasia often have extensive oral ulcerations. Because these occur in childhood, it often is interpreted as a form of major aphthous ulcers (Chapter 4) or other immune deficiency. Loss of periodontal bone and tooth support is not a feature of major aphthous ulcers, so this can be used to help differentiate between the two.

Disorders of the Jaws and Facial Structures

The jaws and facial structures are among the first tissues to develop during fetal life. They are subject to a large number of genetic abnormalities. A few of the most important ones for the dental hygienist will be discussed here.

Hypohidrotic Ectodermal Dysplasia

Ectodermal dysplasia is a group of more than 150 conditions that are characterized by defects in development of two or more tissues of ectodermal origin. These include skin, hair, nails, sweat glands, and teeth. A variety of gene defects cause the different forms of ectodermal dysplasias. Most cases are X-linked recessive. Less commonly, they can have an autosomal dominant or autosomal recessive pattern of inheritance.

Hypohidrotic *ectodermal dysplasia* is one form of ectodermal dysplasia that is of interest to dentistry because it is characterized by congenital hypodontia/oligodontia and hypoplasia of teeth. It is often transmitted in an X-linked recessive mode, but occasionally in an autosomal dominant mode. The teeth are frequently reduced in number (hypodontia) and those that form are hypoplastic. Crowns of incisors appear tapered and conical in shape. Molars tend toward microdontia (Fig. 6-9A). Fingernails may be atrophic (Fig. 6-9B). Hair, another ectodermal structure, is often sparse, light-colored, brittle, and slow-growing, a condition called hypotrichosis. Patients also have distinctive facial features, including a prominent forehead, thick lips, a flattened bridge of the nose, and thin, wrinkled, and dark-colored skin around the eyes (Fig. 6-10).

Patients with hypohidrotic ectodermal dysplasia have a reduced ability to sweat (*hypohidrosis*) because they have few or no functional sweat glands. Sweating is how the body controls its temperature. An inability to sweat can lead to dangerous hyperthermia, particularly in hot weather. In some cases, hyperthermia can be life-threatening. Children with the disease may have difficulty controlling fevers. Mild illness can produce extremely high fevers because the skin cannot sweat and control temperature properly.

Restorative, prosthetic, and/or cosmetic dental treatment is almost always necessary to restore masticatory form and function in patients with ectodermal dysplasia. Children may need dentures as early as 2 years of age, with replacements as the child grows. Dental implants may be an option once the jaw is fully grown. Features of ectodermal dysplasia are summarized in Box 6-1.

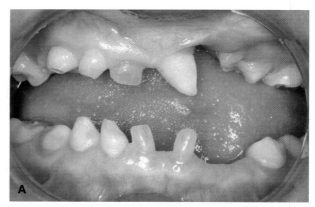

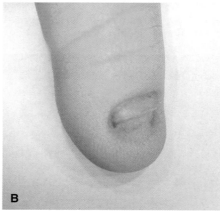

Figure 6–9 **Ectodermal dysplasia. A.** Misshapen and congenitally missing teeth. **B.** Underdeveloped fingernail. (Courtesy of Vladimir Leon Salazar)

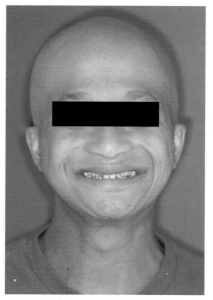

Figure 6–10 **Ectodermal dysplasia: Face.** Patient with sparse hair and underdeveloped permanent teeth.

Box **6-1 Clinical Features of Ectodermal Dysplasia**

Abnormal nails
Dental hypoplasia
Xerophthalmia (lack of tears)
Decreased skin pigment
Heat intolerance
Inability to sweat
Frontal bossing
Hypodontia/oligodontia
Depressed nasal bridge
Hearing loss
Hyperthermia
Poor vision
Alopecia (lack of hair)
Thin skin

Clinical Implications

Affected individuals are unable to tolerate a warm environment and need special measures to keep a normal body temperature. Adjustment of room temperature during a dental appointment may not only increase the patient's comfort, but benefit their health.

Van der Woude syndrome

Van der Woude syndrome is characterized by oro-facial anomalies caused by an abnormal fusion of the palate and lips at 30 to 50 days in utero. Most cases of van der Woude syndrome have been linked to a deletion in chromosome 1q32-q41, which leads to mutations in a gene called the ***IRF6* gene**. This results in a shortage of the IRF6 protein, which affects the development and maturation of tissues in the face. It is inherited in an autosomal dominant pattern, but occasionally an individual who has a copy of the altered gene does not show any signs or symptoms of the disorder. The degree to which individuals who carry the gene are affected varies widely, even within families. Approximately 30% to 50% of all cases arise as a new mutation.

This syndrome occurs in 1 in 35,000 to 1 in 100,000 people worldwide. Patients with this disorder are born with a cleft lip, a cleft palate, or both. Mild cases may present with only a bifid uvula and hypernasal voice. Paramedian lip pits develop near the center of the lower lip. Minor salivary glands rest at the base of the

pits and saliva can be expressed on gentle pressure. The average IQ of patients with van der Woude syndrome is not significantly different from that of the general population.

Clinical Implications

People with van der Woude syndrome who have cleft lip and/or cleft palate, like other individuals with these facial conditions, have an increased risk of delayed language development, learning disabilities, or other mild cognitive problems. Table 6-2 lists a sample of other syndromes that have cleft palate as one of their features.

Table 6.2	Syndromes That Feature Cleft Palate*
Syndrome	**Other Distinguishing Features**
Van der Woude	Paramedian lip pits; hypodontia
Stickler's	Cleft lip; joint pain; myopia
Loeys-Dietz	Hypertelorism; aortic aneurysm
Patau	Intellectual disabilities; microphthalmia; low-set ears
Malpuech facial clefting	Caudal appendage; hypospadias; cryptorchidism, renal agenesis; omphalocele; umbilical hernia
Popliteal pterygium	Paramedian lip pits; webs of skin on the backs of the legs; syndactyly; cryptorchidism
Treacher-Collins	Downward-slanting eyes; notched lower eyelids; underdeveloped midface; deafness
Hardikar	Hydronephrosis; intestinal obstruction
Crouzon's	Premature craniosynostosis
Apert's	Premature craniosynostosis; syndactyly; polydactyly
Waardenberg's	Deafness; partial albinism

Continued

Table 6.2	Syndromes That Feature Cleft Palate—cont'd
Syndrome	**Other Distinguishing Features**
Edward's	Heart defects; microsomia; micrognathia; microcephaly; syndactyly
Hemifacial microsomia	Unilateral underdevelopment of one ear, jaw, and cheek on the same side of the face
Pierre Robin sequence	Micrognathia of mandible; macroglossia; dyspnea

*More than 200 recognized syndromes may include cleft palate as a manifestation.

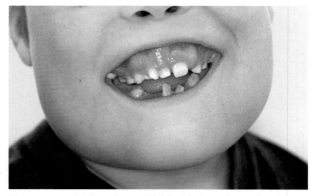

Figure 6–11   Cherubism. Child with 4-quadrant cherubism.

Cherubism

Cherubism is an autosomal dominant condition caused by a defect of the ***SH3BP2* gene**. The proportion of cases caused by new mutations is unknown because of variable expressivity and incomplete penetrance. Each child of an individual with cherubism has a 50 percent chance of inheriting the disease.

Manifestations may begin as early as 1 year, but are clinically apparent by age 5. Cherubism is typically characterized by painless bilateral swelling of the jaws (Fig. 6-11), resulting in widening and distortion of the alveolar ridges. Some cases are so mild that the disease may not be noticeable, whereas others are severe enough to cause problems with vision, breathing, speech, and swallowing. Other facial and skeletal bones usually are not affected. When all four quadrants are affected, the patient typically has a "cherub" appearance, with eyes canted "toward the heavens" and chubby cherubic cheeks; hence, the name of the

disease (Fig. 6-12). These growths often interfere with normal tooth development, causing tooth displacement and failure of eruption of teeth in the region of involvement (Fig. 6-13).

Radiographic examination shows the pathognomonic features of bilateral multilocular radiolucencies and multiple displaced and unerupted teeth (Fig. 6-14). Lesions tend to stabilize after puberty, with the involved sites usually presenting as ground-glass or frosted-glass radiopacities. Figure 6-15 is a three-dimensional (3-D) reconstruction of a child with cherubism that shows the degree of distortion of the jaws and facial bones.

Biopsies of cherubism show replacement of bone by fibrous connective tissue, with accumulation of multinucleated giant cells, histologically identical to those seen in central giant cell granulomas (CGCGs) (see Chapter 2). Radiographic and clinical correlations are necessary to differentiate between the two. There are some reports of "one quadrant involvement" of cherubism; however, these cases actually represent CGCG in young patients.

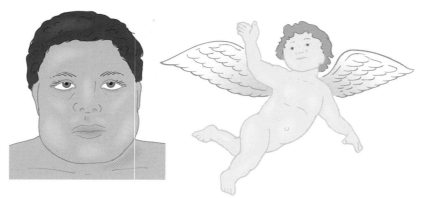

Figure 6–12   Cherubism. Cherubism is named for resemblance to cherubs with chubby cheeks and eyes gazing upward toward heaven.

The clinical alterations of cherubism typically progress until puberty, after which they stabilize and in some patients even show regression. For this reason, surgical treatment is typically delayed until puberty. Surgical curettage of the lesions is usually the preferred treatment. By age 30, facial abnormalities are no longer apparent; residual jaw deformity is rare.

Rarely, cherubism occurs as part of another genetic disorder. For example, cherubism can occur with Ramon syndrome, which also involves short stature, intellectual disability, and gingival fibrosis. In addition to the features of cherubism, patients with Noonan syndrome have short stature and heart defects.

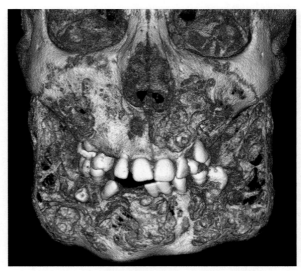

Figure 6–15　Cherubism. A 3-D reconstruction of destructive jaw lesions.

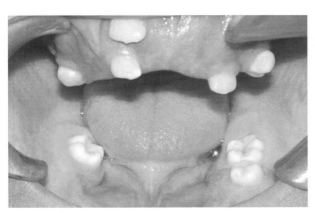

Figure 6–13　Cherubism. Multiple unerupted teeth.

Cleidocranial Dysplasia

Cleidocranial dysplasia is an autosomal dominant condition associated with mutations in the *Runx2* gene, which produces a protein required for osteoblast differentiation. This condition is characterized by bone defects involving the clavicle (*cleido-*) and skull (*-cranial*). Clavicles are absent or underdeveloped and barely functional. The ability of the patient to touch the shoulders together is pathognomonic of cleidocranial dysplasia (Fig. 6-16). Cranial defects in these typically short patients include a relatively large head, ocular **hypertelorism** (wide spacing between eyes), and widened base of the nose with depressed nasal bridge. The large head is because of parietal *bossing*, causing the head to be wider from ear to ear because of delayed closure of the sutures of the skull.

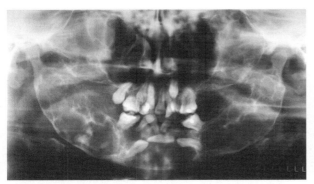

Figure 6–14　Cherubism. Bilateral multilocular jaw enlargement. Multiple unerupted teeth. Note lesions in maxilla. (Courtesy of Vladimir Leon Salazar)

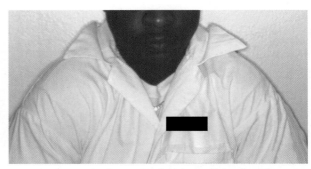

Figure 6–16　Cleidocranial dysplasia. Patient with cleidocranial dysplasia can bring his shoulders together.

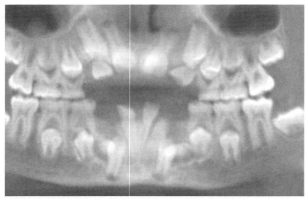

Figure 6–17   Cleidocranial dysplasia. Multiple impacted teeth in the anterior mandible.

Oral manifestations include high-arched palate with increased occurrence of clefting and presence of numerous unerupted permanent and supernumerary teeth (Fig. 6-17). The teeth have distorted crown and root shapes and lack secondary cementum,

resulting in absence of attachment for periodontal ligament fibers. Due to the delay or failure of eruption of permanent teeth, there is prolonged retention of deciduous teeth.

Craniosynostosis Syndromes

Craniosynostosis is a group of syndromes that are characterized by premature closure of cranial (*cranio-*) sutures (*-synostosis*). The two types discussed here are Crouzon syndrome and Apert's syndrome. These syndromes are caused by mutations in a specific gene called the fibroblast growth factor receptor gene (*FGFR*). The type and severity of disease is dependent on the mutation within the *FGFR* gene.

Head shapes in craniosynostosis include brachycephaly, scaphocephaly, trigonocephaly, ranging to the most severe form of "cloverleaf" skull (kleeblattschädel) (Fig. 6-18).

Crouzon syndrome is an autosomal dominant syndrome affecting 1 in 65,000 births. There is wide variation in clinical presentation. When cranial sutures

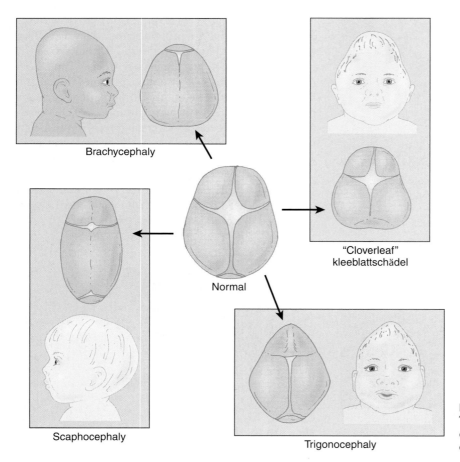

Brachycephaly

"Cloverleaf" kleeblattschädel

Scaphocephaly

Normal

Trigonocephaly

Figure 6–18   Craniosynostosis. The abnormal shape of the head is dependent upon which sutures close prematurely.

close prematurely while the brain is still growing, patients may exhibit *exophthalmos*, a condition in which there is bulging of the eyes due to shallow eye sockets after early fusion of surrounding bones. In addition, cranial nerve disorders such as blindness and hearing deficit may occur. Crouzon syndrome patients have normal intelligence; however, headaches are common. Typical facial features include hypoplastic maxilla with insufficient development of the midface (Fig. 6-19A), crowding of maxillary teeth, a narrow/high-arched palate (Fig. 6-19B), posterior bilateral cross-bite, and relative mandibular *prognathism*, giving the patient a concave facial profile (Fig. 6-19C). Surgery is typically used to prevent closure of sutures of the skull from damaging the brain's development, as well as to improve cosmetic outcomes.

Apert's syndrome (acrocephalosyndactyly) is an autosomal dominant disorder affecting 1 in 65,000 to 160,000 births, making it rarer than Crouzon syndrome. Patients present with similar but more severe head deformity than those with Crouzon syndrome (Fig. 6-20A), but major differences include **syndactyly,** fusion of the second, third, and fourth fingers and toes (Fig. 6-20B, C, and D), and mental developmental delay. Pseudocleft palate formation may be observed in both syndromes (Fig. 6-20E). Swelling is because of abnormal accumulations of glycosaminoglycans, a normal component of connective tissue, in the lateral hard palate. The result may be crowding of teeth.

Treacher-Collins Syndrome

Treacher-Collins syndrome, also called mandibulofacial dysostosis, is an autosomal dominant disorder that affects 1 in 25,000 to 50,000 births, with more than 50 percent representing new mutations. This disorder is caused by mutations in the Treacher-Collins-Franceschetti syndrome 1 (*TCOF1*) gene. The gene encodes a protein that, when missing, allows for defects in first and second branchial arches related to improper migration of neural crest cells. Patients have a narrow face due to hypoplasia of the zygomatic bone (Fig. 6-21A and B). A downward slant of the palpebral fissures and a notch in the lateral aspects of the lower eyelid, called **coloboma**, are noted (Fig. 6-21C). Most patients have external ear defects, including soft tissue ear tags, as well as hearing loss due to defects in the bones of the middle ear (Fig. 6-21D). Condylar and coronoid hypoplasia cause mandibular deficiency and alterations of tooth development. Both cleft palate as well as lateral facial cleft may be noted in some patients.

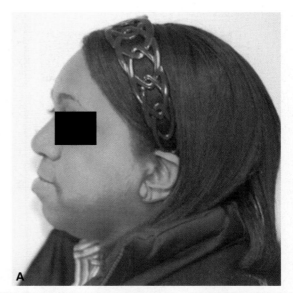

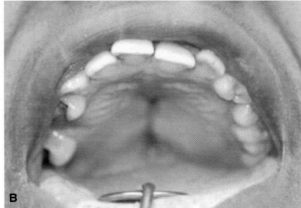

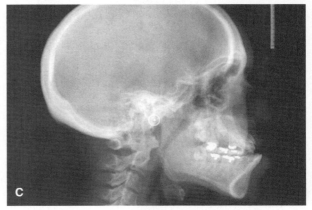

Figure 6–19 **A.** Patient with mid-face deficiency. **B.** Narrow, high-arched palate. **C.** Cephalometric image showing mandibular prognathism. (Courtesy of Rania H. Younis)

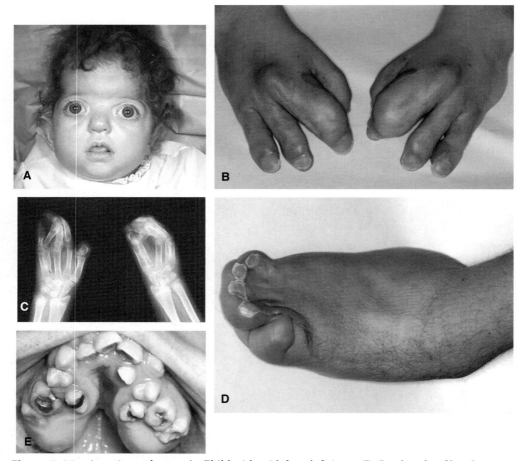

Figure 6–20 **Apert's syndrome**. **A.** Child with mid-face deficiency. **B.** Syndactyly of hands. **C.** Radiograph showing bone fusion. **D.** Syndactyly of toes. **E.** Pseudocleft of maxilla with malpositioned teeth. (A, C, and E from the Gorlin Collection, University of Minnesota; B and D courtesy of Vladimir Leon Salazar)

Nevoid Basal Cell Carcinoma Syndrome (Gorlin Syndrome)

Nevoid basal cell carcinoma syndrome (NBCCS) is an autosomal dominant disorder with variable expressivity caused by mutations in the "patched" gene that is located on chromosome 9. The most significant feature of the syndrome is development of up to several hundred basal cell carcinomas over a lifetime that occur on both sun-exposed and non–sun-exposed skin (Fig. 6-22A). Basal cell carcinomas in the syndrome initially resemble the common melanocytic nevus or "mole," thus the name *nevoid* basal cell carcinoma, but progress to develop central depressions as other basal cell carcinomas (Fig. 6-22B). They begin to appear around the second decade of life and show less aggressive behavior than nonsyndromic basal cell carcinomas (see Chapter 7). Basal carcinomas tend to be fewer and occur less frequently in African Americans than Caucasians who have the syndrome.

Of interest to dentistry is the development of multiple odontogenic keratocysts in the jaws. A typical patient usually develops an average of six to twelve odontogenic keratocysts during their lifetime (Fig. 6-22C). Cysts have been reported in both jaws, with the majority in the mandible. The median age of occurrence for the first odontogenic keratocyst in the syndrome is 15 years. Other lesions characteristic of NBCCS include epidermoid cysts of the skin (see Chapter 5), which can become quite large. In 65 percent of patients, epithelial pits are frequently seen scattered across the palms and soles. Although the etiology is not completely understood, the most widely accepted explanation is a focal reduction in epithelial maturation resulting in a decreased keratin layer, which leads to a depression in the palm and/or sole. Very rarely, basal cell carcinomas may develop from the base of these pits. Other lesions seen in NBCCS are shown in Table 6-3.

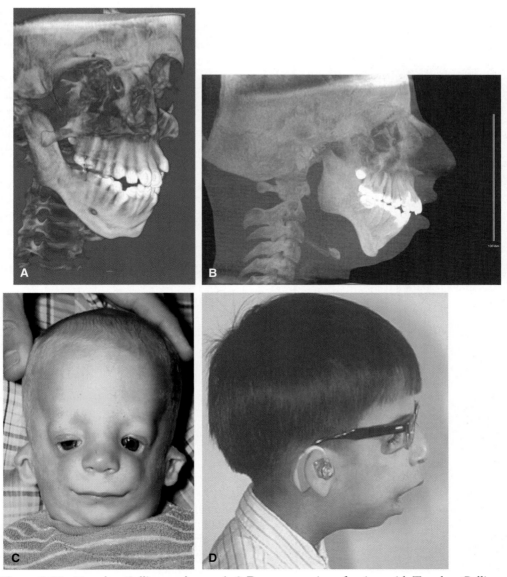

Figure 6–21 **Treacher-Collins syndrome. A.** 3-D reconstruction of patient with Treacher-Collins syndrome showing narrowing of jaws. **B.** Cephalometric image of patient with Treacher-Collins syndrome. **C.** Typical facies seen in Treacher-Collins syndrome. **D.** Child with Treacher-Collins syndrome. Note hearing aid due to deafness associated with this syndrome. (A and B courtesy of Vladimir Leon Salazar; C and D from the Gorlin Collection, University of Minnesota)

Clinical Implications

The basal cell carcinomas in Gorlin syndrome are similar to those observed in nonsyndromic cases and are treated similarly. Syndromic odontogenic keratocysts are similar to nonsyndromic odontogenic keratocysts. However, odontogenic keratocysts associated with Gorlin syndrome have been reported to contain increased daughter cysts in their walls (see Chapter 5), which may be associated with their frequent recurrence.

The prognosis for the NBCCA patients may depend on clinical behavior of the numerous basal cell carcinomas. Some basal cell carcinomas behave aggressively, causing localized invasion of underlying structures, including the brain, which may lead to death. Both sunlight exposure and radiation therapy should be avoided due to the increased propensity to develop basal cell carcinomas. Odontogenic keratocysts are typically enucleated, resulting in jaw deformities because of frequent surgeries.

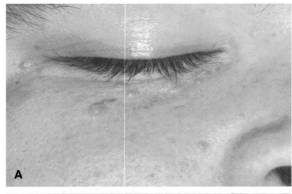

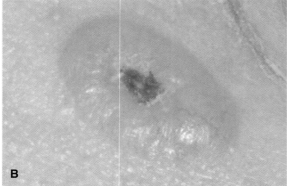

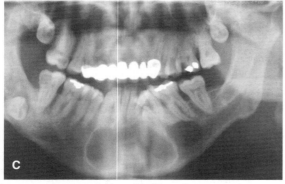

Figure 6–22 Nevoid basal cell carcinoma syndrome.
A. Multiple basal cell carcinomas that resemble common nevi. **B.** Closer view of basal cell carcinoma. **C.** Panoramic radiograph showing multiple odontogenic keratocysts in patient with NBCCS. (A and B from a presentation by Jessica Shireman)

Table 6.3	Features of Nevoid Basal Cell Carcinoma Syndrome
Feature	**Description**
Bifid ribs	Sternal end of the rib is cleaved into two
Calcification of the falx cerebri	Fold of dura mater separating the cerebellar hemispheres
Hypertelorism	Increased distance between the eyes
Strabismus	Eyes do not line up in the same direction; "crossed eyes"
Kyphoscoliosis	Abnormal curvature of the spine in both a coronal and sagittal plane
Short fourth metacarpals	Short finger bones
Ovarian fibromas	Benign growth of ovary frequent during middle age
Fetal rhabdomyomas	Benign muscle tumor of the heart
Medulloblastoma, meningiomas	Brain tumors
Cleft lip/cleft palate	Failure of fusion of the lip/palate
Mental retardation	Lack of normal development of intellectual capacities

dominant, autosomal recessive, or the result of sporadic mutation. Together these forms lead to an occurrence of approximately 1 in 8,000 individuals. The most common genetic defect is mutation in either the *COL1A1* or *COL1A2* genes.

Four major types of OI have been recognized, so the disease is varied in clinical presentation. Patients with type II or III die *in utero*, in the perinatal period, or in early childhood. The main clinical defects seen in those who survive include bone fragility, alterations of teeth, **blue sclera** of the eyes, hearing loss, hyperextension, and increased mobility of joints. There is decreased bone density, which produces deformities such as bowing of the long bones and fractures. Patients with frequent fractures are typically disabled and require use of mobility aids such as a wheelchair.

Dental manifestations present as a form of *dentinogenesis imperfecta (DI)*. (Fig. 6-23) that affects both

Osteogenesis Imperfecta

Osteogenesis imperfecta (OI) is the most common inherited bone disease. It represents a heterogeneous group of disorders characterized by defects in bone, dentin, ligaments, skin, and sclera that are caused by defective collagen synthesis and maturation. It may be autosomal

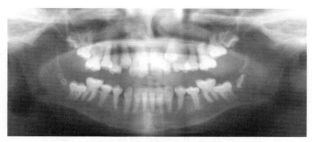

Figure 6–23 Osteogenesis Imperfecta. Lack of proper dentin development seen in patient with osteogenesis imperfecta.

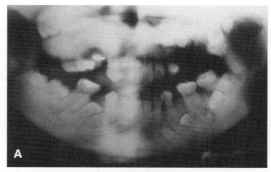

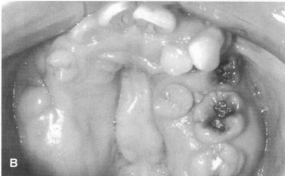

Figure 6–24 Osteopetrosis. **A.** Enlarged dense bone in osteopetrosis. Note loss of bone marrow space. **B.** Bony enlargement of maxilla with malposed teeth.

dentitions. Teeth develop an *opalescent* appearance due to defective dentin, as seen in DI. However, dentin defects due to OI and DI are separate entities, as they are caused by different mutations. Other oral manifestations include pseudo-mandibular prognathism due to hypoplasia of the maxilla and presence of radiolucent, radiopaque, or mixed lesions of the mandible.

Currently, there is no treatment for OI. The main options for control of bone fractures include surgery, physical therapy, and rehabilitation with the primary goal of improving symptoms. Both intravenous and oral bisphosphonates have been reported to decrease frequency of fractures and pain. Orthognathic surgery has been used successfully for mandibular prognathism.

Osteopetrosis (Albers-Schönberg Disease, Marble Bone Disease)

Osteopetrosis is a group of skeletal defects that are caused by a deficiency in or lack of osteoclast function, which leads to a defect in bone remodeling and significant increase in bone density (*-petrosis* = turns to stone). Both autosomal recessive and autosomal dominant forms of osteopetrosis originate from mutations in genes referred to as the *CLCN genes*, which are critical for osteoclast function.

Osteopetrosis variants are classified into two general subtypes: infantile and adult.

The infantile type is an example of an autosomal recessive disease. This severe form leads to generalized dense skeletal bones caused by replacement of the bone marrow by abnormal bone. Patients experience anemia and granulocytopenia that increases susceptibility to infections. The spleen can be recruited to compensate for the need for more red and white blood cells, which results in *hepatosplenomegaly*, a key clinical finding. Although the bones seem dense (Fig. 6-24A), they are brittle and have an increased susceptibility to fractures.

Narrowing of the cranial nerve foramina leads to cranial nerve compression with possible resultant complications of blindness, headaches, and hearing loss. Significant dental findings include failure of teeth to erupt (Fig. 6-24B). Subsequent osteomyelitis is caused by lack of resistance to normal oral flora.

The adult form of osteopetrosis is typically autosomal dominant, less severe, and begins much later in life than the infantile form. Bone marrow failure does not occur and the skeleton shows no sclerosis. Bone pain is the most common symptom. Fractures and cranial nerve compression occur in variable intensity. Dental and maxillofacial findings include osteomyelitis, with fracture of the mandible a rare event.

Adult osteopetrosis patients typically live relatively long lives due to the milder form of the disease, whereas infantile patients may die early in the course of the disease. Bone marrow transplantation, parathyroid hormone, erythropoietin, corticosteroid, interferon gamma, and calcitriol are all treatments that lead to varying control of symptoms. In cases that do not respond, hyperbaric oxygen has also been effective.

Clinical Implications

The role of the dental health-care provider in osteopetrosis may be two-fold: 1) diagnosis of milder adult forms through routine radiographs, and 2) treatment of osteomyelitis. Management must be performed swiftly to avoid unnecessary bone loss. This typically involves antibiotics, debridement/drainage, and surgical management.

Fibrous Dysplasia

Fibrous dysplasia (FD) is a developmental disorder that is characterized by replacement of normal bone by cellular fibrous connective tissue. Mutations in guanine nucleotide-binding protein, alpha stimulating activity polypeptide 1 (*GNAS1*) gene occur within the individual and are not passed from the parents; therefore, the disorder is not hereditary. FD can be classified clinically as *monostotic* (affecting one bone), *polyostotic* (involving multiple bones), or *craniofacial*, involving more than one contiguous craniofacial bone.

Monostotic fibrous dysplasia is the most common form and typically involves the jaws of males and females with equal frequency. Most cases are diagnosed in the early teenage years, when a slow-growing painless swelling of the affected region, usually the maxilla, occurs (Fig. 6-25A). Craniofacial fibrous dysplasia is seen in more than one jaw and/or facial bone concurrently.

The classic radiographic appearance is referred to as "ground glass" or "frosted glass" radiopacity with ill-defined borders (Fig. 6-25B). Early lesions gradually become more radiopaque with age. The natural process of the disease correlates with this radiographic appearance. Early in the disease, normal bone is replaced with dense fibrous connective tissue that expands the bony area. Gradually, this fibrous connective tissue begins to ossify; however, the newly formed bone is abnormal with few or tiny marrow spaces. The lesion is not encapsulated and is directly fused to the surrounding normal bone, giving fibrous dysplasia its characteristic diffuse ill-defined pattern.

Narrowing of the periodontal ligament space with thinning of the lamina dura may be observed in periapical radiographs. Obliteration of the maxillary sinus may be seen with involvement of the maxilla.

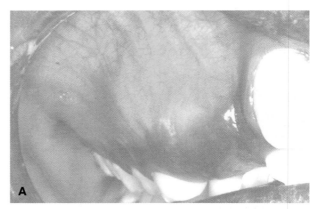

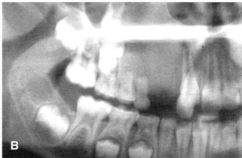

Figure 6–25 Fibrous dysplasia. A. Nontender bony expansion of anterior maxilla. **B.** "Ground" or frosted glass appearance to involved bone in maxilla. (From the Gorlin Collection, University of Minnesota)

Polyostotic fibrous dysplasia is the least common form and is seen as part of a syndrome. *Jaffe-Lichtenstein syndrome* is characterized by polyostotic fibrous dysplasia and café-au-lait pigmentation of the skin. *Café-au-lait pigmentation* is usually present on the skin of the trunk and upper legs. Café-au-lait spots appear as large, light brown macules with irregular borders and are the color of "coffee with cream" (Fig. 6-26). *McCune-Albright syndrome* is characterized by polyostotic fibrous dysplasia, café-au-lait pigmentation of the skin, and endocrine disorders such as hyperthyroidism, pituitary gland dysfunction, and precocious (early) puberty. Polyostotic fibrous dysplasia affects the long bones more often than the craniofacial bones.

Clinical management of fibrous dysplasia can be challenging. Monostotic lesions may be surgically excised and bone malformations recontoured; however, larger lesions, especially in the maxilla, require more extensive and multiple surgeries. Surgical management typically is postponed until after puberty because fibrous dysplasia may stabilize and even

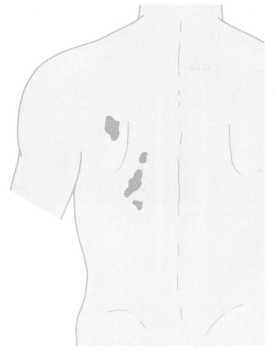

Figure 6–26 **Fibrous dysplasia-café au lait spot.** Large brown macules in patient with polyostotic fibrous dysplasia.

regress after skeletal maturation is complete. However, if rapid expansion occurs, surgical intervention may occur at an earlier age. Approximately 50 percent of lesions regrow and require further surgical management. Both intravenous and oral bisphosphonates have been used successfully to manage symptoms and improve bone strength. Radiation treatment must be avoided because malignant transformation to osteosarcoma has been reported in irradiated bone lesions.

Gardner's Syndrome

Gardner's syndrome is a rare autosomal dominant disorder, with occasional spontaneous mutations reported. It is generally considered as part of the spectrum of **familial polyposis syndromes**, a group of syndromes in which the colon is affected by the overgrowth of colon polyps, some of which have malignant potential. Gardner's syndrome patients have mutations in the adenomatous polyposis coli (*APC*) gene. Several clinical features of the skeleton and teeth are found in this syndrome. However, the most significant manifestation is the colon polyps that develop in 100 percent of cases in the second decade of life, most commonly before age 35. The polyps almost always undergo malignant transformation to adenocarcinoma. Patients with a known family history of Gardner's syndrome often receive prophylactic colectomy upon recognition of the polyps to prevent cancer from developing.

Recognition of Gardner's syndrome in the dental office may help save a patient's life. Classic skeletal defects may affect the skull and maxillofacial bones (Fig. 6-27A). Multiple benign osteomas (bone growths) cause significant facial deformity (Fig. 6-27B). Dental defects include supernumerary teeth, odontomas, and impacted teeth.

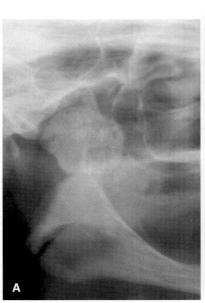
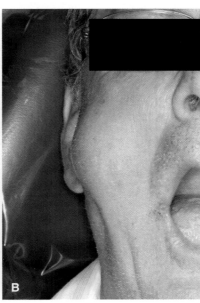

Figure 6–27 **Gardner's syndrome.**
A. Large osteoma in temporomandibular joint area in patient with Gardner's syndrome. **B.** Facial deformity associated with osteoma.

Fortunately, these appear before development of intestinal polyps. If the craniofacial manifestations are detected early, immediate screening for the disorder can be undertaken.

Klinefelter Syndrome

Klinefelter syndrome, also called XXY syndrome, is a disorder in which males have an extra X chromosome. The extra X chromosome is retained because of a *nondisjunction* event during division. Nondisjunction occurs when homologous chromosomes, in this case the X and Y sex chromosomes, fail to separate, producing a sperm with an X and a Y chromosome. Affected individuals experience *hypogonadism, gynecomastia*, and reduced fertility. In childhood, XXY males exhibit weak muscles and reduced strength. Low levels of testosterone are present at puberty, leading to a taller and less muscular body, less facial and body hair, and broader hips compared to unaffected males. By adulthood, XXY males look similar to males without the condition, although they are often taller. They are also more likely to develop autoimmune disorders, breast cancer, vein diseases, and osteoporosis.

Clinical Implications

Approximately 20 percent of patients who have Klinefelter syndrome develop taurodontism (see Chapter 5). Some other syndromes that feature taurodontism include:

- Amelogenesis imperfecta
- Tricho-dento-osseous syndrome
- Down syndrome
- Williams syndrome
- McCune-Albright syndrome
- Van der Woude syndrome

Disorders of the Oral Soft Tissues

Oral soft tissues are affected by genetic abnormalities. These are typically subtle and may escape notice during the oral examination. Selected disorders are presented.

White Sponge Nevus

White sponge nevus is an autosomal dominant mucosal disorder that shows an alteration in keratinization due to mutations in keratin 4 and 13 genes. Lesions usually develop at or immediately after birth and appear as thick, bilateral, white, diffuse, irregular corrugated patches on the buccal mucosa (Fig. 6-28) that are

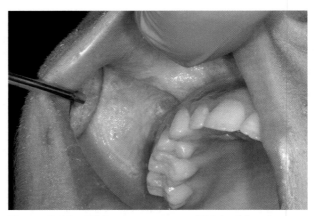

Figure 6–28   White sponge nevus. Thick white plaques that do not wipe off in areas not readily traumatized.

much larger and more widely distributed than morsicatio buccarum (see Chapter 2). The soft palate, labial mucosa, ventral tongue, and floor of the mouth are occasionally affected. Lesions may also affect other mucosal surfaces, including the larynx, esophageal, and genital mucosa. The severity varies from patient to patient. Once the diagnosis is confirmed with a biopsy, treatment is unnecessary. Any surgical or chemical treatment is typically followed by regrowth of the epithelium due to the genetic basis for the condition. Malignant transformation is not reported.

Hereditary Benign Intraepithelial Dyskeratosis

Hereditary benign intraepithelial dyskeratosis (HBID) is an autosomal dominant disorder that shares the clinical appearance of white sponge nevus (Fig. 6-29A). The condition affects an isolate of families of African American/Native American/Caucasian descent that originated in northeastern North Carolina. In addition to the oral mucosal lesions, the eyes develop lesions on the conjunctiva early in life that feature thick, white, jelly-like plaques sometimes affecting the cornea (Fig. 6-29B). The appearance of lesions varies with weather conditions, with active lesions present immediately after winter and during spring. Rarely, blindness may result because of repeated episodes. No treatment is necessary after establishment of diagnosis for oral lesions other than management for candidiasis, if present. Eye lesions that affect vision are surgically removed. Referral to an ophthalmologist is critical.

Peutz-Jegher's Syndrome

Peutz-Jegher's syndrome is an autosomal dominant disorder characterized by freckle-like pigmentations on

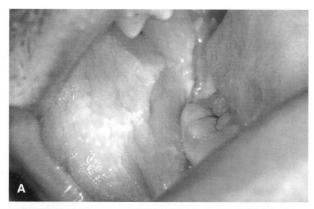

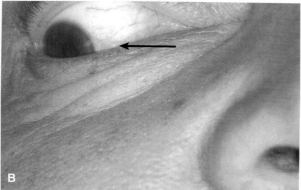

Figure 6–29 Hereditary benign intraepithelial dyskeratosis. A. Thick white plaques on buccal mucosa and tongue in a 50-year-old Native American. **B.** Small yellow gelatinous plaque of the eye.

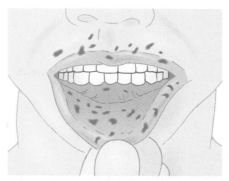

Figure 6–30 Peutz Jegher's syndrome. Peutz-Jegher's syndrome is characterized by an abundance of brown macules (freckles) of the face and oral cavity.

the hands, perioral skin, and intraoral mucosa. Patients develop intestinal polyps that have an increased propensity for malignant transformation to adenocarcinomas. A gene located in chromosome 19, known as *STK11* gene, is mutated in the majority of Peutz-Jegher's syndrome patients.

Typical melanocytic pigmentations of the skin are recognized because they are not altered by or responsive to sun exposure. These develop early in life and typically present around the mouth and inside the oral cavity, including labial mucosa and gingiva (Fig. 6-30). The nose and genitals may also be affected.

Polyps may develop anywhere along the gastrointestinal (GI) tract, but are most frequently observed in the jejunum and ileum. Intestinal obstruction due to intussusception (telescopic folding of a portion of intestine within itself) is a common complication, which can be corrected by surgery, but most cases will self-correct. Adenocarcinoma of the GI tract develops in close to 30 percent of patients. Tumors of the

pancreas, breast, ovary, and genital tract may also develop in affected patients.

Peutz-Jegher's patients need periodic evaluation for intussusception and polyp/tumor development. Recognition of the signs of Peutz-Jegher's syndrome by dental professionals may help the patient seek care that saves his or her life.

Multiple Hamartoma Syndrome (Cowden Syndrome)

Multiple hamartoma syndrome (Cowden syndrome) is an autosomal dominant disorder with a high degree of penetrance, characterized by benign hamartomatous growths and a mild propensity to develop malignancies. Mutation of chromosome 10 (*PTEN*) has been reported.

The term **hamartoma** describes a benign tumor-like growth, made up of normal mature cells in an abnormal number or distribution. Observed in almost all of these patients are small multiple hamartomatous growths of the hair follicles, called trichilemmomas, that appear on the skin of the face, typically around the nose, ears, and mouth. Intraoral hamartomas present as multiple scattered or clustered papules anywhere in the oral cavity, including the tongue (Fig. 6-31A), labial mucosa, and gingiva (Fig. 6-31B). Biopsy shows excess growths of normal tissue. Other skin lesions include *palmoplantar keratosis* (hyperkeratosis of palms and soles), *acral keratosis* (papillary lesions on the dorsal hand), and tumor-like growths such as hemangiomas and neuromas. Patients also develop other significant conditions such as *adenoma* and *adenocarcinoma* of the thyroid gland, fibrocystic disease and carcinoma of the breast, gastrointestinal polyps, and both benign and malignant tumors of the genitourinary system. Patients are advised to have frequent medical examinations due to the risk of malignancies.

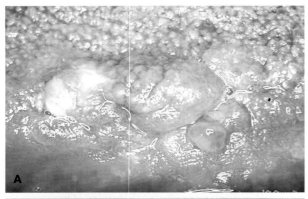
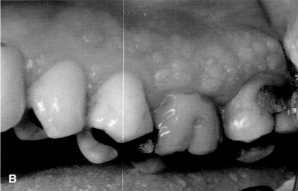

Figure 6–31 Cowden syndrome. A. Nodules of the tongue were made up of normal collagen. **B.** Nodules of the gingiva were made up of normal gingival tissues.

Clinical Implications

The diagnosis may not be conclusive when lesions of multiple hamartoma syndrome are biopsied because microscopically they appear as normal tissue. Patient history and clinical findings must be combined with the microscopic findings when there is a suspicion for this disorder.

INHERITED DISORDERS LIMITED TO THE DENTITION

The teeth are occasionally affected by genetic abnormalities. These differ from developmental disorders of teeth (discussed in Chapter 5) because they are caused by defects in specific genes that are passed from parents to offspring. A few of the most important ones will be discussed here.

Disorders of Enamel: Types of Amelogenesis Imperfecta

Amelogenesis imperfecta is the name given to a group of 14 separate hereditary disorders in which the common outcome is defective enamel formation that cannot be attributed to other systemic disorders, such as excessive fluoride intake, malnutrition, or fever. Etiology is related to the alteration of genes involved in the process of enamel formation and maturation. This is an exclusively ectodermal disorder; mesodermal tissues such as dentin and cementum are not affected.

Genes for most of the subtypes have been identified. Diagnosis and classification of specific amelogenesis imperfecta types are mainly based on morphological characteristics and familial inheritance patterns. The different patterns of inheritance correspond with different genomic sites. Amelogenesis imperfecta may have either an autosomal dominant, autosomal recessive, or X-linked pattern. The specific genetic mutations produce abnormal enamel proteins that are necessary for 1) formation of the enamel matrix, 2) proper mineralization of the matrix, and 3) normal maturation of the enamel. Depending on the gene that has been affected, the resulting amelogenesis imperfecta can be divided into three main types:

1. Hypoplastic
2. Hypomaturation
3. Hypocalcified

Each type has particular clinical features that reflect the stage of formation at which the enamel was affected. A fourth type, hypomaturation/hypoplasia/taurodontism, shows disturbances of more than one stage. Each of these types can be divided into subtypes depending on the mode of inheritance, as well as on the clinical and radiographic aspects of the enamel defects. Overlapping characteristics may make classification difficult. Although it is beyond the scope of this book to provide details about each subtype, there are three basic defects that occur in the amelogenesis imperfecta that can be recognized clinically (Table 6-4).

Hypoplastic types are characterized by incomplete or arrested development of the enamel matrix. The enamel matrix is responsible for the shape of the crown, the thickness of the enamel, and the surface texture. This defect causes alteration in the morphology and thickness of the tooth enamel. Radiographically, the enamel may be absent (Fig. 6-32A). Pitting, grooves, and generally rough surfaces are seen, as well as extremely thin enamel (Fig 6-32B).

Hypomaturation types (Fig. 6-32C) are associated with proper matrix deposition and early mineralization, but the enamel crystalline structure fails to mature. Normal enamel maturation requires the coordinated removal of the enamel matrix and subsequent growth of hydroxyapatite crystals, causing gradual physical hardening of

Table 6.4	Major Types of Amelogenesis Imperfecta
Type	**Clinical Appearance of Teeth**
Hypoplastic	Normal to small teeth; normal to opaque white-yellow brown color
	Thin enamel readily subject to attrition
	Smooth enamel with grooves, furrows, and/or pits
Hypomaturation	Opaque to yellow/brown; enamel soft and rough; dentin sensitivity
	Enamel is the same radiodensity as dentin
	Normal enamel thickness; chips easily
Hypocalcified	Opaque chalky white to yellow-brown; rough surface, dentin sensitivity; open bite; heavy calculus
	Normal enamel thickness; chips easily
Hypomaturation/ hypoplasia/ taurodontism	White/yellow-brown mottled, small teeth; lack proximal contact
	Reduced thickness; hypomineralized pits
	Molars demonstrate taurodontism

newly formed enamel. Failure of this process results in the incomplete maturation of the enamel crystals and the eruption of malformed enamel that is soft and porous. Teeth may appear mottled and opaque because the poorly formed crystals fail to reflect light as normal enamel. Radiographs show enamel is the same radio-density as dentin.

Hypocalcified types (Fig. 6-32D) show normal tooth morphology upon eruption but this becomes rapidly stained. It is soft and undercalcified, giving it an opaque appearance. These chalky-appearing teeth wear down rapidly and are more susceptible to caries. As the underlying dentin is exposed, the teeth take on a yellowish-brown stain.

Hypomaturation/hypoplasia/taurodontism, a fourth and less common type, shows enamel that is both poorly formed and soft and porous. The molars also show taurodontism.

Amelogenesis imperfecta can be a severe disability to the growing individual and dental management can be very difficult. The main clinical problems are aesthetics, dental sensitivity, and loss of tooth structure, which may lead to occlusal disharmony. Treatment depends on the severity of the problem. Early placement of full crowns will improve the appearance of the teeth and protect them from damage. The

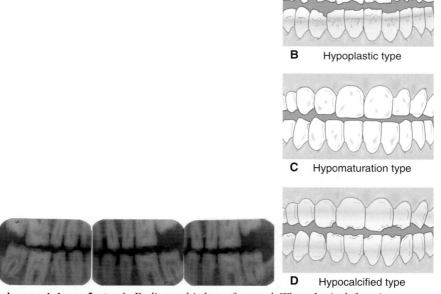

B Hypoplastic type

C Hypomaturation type

D Hypocalcified type

Figure 6–32 **Amelogenesis imperfecta. A.** Radiographic loss of enamel. Three basic defects in amelogenesis imperfecta. The specific types feature one or more of these patterns. **B.** Hypoplastic type. **C.** Hypomaturation type. **D.** Hypocalcified type.

primary dentition is protected by the use of preformed metal crowns on posterior teeth and composite restorations on anterior teeth. As permanent teeth erupt, they can be preserved with crowns as well.

Clinical Implications

Amelogenesis imperfecta often has similar clinical features as fluorosis. To distinguish amelogenesis imperfecta from fluorosis, one needs a detailed medical, dental, and family history. This should include the condition of family members' teeth as well as their history of fluoride exposure.

Hereditary Disorders of Dentin Formation

Table 6-5 lists the major genetic disorders that affect the dentin and pulp. They represent hereditary disorders that affect the dental papilla of the developing tooth. The dental papilla gives rise to the dentin and pulp of the normal tooth. When these tissues are affected, disorders of dentin and pulp result.

Dentinogenesis Imperfecta

Dentinogenesis imperfecta is an autosomal dominant disorder characterized by abnormal tissues formed from the dental papilla. The dental papilla is the portion of the tooth germ responsible for dentin and pulp formation. Therefore, the disorder is characterized by abnormal pulp formation and defective mineralization of dentin. Enamel and cementum are unaffected. Both the primary and permanent dentitions may be affected, but commonly both are involved.

Dentinogenesis imperfecta occurs alone or with osteogenesis imperfecta (see earlier discussion of OI in this chapter). These are often referred to as type I and type II, respectively. Both types have the same dental features that appear upon tooth eruption. The principal feature is an abnormal discoloration of the teeth due to the involved dentin showing through the normal unaffected enamel (Fig. 6-33A). The dentin lacks its normal tubular structure and the teeth have a variable blue-purple or gray-to-yellow-brown discoloration that causes the teeth to appear opalescent (Fig. 6-33B).

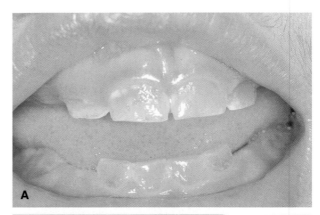

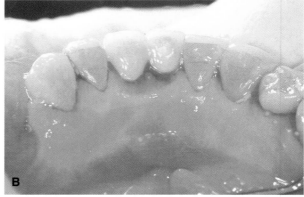

Figure 6–33 Dentinogenesis imperfecta. A. Child with dentinogenesis imperfecta with opalescent discoloration due to altered dentin. **B.** Her mother with similar-appearing teeth, some of which have been treated cosmetically.

Table 6.5	Comparison of Dentinogenesis Imperfecta and Dentin Dysplasia		
	Hereditary Pattern	**Clinical Features**	**Radiographic Featurese**
Dentinogenesis imperfecta	Autosomal dominant	Opalescent crowns; severe attrition	Obliterated pulp canal; constricted cementoenamel junction; thistle-shaped root
Dentin dysplasia	Autosomal dominant	Normal crown color; severe hypermobility; premature tooth loss; easy fracture on extraction	Short roots; crescent-shaped horizontal pulps; multiple periapical dental abscesses or cysts

Excessive amounts of this poorly formed dentin cause abnormal root shape and bulbous crowns with cervical constriction, giving the tooth a "thistle-shape." Excess abnormal dentin formation leads to alteration or obliteration of the pulp chamber (Fig. 6-34). The blood vessels and nerves of the pulp are present and the teeth are vital, but the pulp chamber is not visible radiographically.

Because the dentin is defective, the overlying normal enamel is poorly supported and eventually fractures away, leading to rapid wear and attrition of the teeth. The severity of discoloration and enamel fracturing is highly variable even within the same family. Treatment is restoration of the clinical crowns. With the advent of dentin bonding systems, these treatments are more successful than in the past. If left untreated, it is not uncommon to see the entire dentition worn down level with the gingiva at an early age.

Clinical Implications

Not everyone with dentinogenesis imperfecta may have a family member with the condition. The condition may present as a spontaneous "mutation." Detailed family history along with complete documentation of all clinical dental features is essential in arriving at a diagnosis.

Dentin Dysplasia

Dentin dysplasia is an autosomal dominant hereditary disorder that also affects tissues derived from the dental papilla, but it varies from dentinogenesis imperfecta in several important ways. Genetic evaluation shows that dentin dysplasia arises from a different mutation of the gene responsible for dentinogenesis imperfecta (*DSPP* gene). It is characterized by clinically normal appearing crowns, malformed roots, severe hypermobility, and spontaneous dental abscesses or cysts without obvious cause. Root dentin is weak, often leading to fracture during extraction. The pathogenesis of dentin dysplasia is unknown, but it has been suggested that the dental pulp becomes calcified, leading to reduced growth and final obliteration of the pulpal space.

Because teeth in dentin dysplasia erupt with a normal clinical appearance of the crown (Fig. 6-35A), the diagnosis is based on radiographic findings of the roots. Both dentitions are affected. Roots are short, blunt, and conical. The teeth lack pulp chambers or have pulp chambers that are horizontally oriented with a crescent shape and roots that are only a few millimeters in length. Frequently, periapical radiolucencies are observed (Fig. 6-35B). The extremely short roots give dentin dysplasia the name "rootless teeth." Premature loss of teeth may occur. Occasionally, there is a visible normal pulp with large pulp stones that creates localized obstructions within the pulp chambers (Fig. 6-35C).

Management of patients with dentin dysplasia includes extraction of teeth with necrotic pulp and apical abscess. Because these patients usually have early tooth exfoliation and alveolar bone atrophy, treatment with a combination of bone grafting and/or sinus lift may be needed for implant placement. Alternately, apical surgery with root end resection/root end fill may save teeth if they have long roots.

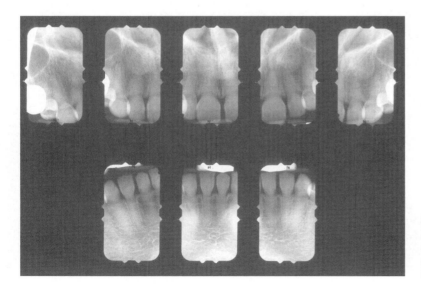

Figure 6–34 Dentinogenesis imperfecta. Portions of a full mouth series that show obliteration of pulp chambers and constricted cementoenamel junctions. Pulp is present but is embedded within the poorly formed dentin.

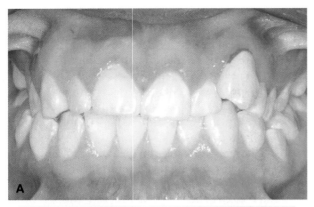

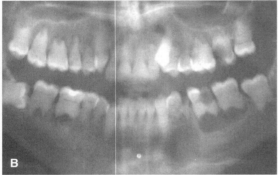

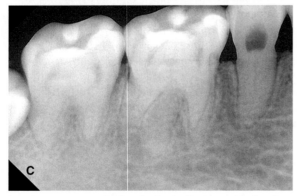

Figure 6–35 Dentin dysplasia. A. Patient with dentin dysplasia displays normal clinical appearance. **B.** Same patient with abnormal horizontal crescent-shaped pulp chambers, "rootless teeth," and periapical pathology. **C.** Obliteration of the pulps by large pulp stones.

Disorders of Cementum: Odontohypophosphatasia

Hypophosphatasia is a rare inherited metabolic bone disorder that affects the development of bones as well as cementum and periodontal ligament. Systemically, there is a deficiency of serum and bone alkaline phosphatase activity that is essential for proper bone and cementum formation. The etiology is mutations in a gene referred to as the *ALPL* gene that directs production of alkaline phosphatase, which is essential for mineralization of the skeleton and teeth. Disruption of mineralization of bones and cementum occurs.

The signs and symptoms of hypophosphatasia vary widely and may appear anywhere from before birth to adulthood. There are childhood and adult forms. Severe forms of hypophosphatasia that appear early in life are inherited in an autosomal recessive pattern. Before birth and in early infancy, severe hypophosphatasia weakens and softens the bones, causing skeletal abnormalities similar to rickets (see Chapter 9). Affected infants are born with short limbs, an abnormal-shaped chest, soft cranial bones, failure to gain weight, respiratory problems, and high levels of calcium in the blood (**hypercalcemia**). This may lead to recurrent bouts of vomiting and kidney problems as well as complications that are life-threatening in some cases.

Milder forms of hypophosphatasia that appear in childhood or adulthood are typically less severe than those that appear in infancy. Early loss of deciduous teeth is one of the first signs of the condition in children. Affected adults may lose their teeth and are at increased risk for joint pain and inflammation.

The mildest form of this condition, called *odontohypophosphatasia*, only affects the teeth. People with this disorder typically experience abnormal tooth development and premature tooth loss (Fig. 6-36A), but do not have the skeletal abnormalities seen in other forms of hypophosphatasia. Odontohypophosphatasia is characterized by premature exfoliation of fully rooted teeth (Fig. 6-36B) due to the lack of cementum, which serves as an anchor for the periodontal ligament (Fig 6-36C). Without cementum, the periodontal ligament fails to support the tooth in the socket. The anterior deciduous incisors are more likely to be affected. Radiographs show reduced alveolar bone, enlarged pulp chambers, and root canals. Although the only clinical feature is the dental findings, biochemical values are generally indistinguishable from those in patients with mild forms of hypophosphatasia, either adult or childhood forms. Odontohypophosphatasia should be considered in any patient with a history of early, unexplained loss of teeth, or abnormally loose teeth on dental examination. Box 6-2 lists other genetic causes for premature tooth loss.

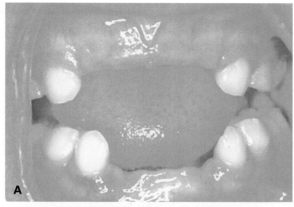

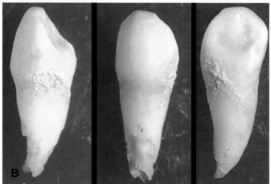

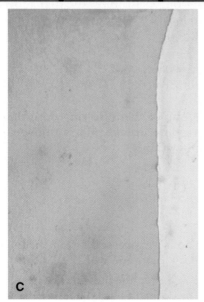

Figure 6–36 Hypophosphatasia. A. 7-year-old child with hypophosphatasia after early exfoliation of primary teeth. **B.** Canine tooth showing no cementum. **C.** Histology shows no cementum along the root surface. (From the Gorlin Collection, University of Minnesota)

Box 6-2 Hereditary Causes of Premature Tooth Loss

Acatalasia
Chediak-Higashi syndrome
Chronic neutropenia
Cyclic neutropenia
Dentin dysplasia
Hypophosphatasia
Hypophosphatemic vitamin D-resistant rickets
Lesch-Nyhan syndrome
Papillion-Lefèvre syndrome

Critical Thinking Questions

Case 6-1: Your 28-year-old female patient reports that her new husband had mild cherubism as a child. His lesions regressed after puberty and a minor surgery restored his normal facial contours. He is going to be a new patient in your practice soon.

• • •

What dental problems might you expect to find when he comes in for his new patient examination?

Your patient wonders if her children will have cherubism. What is the risk for each of her future children?

Case 6-2: Your 22-year-old female patient presents with diffuse thick white plaques of the buccal mucosa and lateral tongue. They have been present for as long as she can remember. They are not painful but she thinks they look unattractive. She wants to have them removed. She said her mother and grandmother have similar lesions.

• • •

She wonders if it is related to something she eats or drinks. How do you respond to her concerns?

What most likely will happen if the lesions are removed?

She wonders why her sister and brother do not have this condition. What do you know about the inheritance of this disorder?

Case 6-3: Your 6-year-old patient presents with several loose teeth. He has experienced early exfoliation of all his primary teeth and now his few permanent teeth are mobile.

• • •

List some possible causes of premature tooth loss in a child.

In addition to a complete medical history and family history, what supplementary information should be obtained to help differentiate among these causes? What data can be obtained during the dental appointment?

Case 6-4: A new family presents to your practice for routine dental care. You have the opportunity to examine four of the six family members. Three of them, including one of the parents, have mottled enamel and severe attrition. X-rays show thinning of the enamel and numerous open contacts. When questioned, the parents report that they believe their well water is the source of the problem. All the children have lived in the same location since birth: however, only two of them show the tooth abnormality.

• • •

Do you believe that the well water is the source of the problem?

If not, what condition do you believe this family has? What is your evidence?

Review Questions

1. **All of the following are true about DNA EXCEPT:**
   A. It is present in the cytoplasm of every cell.
   B. Strands of DNA are arranged in a double helix.
   C. Chromosomes are tiny units of organization.
   D. It can replicate or make copies of itself.

2. **Segments or sequences of DNA that determine specific traits or characteristics are called**
   A. euploid.
   B. aneuploid.
   C. genes.
   D. centromeres.

3. **If a cell has a missing chromosome, that cell is referred to as**
   A. autosomic.
   B. euploid.
   C. aneuploid.
   D. haploid.

4. **Which one of the following is an "address" of a gene along a chromosome that allows geneticists to locate a defective gene?**
   A. 10p12
   B. 23n-33m
   C. 1600der
   D. 46j38

5. **Which one of the following describes when a chromosome breaks and is reinserted in the wrong location?**
   A. Deletion
   B. Euploid
   C. Aneuploid
   D. Inversion

6. **If a gene is "expressed," that means the trait carried by that gene will**
   A. be seen in the individual.
   B. lie dormant until the next generation.
   C. be passed on to the next generation.
   D. cause the person to be outgoing and eloquent.

7. Many genetic disorders demonstrate signs and symptoms that differ among affected individuals. This is known as

    A. penetrance.
    B. syndromism.
    C. mutation.
    D. variable expressivity.

8. All of the following are true about autosomal recessive disorders EXCEPT:

    A. There must be two copies of the disease allele for the person to be affected.
    B. Affected individuals usually have one un-affected parent.
    C. There is a 25 percent chance that a child will inherit the mutated gene.
    D. There is a 50 percent chance that a child will be an asymptomatic carrier.

9. What term is used to describe the visible characteristics that are created by the gene codes?

    A. Phenotype
    B. Genotype
    C. Penetrance
    D. Carrier

10. A collection of signs and symptoms that occur together and when concurrent lead to the diagnosis of the condition is called a(n)

    A. mutation.
    B. epinonymous.
    C. syndrome.
    D. malformation.

11. All of the following are characteristics of Papillon-Lefèvre syndrome EXCEPT:

    A. It is characterized by the lack of an enzyme called catalase.
    B. There are both dermatological and oral manifestations.
    C. Mutation occurs in the cathepsin C gene.
    D. Palmoplantar keratosis and advanced peri-odontitis are features.

12. Patients with ectodermal dysplasia

    A. have scant eyebrows and sparse fine hair.
    B. develop fevers of unknown origin.
    C. have conical shaped and numerous missing teeth.
    D. All of the above

13. Which one of the following is associated with paramedian lip pits?

    A. Cherubism
    B. Papillon-Lefèvre syndrome
    C. Hypohydrotic ectodermal dysplasia
    D. van der Woude syndrome

14. How is cherubism transmitted?

    A. Autosomal dominant
    B. Autosomal recessive
    C. X-linked recessive
    D. Mutation only

15. All of the following are true about Cleidocranial dysplasia EXCEPT:

    A. It is also known as Crouzon's syndrome.
    B. There is delayed closure of the sutures of the skull.
    C. Individuals are usually short with large heads.
    D. Ability of the patient to touch the shoulders together is pathognomonic.

16. Craniosynostoses

    A. involve premature closure of cranial sutures.
    B. are characterized by accumulations of mult-inucleated giant cells.
    C. are characterized by delayed closure of cranial sutures.
    D. patients have a reduced ability to sweat.

17. All of the following characterize Treacher-Collins syndrome EXCEPT:

    A. It is an autosomal dominant disorder.
    B. There is hyperplasia of the zygomatic bone.
    C. Colobomas are a feature.
    D. Most patients have hearing loss due to defects in the bones of the middle ear.

18. **Which of the following is not a feature of nevoid basal cell carcinoma syndrome?**
    A. Basal cell carcinomas
    B. Bifid ribs
    C. Odontogenic keratocysts
    D. Coronoid hyperplasia

19. **Which one of the following is false regarding osteogenesis imperfecta?**
    A. Dental manifestations include supernumerary and conical teeth.
    B. Teeth develop an opalescent appearance because of defective dentin.
    C. It is the most common inherited bone disease.
    D. Blue sclera of the eyes and hearing loss can occur.

20. **What group of inherited skeletal defects, caused by a deficiency in osteoclast function, results in defective bone remodeling and a significant increase in bone density?**
    A. van der Woude syndrome
    B. Cleidocranial dysplasia
    C. Osteopetrosis
    D. Cherubism

21. **Café-au-lait pigmentation (spots) is**
    A. a feature of cherubism.
    B. present in McCune-Albright syndrome.
    C. associated with mutation of the *TCOF1* gene.
    D. caused by mutations in the "patched" gene

22. **The most significant manifestation of Gardner's syndrome is**
    A. colon polyps that develop in the second decade of life.
    B. high arched palate with clefting.
    C. dentinogenesis imperfecta.
    D. tendency to develop malignant bone tumors.

23. **Peutz-Jegher's syndrome is characterized by all of the following EXCEPT:**
    A. Adenocarcinoma of the GI tract develops in close to 30 percent of patients.
    B. Freckle-like pigmentations occur on the hands, perioral skin, and intraoral mucosa.
    C. Intestinal obstruction due to intussusception is a common complication.
    D. There is mutation of the keratin 4 and 13 genes.

24. **A benign tumor-like growth made up of normal mature cells in an abnormal number or distribution is known as a(n)**
    A. granulocytopenia.
    B. kleeblattschädel.
    C. hamartoma.
    D. nondisjunction.

25. **Which of the following statements concerning amelogenesis imperfecta is incorrect?**
    A. It is an exclusively ectodermal disorder.
    B. This condition results from a defective formation, mineralization, or maturation of enamel.
    C. Dentin develops abnormally as part of this condition.
    D. The enamel of these teeth is very soft and abrades away or chips off easily.

26. **Which condition is characterized by gray to violet opalescent teeth and obliterated pulp chambers and canals, and may occur in conjunction with osteogenesis imperfecta?**
    A. Dentin dysplasia
    B. Dentinogenesis imperfecta
    C. Hypophosphatasia
    D. Amelogenesis imperfecta

27. **Which statement about dentin dysplasia is incorrect?**
    A. This condition is also called "rootless teeth."
    B. It is sex-linked recessive.
    C. The roots of these teeth appear short, blunted, or conical.
    D. Premature loss of teeth may occur.

28. **Which one of the following is a metabolic bone disorder that affects the development of bones, cementum, and periodontal ligament?**
    A. Peutz-Jegher's syndrome
    B. Amelogenesis imperfecta
    C. Cherubism
    D. Hypophosphatasia

SUGGESTED READINGS

Books

Abouelmagd, A, Agreely, H: Basic Genetics: Textbook and Activities, ed. 1. University-Publishers, Boca Raton, 2009.

Lewis, R: Human Genetics: The Basics, ed. 1. Routledge, Francis and Taylor, New York, 2011.

Raoul, CM, Hennekam, JE, Allanson, DK, et al: Gorlin' Syndromes of the Head and Neck, ed. 5. Oxford University Press, New York, 2010.

Journal Articles

Allam, KA, Wan, DC, Kawamoto, HK, Bradley, JP, Sedano, HO, Saied, S: The spectrum of median craniofacial dysplasia. Plastic Reconstructive Surgery 127(2):812–821, February 2011.

Blumberg, B: Syndromes of the head and neck. American Journal of Human Genetics 49(1):246–247, July 1991.

Cai, R, Zhang, C, Chen, R, Bi, Y, Le, Q: Clinicopathological features of a suspected case of hereditary benign intraepithelial dyskeratosis with bilateral corneas involved: A case report and mini review. Cornea 30(12):1481–1484, December 2011.

Chacon, GE, Ugalde, CM, Jabero, MF: Genetic disorders and bone affecting the craniofacial skeleton. Oral and Maxillofacial Surgery Clinics of North America 19(4):467–474, v. Review, November 2007.

Dixon, J, Trainor, P, Dixon, MJ: Treacher Collins syndrome. Orthodontics and Craniofacial Research 10(2):88–95, May 2007.

Horbelt, CV: A review of physical, behavioral, and oral characteristics associated with Treacher Collins syndrome, Goldenhar syndrome, and Angelman syndrome. General Dentistry 56(5):416–419, July-August 2008.

Johnson, JM, Moonis, G, Green, GE, Carmody, R, Burbank, HN: Syndromes of the first and second branchial arches, part 2: Syndromes. American Journal of Neuroradiology 32(2):230–237, February 2011.

Kim, JW, Simmer, JP: Hereditary dentin defects. Journal of Dental Research 86(5):392–399, Review, May 2007.

Michou, L, Brown, JP: Genetics of bone diseases: Paget's disease, fibrous dysplasia, osteopetrosis, and osteogenesis imperfecta. Joint Bone Spine 78(3):252–258, Epub 2010 Sep 19, Review, May 2011.

Ng, FK, Messer, LB: Dental management of amelogenesis imperfecta patients: A primer on genotype-phenotype correlations. Pediatric Dentistry 31(1):20–30, Review, January-February 2009.

Passos-Bueno, MR, Ornelas, CC, Fanganiello, RD: Syndromes of the first and second pharyngeal arches: A review. American Journal of Medical Genetics Part A 149A(8):1853–1859, August 2009.

Sarda, D, Kothari, P, Kulkarni, B, Pawar, P: Cherubism in siblings: A case report. Journal of Indian Society of Pedodontics and Preventive Dentistry 25(1):27–29, Review, March 2007.

Neoplasms of the Oral Soft Tissues and Facial Skin

Learning Outcomes

At the end of this chapter, the student will be able to:

7.1. Define all key terms in the chapter.

7.2. Explain how neoplasms differ from reactive lesions.

7.3. Describe the characteristics that distinguish benign neoplasms from malignant neoplasms.

7.4. Describe the standard method of tumor nomenclature and list exceptions to the method.

7.5. List known and suspected risk factors for oral squamous cell carcinoma.

7.6. Explain the significance of dysplasia of oral epithelium.

7.7. List the most common locations for intraoral squamous cell carcinoma.

7.8. Explain the use of the TNM Classification of Malignant Tumors.

Continued

7.9. Describe the treatment for oral squamous cell carcinoma and its side effects.

7.10. Give examples of the most common benign and malignant salivary gland tumors.

7.11. Describe the clinical features as well as prognosis for neoplasms affecting the oral cavity.

7.12. Describe epithelial neoplasms commonly seen on the facial skin.

BASIC PRINCIPLES OF NEOPLASIA

Neoplasia comes from the Greek word meaning "new growth." In neoplasia, the growth of cells is not coordinated with growth of adjacent normal tissues. This typically causes a lump referred to as a **tumor**. The word tumor literally means "swelling" but has become accepted to be synonymous with **neoplasm**. However, contrary to common belief, tumor and neoplasm are not synonymous with cancer. This chapter reviews a variety of tumors, some **benign** (noncancerous) and some **malignant** (cancerous), that are encountered in dental hygiene practice.

In the 1960s, R. A. Willis defined a neoplasm as "an abnormal mass of tissue, the growth of which exceeds and is uncoordinated with that of normal tissues and persists after cessation of the stimuli that evoked the change." The resulting mass is purposeless. For example, a neoplastic osteoblast (bone-forming cell) may continue to lay down bone, but the bone is abnormal in form and function. Tumors grow autonomously (independently) and may be life-threatening, invading vital structures.

All benign or malignant tumors originate from a single cell that was injured. If injury does not kill a cell, it may recover and/or adapt to its new environment. Alternately, its DNA may be damaged to the extent that the cell can no longer recover sufficiently to carry out its normal functions.

DNA contains genes that regulate the growth and functions of the body. When DNA is damaged, one of several outcomes occurs: the cell dies; the cell recovers with the help of specialized repair genes; portions of the DNA that regulate the life cycle of the cell are permanently damaged. Neoplasia results from damage to the cell's DNA. When cells undergo change as a result of DNA damage, they are known as **neoplastic.** These cells form a neoplasm, or tumor. A unique feature of neoplastic cells is that if the injurious agent is removed, the cells continue to grow on their own without further provocation or stimulation. This is one of the major differences between a *neoplasm* and a *reactive process*: reactive lesions generally resolve when the originating stimulus is removed; neoplasms do not.

Damage to a cell's genes, within the DNA, may be caused by both known and unknown etiologic agents. The etiology of most neoplasms is unknown. Damage that results in neoplasia includes but is not limited to environmental agents and **oncogenic viruses** (Table 7-1).

Table 7.1	Known Carcinogens and Associated Cancers	
	Etiologic Agent	**Cancer Type**
Environmental Agents	Asbestos	Lung, mesothelioma, esophagus
	Benzene	Leukemia, Hodgkin's lymphoma
	Cadmium	Prostate
	Nickel	Nose, lung
	Radon	Lung
	Second-hand tobacco smoke	Oropharyngeal, lung, breast, kidney
	Wood dust; leather dust	Maxillary sinus
	Ultraviolet light	Skin
	Therapeutic radiation	Sarcomas of tissue in field of radiation: osteosarcoma, fibrosarcoma, etc.

Table 7.1	Known Carcinogens and Associated Cancers—cont'd	
	Etiologic Agent	**Cancer Type**
Oncogenic Viruses	Human papilloma virus 16 and 18	Cervical, oropharyngeal
	Epstein-Barr	Burkitt's lymphoma, nasopharyngeal carcinoma
	Hepatitis B and C	Hepatocellular (liver)
	HTLV-1	T-cell leukemia
	Human herpes virus 8	Kaposi's sarcoma

An altered gene capable of causing a neoplasm is called an **oncogene**. The prefix *onco-* means neoplasm or tumor. Cells have the ability to repair this damage through the action of DNA repair genes. If damage occurs rapidly and repair genes are overwhelmed, the cells may continue to divide and transfer genetic damage to future generations of cells. Cells also have a mechanism to eliminate abnormal or damaged cells, a process called **apoptosis**. If the gene that regulates apoptosis is damaged, cell death may not occur. Affected cells then continue to live and transmit defective genetic material to future generations of cells. This type of transformation is the first step in tumorigenesis (tumor development) (Fig. 7-1).

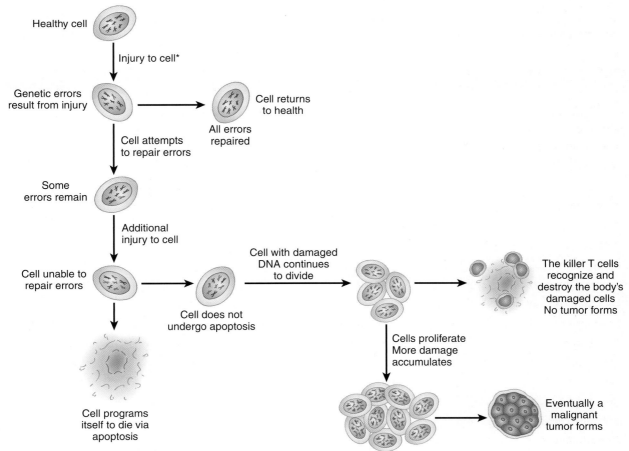

* See Table 7-1 for injurious agents.

Figure 7–1 **Carcinogenesis.** When the DNA of cells is exposed to a carcinogen, the cells either die (apoptosis) or carry on the defect to form a tumor mass.

Tumor Nomenclature

Understanding tumor nomenclature helps communicate whether the tumor is benign or malignant and also its tissue of origin. All tumors are named based on the cell or tissue that has been altered. If the tumor is benign, the suffix *-oma* is added to the end of the cell or tissue name. An example is neuroma, a benign tumor of nerve tissue. If the tumor is malignant, the suffix *-carcinoma* or *-sarcoma* is added. Malignant tumors arising from cells that originated from embryonic ectoderm are termed **carcinomas**. An example of a carcinoma is malignant transformation of the squamous epithelium lining of the oral cavity to *squamous cell carcinoma*. The Greek term for glands is *adenas*; therefore, any benign tumor that arises from glandular tissue is called an **adenoma.** Because glands originate from embryonic ectoderm, any malignant glandular tumor is called an **adenocarcinoma**. The name of the specific gland is added. Examples are salivary gland adenocarcinoma and thyroid adenocarcinoma. Malignant tumors arising from cells that originated from embryonic mesoderm or neural crest are termed **sarcomas**. An example of a sarcoma is malignant transformation of the fibroblasts of fibrous connective tissue to *fibrosarcoma*. See Table 7-2 for more examples of tumor nomenclature. Please note that there are important exceptions to the tumor nomenclature rule.

Benign Versus Malignant

Clinical behaviors and outcomes of benign tumors differ significantly from malignant tumors. Benign tumors are most often not life threatening and patients generally do not die as a direct result from them or suffer long-term ill effects. Exceptions are benign tumors growing in or near vital structures such as the brain or heart.

Malignant tumors, on the other hand, cause significant **morbidity**. Patients often suffer long-term effects and many do not recover even after treatment. However, the long-term outcome for certain malignant tumors is more positive with high survival rates.

Microscopic characteristics are important in determining whether a tumor is benign or malignant.

Table 7.2	Tumor Nomenclature	
Tissue of Origin	**Benign**	**Malignant**
Squamous epithelium	None common	Squamous cell carcinoma
Basal epithelium	Seborrheic keratosis	Basal cell carcinoma
Melanocytes	Nevus	*Melanoma
Glands	Adenoma	Adenocarcinoma
Connective tissue proper	Fibroma	Fibrosarcoma
Bone	Osteoma	Osteosarcoma
Bone marrow leukocytes	None common	Leukemia
Blood vessels	Hemangioma	Angiosarcoma
Lymphatic vessels	Lymphangioma	Lymphangiosarcoma
Lymph nodes and tonsils	None common	*Lymphoma
Enamel organ	Ameloblastoma	Ameloblastic carcinoma
Dental papilla	Odontogenic myxoma	Odontogenic myxosarcoma
Cartilage	Chondroma	Chondrosarcoma
Fat	Lipoma	Liposarcoma
Nerve	Neuroma	Neurosarcoma
Schwann cells	Schwannoma	*Malignant peripheral nerve sheath tumor
Smooth muscle	Leiomyoma	Leiomyosarcoma
Skeletal muscle	Rhabdomyoma	Rhabdomyosarcoma

*By convention, these malignancies are not termed melanocarcinoma, lymphosarcoma, or schwannosarcoma.

The most common defining characteristic is cell appearance. Cells from benign tumors resemble the cells from which the tumor arose, but they comprise a disorganized, purposeless mass. For example, benign smooth muscle tumors called leiomyomas are made up of cells that look the same as normal smooth muscle cells.

Cells change appearance due to damage to their DNA. The term used to describe the degree to which they appear different from their normal counterparts is **differentiation**. The range of differentiation is from *well-differentiated* (closest to normal appearance) to *poorly differentiated* (harder to recognize normal appearance) to *undifferentiated* (change so great that origin of cells cannot be determined by visual inspection). Cells that do not appear like their normal counterparts are termed **anaplastic**. Anaplastic cells with DNA damage display one or more of the following features:

- **Pleomorphism:** wide range in cell size and shape (cells are dissimilar to the size and shape of normal cells; *pleo* = many; *morphism* = shape)
- **Hyperchromatism (hyperchromasia):** intense deep blue coloration to nucleus
- **Altered nuclear/cytoplasm ratio:** nucleus may appear extra large or extra small

- **Increased or bizarre mitosis:** mitotic activity that is increased and abnormal (Cancer cells often divide at a faster rate so more dividing cells than normal may be seen; because their division is out of control, the dividing cells may show bizarre shapes, as shown in Figure 7-2.)
- **Disordered maturation:** normal growth and development of cells is altered; they do not mature properly (Normal cells form layers or exhibit patterns necessary for the functions of a specific tissue. An example of altered development is epithelium that is undergoing malignant change. Basal cells normally located along the basement membrane may be seen near the surface; Keratin normally located on the surface may be seen forming in the basal layer.)

Besides alteration in individual cells, the tumor as a whole may display features that can predict whether it is benign or malignant:

1. **Rate of growth:** Most, but not all, benign tumors grow slowly over several years; malignant tumors tend to grow more quickly, often with sporadic growth spurts.
2. **Encapsulation:** Because benign tumors grow slowly, they have time to form an outer fibrous capsule or "shell" (Fig. 7-3). This keeps the cells

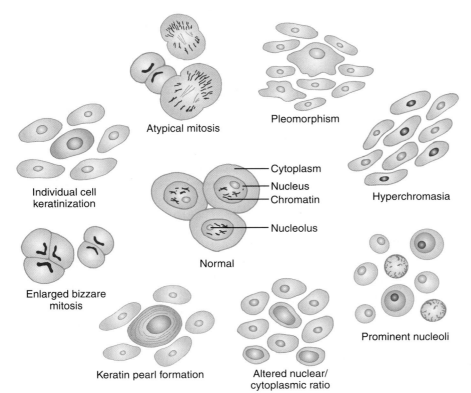

Atypical mitosis

Pleomorphism

Individual cell keratinization

Cytoplasm
Nucleus
Chromatin

Nucleolus

Hyperchromasia

Normal

Enlarged bizzare mitosis

Prominent nucleoli

Keratin pearl formation

Altered nuclear/ cytoplasmic ratio

Figure 7–2 Anaplasia. Cells undergoing malignant change show a variety of atypical cellular features.

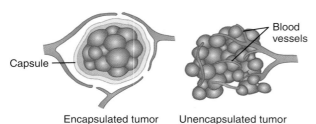

Figure 7–3 Encapsulated versus unencapsulated tumors. Encapsulation is a feature of tumors that helps limit their spread.

bound tightly together so they do not spread or infiltrate into surrounding normal tissue. It also makes most benign tumors easy to remove. Malignant tumors tend to grow quickly and do not have time to form a capsule. Malignant cells are free to wander and infiltrate or invade adjacent normal tissue. This makes removal of malignant tumors more difficult.

3. **Metastasis:** With rare exception, only malignant tumors metastasize. Metastasis differs from infiltration in that tumor cells travel to distant sites, such as lymph nodes (Fig 7-4A) or lungs (Fig 7-4B). When a tumor metastasizes, the cells most often resemble the original tumor. For example, a squamous cell carcinoma (SCC) of the oral cavity that metastasizes to the liver resembles an SCC, not liver cancer. Depending on the type of tumor, metastasis may occur via the lymphatic system, the bloodstream, or along nerves. The presence of metastasis often dramatically alters treatment and prognosis.

> **Clinical Implications**
>
> If a tumor from the oral cavity metastasizes to the lung, it is incorrect to state that the patient now has lung cancer. The patient has metastatic cancer to the lung.

ORAL SQUAMOUS CELL CARCINOMA (ORAL CANCER)

Comprehensive head and neck examination is a vital tool in detection of early **squamous cell carcinoma (SCC)**. The dental team possesses a combination of unique expertise and opportunity to thoroughly examine the head and neck, and oral cavity. Diligent examination and evaluation of suspicious lesions saves lives. This section begins with a detailed discussion of SCC, the most common cancer found in the oral cavity.

Epidemiology and Risk Factors of Oral Cancer

Epidemiology refers to the study of disease within a population rather than in an individual person. Ninety percent of all oral cancers arise from stratified squamous epithelium. This type of cancer is the sixth most common malignancy worldwide. Observing disease patterns within a population provides important information to health professionals on causes, risk factors, and prevention. A classic example is the observation that the incidence of oral cancer is higher in smokers than in nonsmokers. This observation has led to a better understanding of oral cancer prevention. **Incidence** refers to the number of newly diagnosed cases during a specific time period. For example, the incidence of oral cancer each year in the United States is 36,000 new cases. Another term used in discussing epidemiology is **prevalence,** which refers to the number of people with a disease at any point in time. For example, currently in the United States there are approximately 240,000 people living with oral cancer.

A **risk factor** is a characteristic or behavior that may increase the chances that a particular disease will occur. Risk factors may predispose a patient to develop disease. They are most often not the sole cause of the disease, in spite of their close association with it. Risk factors are either extrinsic or intrinsic. **Extrinsic** risk factors are related to the patient's environment or personal habits, such as smoking. Risk factors for SCC have been identified in approximately 75% to 85% of oral cancer patients, which leaves approximately 15% to 25% of patients with oral cancer who have no known risk factors.

Known risk factors for oral cancer include tobacco smoking, alcohol consumption, syphilis, smokeless tobacco use, radiation therapy to the head and neck, industrial carcinogens, and sunlight to the lips. In some cultures, oral habits may be harmful to the oral tissues and predispose the patient to oral cancer. In populations in which **betel quid** is chewed (betel quid is composed of palm nuts, shredded tobacco, clay, and slaked lime wrapped in a betel palm leaf), rates of oral cancer tend to be high.

Oncogenic (tumor-producing) viruses, such as human papilloma virus (HPV) strains 16 and 18, are considered a major risk factor for posterior oropharyngeal cancer but not for intraoral cancer. Another example is Epstein-Barr virus, which is the etiologic agent of a specific type of nasopharyngeal cancer found most commonly in Asia.

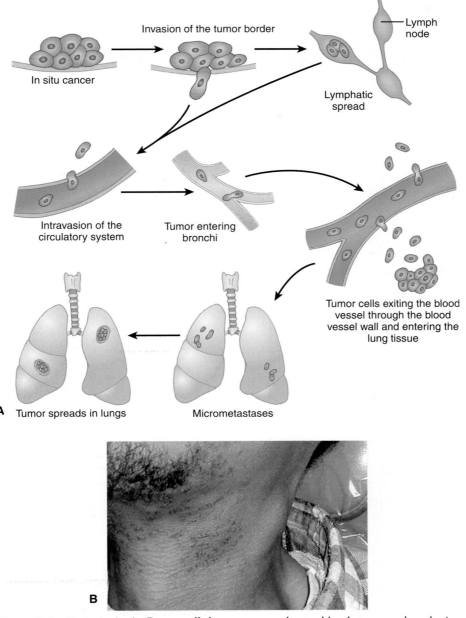

Figure 7–4   Metastasis. A. Cancer cells leave tumor and enter blood stream or lymphatics, eventually spread to the lungs. **B.** Patient with indurated lymph node of left neck indicating metastasis of oral cancer.

Other risk factors for oral cancer are *intrinsic*, which means they are not related to the patient's habits or environment. Intrinsic risk factors include age, gender, iron-deficiency anemia, immunosuppressive diseases such as HIV/AIDS, and therapeutic immune suppression for organ transplantation.

Clinical Implications

Clinicians must be aware of a phenomenon known as **field cancerization.** This involves the exposure of a wide area to a cancer-promoting agent. For example, all mucosal surfaces that are

Continued

exposed to tobacco smoke comprise a field of exposure. One or more sites in this field can develop oral cancer over time. Patients with one tumor may go on to develop additional tumors in different parts of the mouth in the future.

Heredity has not been shown to be a strong risk factor in oral cancer development; oral cancer tends not to "run in families." There is also a misconception that chronic irritation is a cause of oral cancer. Research has not proven a causal relationship between chronic irritation, such as a rough tooth, denture, or cheek-chewing habit, and the development of oral cancer. However, some researchers have observed an association between chronic inflammation and oral cancer. A new area of research is the association between mediators of inflammation and cellular changes that may predispose a person to cancer. Many of these factors are yet unknown.

Knowledge of oral cancer is important in understanding the:
- Known risk factors: This is useful in counseling patients on social habits such as alcohol use and smoking.
- Concept that *association* does not imply *causation*. For example, it is incorrect to tell a patient that smoking will cause him or her to develop oral cancer. However, it is correct to tell the patient that smoking will increase his or her *risk* for developing oral cancer.
- Importance of a comprehensive head and neck examination for all patients, regardless of the presence or absence of known risk factors.

Not all risk factors for oral cancer are known. Early lesions in patients may escape detection if thorough extraoral and intraoral exams are not performed, simply because a patient does not appear to be "at risk."

Clinical Features of Oral Cancer

Cancer may develop in all oral tissues, including lining and masticatory mucosa, salivary glands, blood vessels, or tonsils. In addition, cancers from other areas in the body may metastasize to the oral cavity. However, the term *oral cancer* is reserved in this text to describe malignancies that develop within the squamous epithelium of the oral mucosa. This results in visible and detectable changes to the surface appearance. The next

section explores what these precancerous and cancerous changes look like.

Precancerous Changes in the Oral Cavity

The development of oral cancer is often progressive. Under the influence of a carcinogen, the basal cells of the epithelium produce abnormal cells that divide at a rapid rate. This can vastly increase the numbers of cells within the epithelial layer, resulting in excess keratin production at the surface. The excess keratin appears clinically as a white plaque. In some cases, the rapidly produced abnormal cells lose their ability to produce keratin and surface breakdown occurs. The lack of keratin appears clinically as ulceration. Therefore, precancerous changes may appear clinically with excessive keratin, lack of keratin production, or a combination of both.

Clinical Implications

Many white lesions occur in the oral cavity, the most common of which is *frictional keratosis*, a benign condition caused by chronic irritation (see Chapter 2). Often, it is impossible to tell by appearance alone which white lesions are precancerous and which ones are not. All white lesions are considered suspicious until the diagnosis is confirmed. Eighty to ninety percent of white lesions in the oral cavity are *not* precancerous or cancerous. Biopsy is often the only way to differentiate between nonmalignant, premalignant (precancer), or malignant (cancer) changes. Look at Figure 7-5A and B. Can you identify which one is oral cancer?

Dysplasia

Dysplasia means ~~loss of normal maturation~~. Normal oral squamous epithelium is ~~composed of a cuboidal basal layer, a spinous layer that flattens near the surface, and a keratin layer.~~ Dysplasia means that the cells have an altered ability to mature from basal cells into keratinocytes that produce keratin. This may result in loss of the stratified (layered) structure. ~~Dysplastic oral epithelium is considered *precancerous*,~~ meaning there is a *risk* that it will develop into oral cancer. Dysplasia may be mild, moderate, or severe depending on the extent of altered maturation. Mild dysplasia is cellular change confined to the basal cell layer. This can revert to normal epithelium if the suspected carcinogenic agent, such as tobacco, is

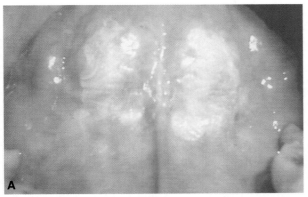
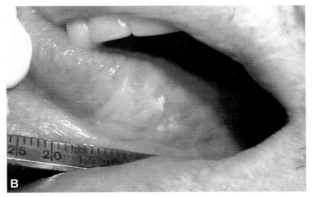

Figure 7–5   Comparison of two white plaque of unknown diagnosis. Which of these white lesions is cancerous and which one is benign? Can you tell?

removed or eliminated. Moderate and severe dysplasia affect the basal, spinous, and keratin layers. Here the cells cannot revert to normal even if the suspected carcinogenic agent is removed. Mild, moderate, or severe dysplasia can only be determined by a biopsy and examination under the microscope (Fig. 7-6).

Clinical appearance of oral epithelial dysplasia varies depending on the extent of cellular changes. If abnormal cells "pile up" and produce a thick layer of keratin, the lesion will appear as a white plaque that does not wipe off. White lesions that do not wipe off are called **leukoplakia** (*white plaque* in Greek) (Fig. 7-7A). If the cells fail to produce keratin and the surface epithelium becomes thinned (atrophic) or is lost, then the lesion will appear erythematous (red). Erythematous lesions are called **erythroplakia** (*red plaque* in

Greek). Often, there is a mixture of red and white in dysplastic lesions. **Erythroleukoplakia** is a patch with both red and white features (Fig. 7-7B). These are clinical descriptive terms and do not imply any specific diagnosis. Diagnosis is determined microscopically with a biopsy.

Progression to Oral Cancer

Carcinoma-in-situ (CIS) is the earliest form of oral cancer. **In-situ** means "in the original place"—not having been moved or transferred to another location. In CIS, all layers of the squamous epithelium demonstrate lack of proper maturation. There is no invasion into the underlying connective tissue (Fig. 7-8).

When oral cancer cells invade the underlying connective tissue, the lesion may become **indurated or**

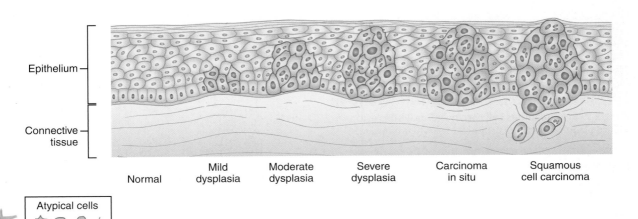

Figure 7–6   Grades of dysplasia to SCC. Epithelial dysplasia is considered a precancerous condition that can develop through stages from mild to severe, leading to carcinoma.

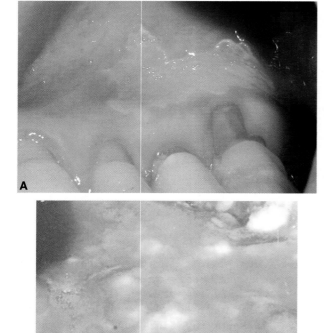

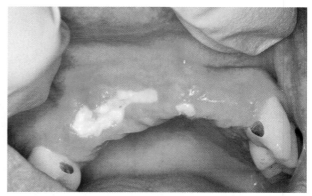

Figure 7–9   White plaque. Flat white plaque.

- **Flat red plaque:** Loss of normal keratin production in early lesions that have not formed a solid mass (Fig. 7-10).
- **Combined red and white plaque:** Alternating areas of increased and decreased keratin production result in a speckled appearance, seen in early lesions that have not formed a solid mass (Fig. 7-11).
- **Exophytic mass:** White and/or red solid mass that grows outward, proliferating off the epithelial

Figure 7–7   Clinical appearance of dysplasia.
A. Leukoplakia. **B.** Erythroleukoplakia. Both are clinical descriptive terms, not diagnoses.

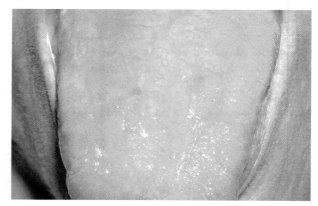

Figure 7–10   Red plaque. Flat red plaque.

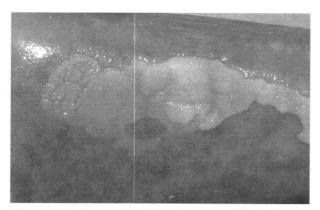

Figure 7–8   Squamous cell carcinoma as white lesion.
White plaque shows cancerous change when biopsied.

firm to palpation. This can be detected during the intraoral or head and neck examination.

Oral epithelium undergoing malignant transformation may produce the following clinical appearances:

- **Flat white plaque:** Excess abnormal keratin formation in early lesions that have not formed a solid mass (Fig. 7-9).

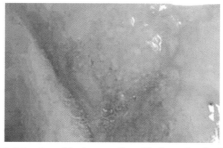

Figure 7–11   Speckled mass. Speckled erythroleukoplakia (red and white plaque).

surface; may appear warty or papillary (Fig. 7-12). Malignant cells may invade from the epithelium into the underlying connective tissues. The mass may be indurated (firm) to palpation.

- **Endophytic mass**: White and/or red mass that grows inward, proliferating down from the epithelial surface. These often appear as chronic ulcerations with a central depressed area surrounded by raised borders. Malignant cells have invaded from the epithelium into the underlying connective tissue (Fig. 7-13). The mass is often indurated (firm) to palpation.

High-Risk Locations for Oral Cancer

Oral cancer may occur in any intraoral anatomic location but some locations are at higher risk. The following list highlights areas of highest to lowest risk:

- **Vermillion of the lip.** SCC of the lip is the most common form of oral cancer. Fair-skinned individuals who have outdoor occupations or hobbies are at increased risk of excessive sun exposure and damage to the lips. **Actinic damage** (change produced by radiant energy, i.e., sun exposure) can predispose the lower lip to dysplastic and cancerous alterations (Fig. 7-14). Atrophy (thinning) of the vermillion

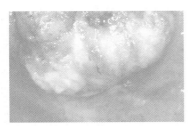

Figure 7–12   Exophytic mass. Papillary exophytic mass (red and white mass).

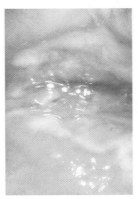

Figure 7–13   Enodophytic mass. Endophytic mass with rolled borders.

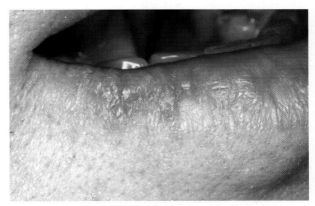

Figure 7–14   Actinic cheilitis. Dry crusted change to lower lip indicating premalignant lesion.

border of the lip is characterized by loss of normal fine wrinkling and loss of a well-defined vermillion-skin interface. Individuals who smoke a pipe or cigar may experience similar localized alterations of the lip. These changes predispose for development of SCC. SCC of the lip initially presents as a crusted, nontender, indurated area. This often mimics "chapped" lips and lesions may grow unattended for many months. SCC of the lower lip can be destructive, resulting in significant lip deformity. Metastasis occurs in advanced lesions.

Clinical Implications

Individuals spending a great deal of time outdoors should be counseled on how to avoid sun damage to the lips, especially the lower lip. Sun-blocking lip balm is recommended, along with wearing a hat. Hats with a brim shade and protect the face and lower lip from sun exposure. Close surveillance is indicated for sun-damaged lips with a mottled chapped appearance and indistinct vermillion-epithelial interface.

- **Lateral and ventral tongue.** The most common intraoral site for development of SCC is the posterior lateral border of the tongue (Fig. 7-15A). This site, along with the anterior lateral and ventral tongue (Fig. 7-15B), account for approximately 50 percent of all intraoral cancers in the United States. Lesions will vary from flat or pebbly white plaques (Fig. 7-15C) to large ulcerated exophytic indurated masses (Fig. 7-15D). During the oral examination, the tongue must be extended completely and turned from side to side so that the posterior borders may be fully inspected. The dorsum of the tongue is rarely affected (Fig. 7-15E).

- **Floor of the mouth.** The floor of the mouth is continuous with the ventral tongue. This makes the rates of occurrence for SCC between floor of

mouth and ventral tongue difficult to determine and compare. However, approximately 35 percent of all oral cancer is reported to occur in the floor of mouth (Fig. 7-16). Oral cancers of the lateral border of the tongue and floor of mouth occur with greatest frequency in tobacco smokers, more than in any other known risk group. SCC in this

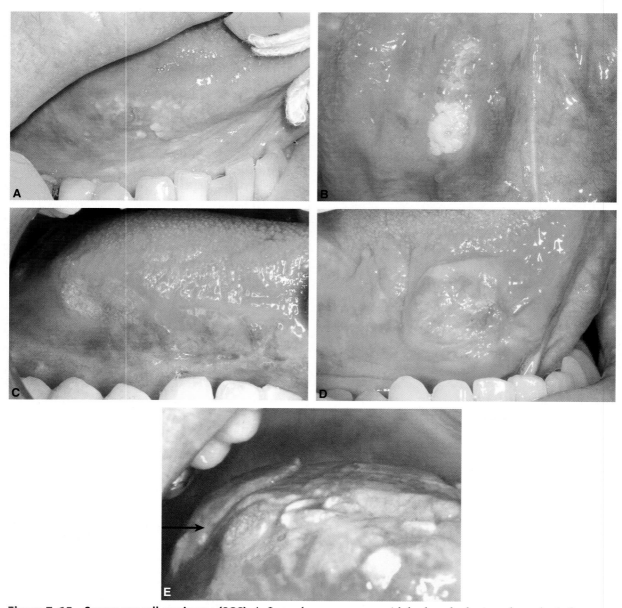

Figure 7–15   Squamous cell carcinoma (SCC). A. Lateral tongue cancer with both endophytic and exophytic features. **B.** SCC ventral tongue. Indurated thick, white plaque with raised rolled borders. **C.** SCC latero-ventral tongue. Lateral tongue cancer with pebbly red and white surface, extending to ventral tongue. **D.** SCC ventral tongue. Large exophytic mass with ulcerated surface. **E.** SCC dorsal tongue. Red and white change with pebbly exophytic mass on dorsal tongue.

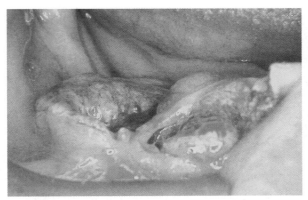

Figure 7–16 Squamous cell carcinoma-floor of mouth. Fungating red and white indurated mass encroaching upon the alveolar ridge.

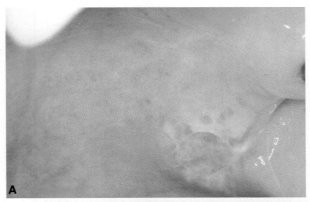

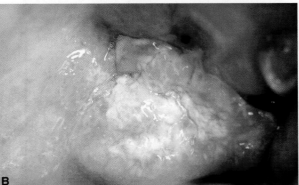

Figure 7–17 Squamous cell carcinoma: Soft palate. **A.** Painless ulcer of soft palate with indurated rolled border. **B.** Large fungating mass with necrotic surface causing dysphagia.

region may extend to the alveolar ridge and destroy bone.

- **Soft palate and oropharynx.** Because of their posterior location, cancers that develop in these areas often go undetected in early stages (Fig. 7-17A). They often increase significantly in size before the first signs appear, including dyspnea or dysphagia (Fig. 7-17B). Metastasis may already have occurred before the initial diagnosis is made.

Clinical Implications

Tumors of the soft palate and oropharynx often test positive for HPV types 16 and 18. These oncogenic viruses have been implicated as likely etiologic agents in some types of cancer.

- **Gingiva and alveolar ridge.** SCC of the gingiva often mimics benign non-neoplastic processes such as oral lichen planus and traumatic ulcers. However, on close inspection these SCCs tend to have a speckled pattern not seen in the other conditions (Fig. 7-18A). SCC in these locations may take on the appearance of a pyogenic granuloma as they enlarge (Fig. 7-18B). They may also resemble an isolated periodontal defect (in an otherwise healthy mouth) as the tumor begins to invade underlying alveolar bone; tooth mobility may result (Fig. 7-18 C and D).

    SCC of the edentulous alveolar ridge may mimic injury from full or removable partial dentures (Fig. 7-19A). The clinical impression may be that of an epulis fissuratum or traumatic denture ulcer

(Fig. 7-19B). Persistent changes in the fit of removable, full, or partial dentures occur as the tumor mass steadily increases in size.

- **Retromolar pad and buccal mucosa.** SCC of the retromolar pad (Fig. 20A) and buccal mucosa may appear as a white exophytic plaque, a red and white granular or pebbly lesion, or an ulcerated lesion with raised rolled borders. On the retromolar pad, early SCC may be interpreted as irritation from masticatory forces. Lesions on the buccal mucosa may present as plaque-like lesions, often misinterpreted as oral lichen planus (Fig. 7-20B).
- **Hard palate.** SCC of the hard palate occurs most often under a full or removable partial denture. It may be mistaken clinically as hyperplastic candidiasis or denture stomatitis. Occasionally, lesions may mimic inflammatory papillary hyperplasia (Fig. 7-21A). Dysphagia often occurs with larger tumors (Fig. 7-21B).

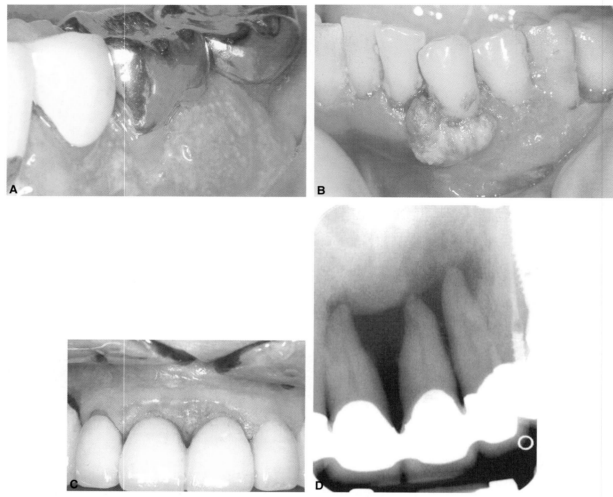

Figure 7–18 Squamous cell carcinoma: Gingiva. A. Exophytic pebbly red and white mass, thought to be lichen planus until it became indurated. **B.** Painless exophytic red and white mass thought to be a pyogenic granuloma. **C.** Granular red and white change to the gingiva; teeth became mobile over a 3- to 4-month period. **D.** Radiograph of C. Posteroanterior film shows dramatic bone loss of short period of time as tumor invades the alveolar bone.

Verrucous Carcinoma

Verrucous means "wart-like." Verrucous carcinoma is characterized by a thick, wart-like surface texture. It is seen most commonly in smokeless tobacco users who develop lesions where the tobacco is placed, but it may be seen in those who do not have this habit. Verrucous carcinomas tend to be red and white, thick, mushrooming (fungating), exophytic papillary masses that are soft and sometimes **friable** (Fig. 7-22A). Some lesions may present with a more subtle appearance (Fig. 7-22B). Verrucous carcinoma is a very low-grade tumor that rarely invades the

underlying connective tissue, metastasizes, or causes death. However, verrucous carcinoma predisposes for the development of SCC, which has a more ominous prognosis.

Clinical Implications

Approximately 7 percent of adults, 8 percent of high school students, and nearly 3 percent of middle school students currently use smokeless tobacco in the United States. This may predispose for the development of verrucous carcinoma. Smokeless tobacco products come in various forms, such as finely ground, shredded, or powdered. They often contain more than 28 known carcinogens, in addition to sugared flavoring agents. Users are not only at risk for developing oral cancer, but also for developing periodontitis and caries. Occasionally, because of social stigma attached to smokeless tobacco use, users hide the tobacco out of sight, including under dentures.

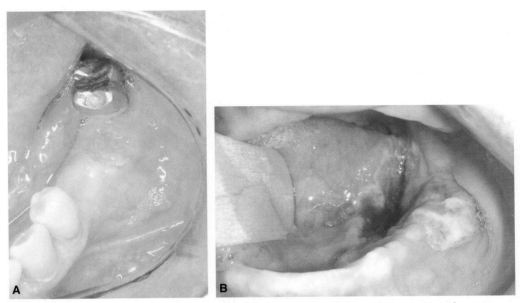

Figure 7–19   Squamous cell carcinoma: Alveolar ridge. A. Mobile tooth was extracted; tumor grew into socket. **B.** Patient's denture became unstable as tumor spread from alveolar ridge to floor of mouth and lateral tongue.

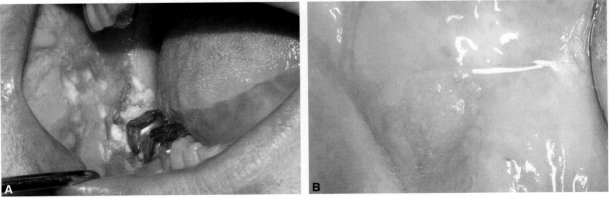

Figure 7–20   Squamous cell carcinoma: Buccal mucosa. A. Extensive firm, indurated tumor extends from buccal mucosa to retromolar pad and gingiva. **B.** Stippled red and white patch with ill-defined borders.

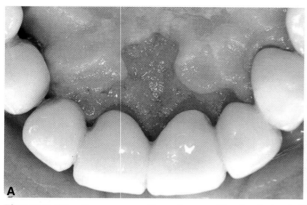
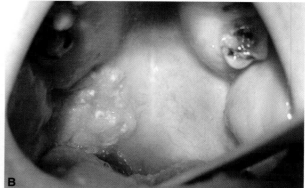

Figure 7–21 **Squamous cell carcinoma: Hard palate. A.** Depressed granular center with raised indurated borders with white surface alteration. **B.** Nonpainful exophytic red and white tumor extending to involve soft palate.

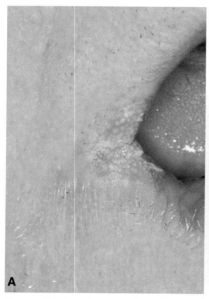
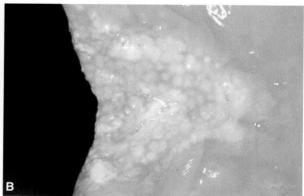

Figure 7–22 **Verrucous carcinoma. A.** Firm verruco-papillary surface texture. **B.** On close inspection, early verrucous carcinoma shows fine verruco-papillary surface.

Staging of Oral Cancer

The **TNM Classification of Malignant Tumors** (**TNM**) is a cancer staging system developed by the American Joint Committee on Cancer (AJCC). **Staging** describes the extent to which cancer has spread in a patient's body and is determined after a thorough physical examination and diagnostic testing, including imaging studies and biopsy. Separate staging systems have been developed for each organ system, with criteria specific to the location. Some factors are similar among all systems and include:

■ Tumor size (measured in centimeters)
■ Node (lymph node) involvement

■ Metastasis: spread of the cancer to distant organs, away from the original tumor

See Table 7-3 for the specific parameters for determining TNM for oral and oropharyngeal cancer.

Once TNM values have been determined, staging is calculated, treatment is planned, and prognosis is determined. Higher stages tend to have a poorer prognosis and often require more aggressive treatments. Oral cancers found in Stages 1 or 2 have a better prognosis and tend to require less treatment than those found in Stages 3 or 4.

When discussing cancer survival, the phrase **5-year survival rate** is often used. This indicates the percentage

Table 7.3 TNM System for Staging of Oral and Oropharyngeal Cancer

TNM System

T = tumor size and invasion
- TX - primary tumor cannot be assessed
- T0 - no evidence of primary tumor
- Tis - carcinoma in situ
- T1 - tumor less than 2 cm in greatest dimension
- T2 - tumor more than 2 cm but not more than 4 cm in greatest dimension
- T3 - tumor more than 4 cm in greatest dimension
- T4 - tumor invades adjacent structures (mandible, tongue musculature, maxillary sinus, skin)

N = node involvement)
- NX - regional lymph nodes cannot be assessed
- N0 - no regional lymph node metastasis
- N1 - metastasis in a single ipsilateral lymph node, less than 3 cm in greatest dimension
- N2a - metastasis in a single ipsilateral lymph node, more than 3 cm but not more than 6 cm in greatest dimension
- N2b - metastasis in multiple ipsilateral lymph nodes, none more than 6 cm in greatest dimension
- N2c - metastasis in bilateral or contralateral lymph nodes, none more than 6 cm in greatest dimension
- N3 - metastasis in a lymph node, more than 6 cm in greatest dimension

M = metastasis
- M0 - no distant metastasis
- M1 - distant metastasis

Staging

Stage I: T1N0M0
Stage II: T2N0M0
Stage III: T3N0M0 T1 *or* T2 *or* T3N1M0
Stage IV: T4N0 *or* N1M0 *or* Any T, N2, *or* N3M0 *or* Any T, any N, M1

Reprinted with permission from AJCC: Pharynx. In: Edge, SB, Byrd, DR, Compton, CC, et al., Eds.: AJCC Cancer Staging Manual, ed. 7. Springer, New York, 2010, pp 41–56.

of patients who will survive 5 years after the initial diagnosis. On average, for all stages and locations of oral cancer, the 5-year survival rate is 52 percent. This means that 52 percent of all patients who are diagnosed with all stages oral cancer combined will be alive after 5 years. However, if a patient is diagnosed with Stage 1 oral cancer, the 5-year survival rate approaches 80 percent. The overall 5-year survival rate has improved only slightly in the past 30 years, with the greatest improvement seen in tonsillar and tongue cancers. Patients who survive beyond 10 years have

a relatively good prognosis. See Table 7-4 for current 5-year-survival data on oral cancer.

Clinical Implications

A patient presents with a tumor of the right posterior lateral border of the tongue. It measures greater than 2 cm in greatest dimension. One small, firm, palpable fixed cervical lymph node is present in the right neck. There is no evidence of metastasis to distant sites in the body. TNM values are T2 N1 M0; the patient has Stage 3 oral cancer. The 5-year survival rate is 20 percent, meaning there is a 20 percent chance of being alive in 5 years.

Oral Cancer Treatment and Side Effects

The treatment for oral cancer varies and is determined by such factors as:

- Patient's age, general health, and past medical history
- Cancer type, size, location, and stage
- Patient's ability to withstand treatment
- Need to preserve oral function (affects quality of life)

Table 7.4 Oral Squamous Cell Carcinoma: 5-year Survival by Stage at Diagnosis

Site	Stage I	Stage II	Stage III	Stage IV
Posterior tongue	60%	50%	20%	20%
Anterior tongue	71%	59%	47%	37%
Floor of mouth	73%	60%	36%	30%
Gingiva	90%	90%	90%	35%
Retromolar area	90%	90%	90%	60%
Soft palate	90%	80%	50%	50%
Buccal mucosa	90%	90%	70%	60%
Lip	96%	83%	57%	48%
Tonsil	70%	50%	30%	14%
Maxillary sinus	70%	60%	30%	18%

Retrieved August 2012 from http://www.cancer.org/cancer/oralcavityandoropharyngealcancer/detailedguide/oral-cavity-and-oropharyngeal-cancer-survival-rates

Surgery, radiation therapy, and chemotherapy are the most common treatments available to help treat and manage oral cancer. Although each type of therapy has the potential to increase the chance of survival, each has side effects.

Surgery and Side Effects

Surgery offers the greatest chance of survival for many types of cancer, especially those that have not yet metastasized. Tumors are removed while preserving as much normal structure and function as possible. The ideal situation occurs when the tumor is relatively small and can be completely excised during surgery.

Surgical alternatives include **debulking** in which only a portion of a large tumor is removed because it impinges on vital structures, or is not totally **resectable** (removable). The residual tumor is then treated with **radiation** or **chemotherapy**. **Palliative** surgery is used to treat complications of advanced disease to help ease the patient's symptoms, but is not intended to be curative.

Surgery for oral cancer may be disfiguring, leaving patients with functional difficulties. **Obturators** are sometimes constructed to cover large intraoral defects so patients can function as normally as possible (Fig. 7-23A and B). Reconstructive surgery may be necessary once the cancer is removed so that the patient's appearance and function can be restored. Speech and swallowing may be affected and require specialized therapy. Customized oral hygiene and home care may be needed to maintain optimal oral health.

Radiation and Side Effects

Radiation therapy is a painless treatment that uses ionizing radiation to destroy tumor cells by damaging their DNA, making it impossible for them to continue dividing. The total dose of radiation is broken down into small increments. It is often delivered daily over 6 to 8 weeks with breaks to allow for normal tissues to undergo repair. The daily dose must be great enough to destroy cancer cells while sparing normal cells. Most normal, healthy cells in the path of radiation are able to repair themselves and return to proper functioning, but some cannot.

When radiation is delivered directly to the head and orofacial region, patients experience side effects. These are related to tissues and glands in the path of the radiation and include:

1) Radiation-induced xerostomia
2) Radiation-induced mucositis
3) Osteoradionecrosis

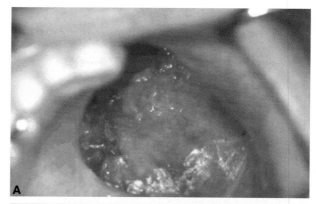

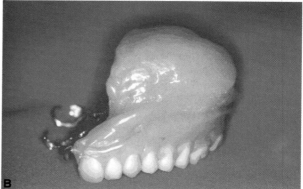

Figure 7–23 Obturator. A. Patient treated with surgery to remove squamous cell carcinoma of the palate **B.** The patient now wears an obturator to cover defect and restore function.

Radiation-induced xerostomia is defined as severe mouth dryness resulting when the beam of radiation passes through the salivary glands to reach the tumor. Salivary glands are **radiosensitive** and are easily injured or destroyed. Only cancers of the head and neck have this complication from radiation. Every attempt is made to shield salivary glands but this may not be possible because of tumor location. Resulting xerostomia is often temporary but may be permanent depending on the amount and duration of radiation treatment.

After 2 weeks of radiation therapy, the production of saliva by the parotid and submandibular/sublingual salivary glands may be reduced by as much as 80 percent. Typically, the watery serous saliva of the parotid gland is lost first, leaving only thick mucus saliva. Function may not recover until 6 weeks following radiation therapy. However, after long-term high-dose radiation therapy for extensive disease, loss of both serous and mucous saliva may become permanent due to obliteration of saliva-producing cells. The following important functions of normal saliva are compromised or lost:

- Diluting and clearing dietary sugars
- Buffering acids generated by bacterial fermentation
- Remineralizing enamel
- Producing secretory IgA
- Producing antimicrobial peptides and proteins
- Lubricating

A variety of problems arise when salivary gland function is compromised, including development of rampant caries (Fig. 7-24), oral infections including candidiasis (see Chapter 3), difficulty eating and speaking, loss of taste, and mucositis. Increased caries control measures may be required that include daily fluoride application via custom trays and dietary counseling to reduce or eliminate sugar exposure.

Prevention of radiation-induced xerostomia has been the subject of research for many years. Surgery to move salivary glands out of the path of radiation before therapy has been used with some success. Administration of medications before radiation to protect the salivary glands from damage has also been attempted.

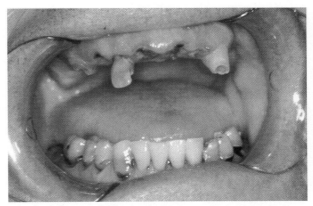

Figure 7–24   Radiation caries. Patient with rampant caries after radiation for floor of mouth tumor damaged salivary glands.

Clinical Implications

For patients who have reduced or complete loss of saliva, an increase in oral moisture can be supplied by sialogogues or saliva substitutes. **Sialogogues** are agents that stimulate salivary flow in glands that are still functional. These include prescription medications such as pilocarpine or over-the-counter sugar-free, buffered lozenges. **Saliva substitutes** are sprays and rinses that temporarily replace lost saliva and provide relief from the physical discomfort of dry mouth. Lubricating gels or a drop of olive oil on the tongue can help reduce oral discomfort.

For dentate patients, the addition of daily fluoride in custom-fabricated gel carriers and regular dietary counseling are important to reduce the risk of caries.

Radiation-induced mucositis is an acute injury to the oral and pharyngeal mucosal lining caused by the harmful effects of ionizing radiation (Fig. 7-25). Treatments for mucositis include basic oral care, use of oral moisturizing products, and periodic dental evaluations

and cleanings. Because the tissues are tender, coating them with a muco-adherent agent may bring enough relief so that the patient can eat comfortably. Current recommendations for mucositis focus on prevention as well as supportive and palliative care, including aggressive use of analgesics, use of feeding tubes, and swallowing therapy. Unlike radiation-induced xerostomia, radiation-induced mucositis is not permanent.

Osteoradionecrosis is an unfortunate side effect seen in the jaws when the beam of radiation damages bone. This occurs in bone that was in the path of radiation. Bone out of the field of radiation is not affected. The blood supply to irradiated alveolar bone is irreparably damaged and it loses the ability to repair itself or respond to common injury or infection. Innocuous forms of trauma such as denture injury or tooth extraction can result in bone death (osteonecrosis)

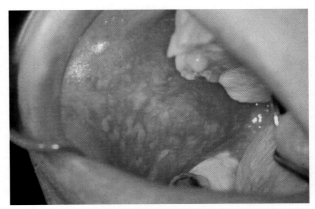

Figure 7–25   Radiation mucositis. Severe ulceration of the buccal mucosa following radiation therapy for oral cancer.

and loss of the overlying oral mucosa. The soft tissue sloughs, exposing areas of dead bone to the oral cavity (Fig. 7-26). The threat of developing osteoradionecrosis is lifelong and preventive measures must continue throughout life.

Clinical Implications

Figure 7-27 shows a young patient who received radiation therapy to treat cancer during childhood to the left side of the head. Tooth follicles developing at that time received radiation damage, resulting in dental hypoplasia.

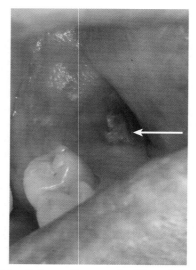

Figure 7–26 Osteoradionecrosis. Necrotic bone in patient who received radiation therapy for tumor in posterior tongue.

Chemotherapy and Side Effects

Chemotherapy involves the use of drugs that interfere with cancer cells' ability to divide or grow. The types of drugs used depend on what type of tumor is being treated. Not all tumors are sensitive to chemotherapy so not all patients receive it.

The severity of chemotherapy side effects differs from person to person. Typical side effects include gastrointestinal tract irritation leading to nausea and vomiting, alopecia (hair loss), *anemia* and *leukopenia*, *thrombocytopenia*, *dermatitis*, *mucositis*, fatigue, and delayed wound healing. During chemotherapy, patients may be unable to mount a normal immune response to common injuries and infections. Mucositis may affect eating and maintaining good nutrition. Erosion of the teeth may result from prolonged periods of nausea and vomiting.

Chemotherapy-induced mucositis is typically less severe and of shorter duration than radiation-induced mucositis. However, patients receiving concurrent radiation and chemotherapy treatment have increased severity and duration of mucositis. Mucositis has recently become more problematic as the combination of treatment with chemotherapy and radiation have become more common.

Oral mucositis is painful, making eating and swallowing difficult. Oral ulcerations commonly develop (Fig. 7-28) and when they are extensive, there is an increased risk of a developing **septicemia.** Prophylactic antibiotics may be indicated. Oral care is difficult during an episode of oral mucositis. Severe pain may make brushing and flossing difficult and unpleasant, leading to compromised oral hygiene.

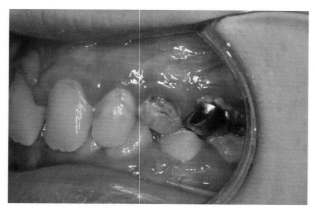

Figure 7–27 Dental hypoplasia in patient irradiated for cancer as a child; the developing tooth buds in the path of radiation were damaged.

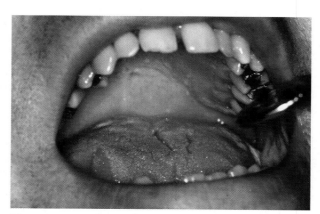

Figure 7–28 Chemotherapy mucositis. Severe inflammation of palate, tongue, and gingiva causing problems with proper nutrition and hydration.

Spontaneous healing of chemotherapy-induced mucositis occurs within 2 to 3 weeks after completion of treatment. Healing of ulcers usually takes 7 to 10 days. Because oral mucositis is self-limiting, management of lesions should include oral debridement, antifungal and antibacterial rinses, pain management, and control of bleeding. Palliative care with topical bio-adherent oral gels may help the patient for the duration of the therapy. A protocol consisting of regular rinsing with bland agents, brushing with a soft toothbrush, using water-based moisturizers, and flossing, if tolerable, is indicated. Cryotherapy (sucking on ice chips) and topical anesthetics may be helpful.

EPITHELIAL NEOPLASMS OF THE ORAL MUCOUS MEMBRANES AND FACIAL SKIN

Oral cancer is the epithelial neoplasm of most concern in the oral cavity; however, additional benign neoplasms do occur in the oral cavity and on the facial skin. Some of these are presented in the next section.

Benign Tumors

Acquired Melanocytic Nevus (Common Mole)

Nevus (plural *nevi*) refers to a **congenital** (present at or shortly after birth) circumscribed malformation of the skin composed of nevus cells. The **acquired melanocytic nevus** (common mole) is a benign collection of nevus cells that have the ability to produce melanin pigment. Nevus cells have an embryonic origin similar to melanocytes cells of the epidermis. Nevi develop early in childhood, most commonly on skin of the head and neck region. They begin as a sharply delineated brown macule that gradually evolves into a smooth exophytic papule as cells proliferate in the dermis (Fig. 7-29). Lesions rarely exceed 6 mm in diameter. As the lesion ages, pigment tends to fade. The surface becomes less smooth and occasionally a

hair may be observed growing in the center. Many regress with age, so few may be seen in older adults. No treatment is needed unless the patient elects to have the lesions removed for cosmetic reasons or they become irritated. Few ever progress to cancer.

Intraoral Melanocytic Nevus

Intraoral melanocytic nevi may be seen on any mucosal surface. They tend to be less pigmented than nevi of the skin (Fig. 7-30); however, when they are pigmented they can mimic the rare intraoral melanoma (discussed below). Unlike the skin, there are few distinguishing clinical features to differentiate between intraoral nevus and intraoral melanoma, so surgical excision is often undertaken.

The unusual **blue nevus** has been reported in the oral cavity. It most often occurs as a macular lesion on the palate. Blue nevi have a characteristic blue to blue-black color produced by abundant melanin particles located deep in the submucosa. The overlying tissues cause a change in light reflectance, causing these nevi to appear blue rather than brown.

Clinical Implications

With the exception of an x-ray–confirmed amalgam tattoo (Chapter 2), it is not possible to differentiate among most intraoral pigmented lesions by visual inspection alone. All pigmented lesions in the oral cavity that cannot be clearly identified should be considered for biopsy.

Seborrheic Keratosis

Seborrheic keratosis (SK) is a benign proliferation of basal cells, which is common on sun-exposed areas of

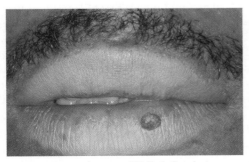

Figure 7–29   Dermal nevus. Well-defined pigmented nodule of the lower lip.

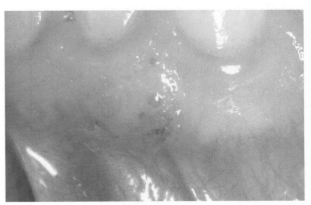

Figure 7–30   Intramucosal nevus. Exophytic pigmented mass of the gingiva.

the skin as an individual ages. SK is not seen inside the oral cavity. Lesions are caused by a proliferation of normal basal cells of the epithelium in response to sunlight or because of a genetic mutation in one of the growth factor genes. Because melanocytes reside among the basal cells, SKs tend to be pigmented. They appear as pigmented soft tissue masses that may occur singly but often occur in clusters. SKs rarely exceed 2 mm in diameter though they may gradually increase in size and eventually flatten. The surface can vary from rough to smooth. The lesions have been described as having a "stuck-on" raisin-like appearance in the early stages. Occasionally, patients report they are pruritic (itchy).

A variant of seborrheic keratosis is seen in patients of African descent. *Dermatosis papulosa nigra* is seen as multiple small pigmented papules of the face, usually in the **malar** and infraorbital areas (Fig. 7-31).

Seborrheic keratosis is rarely of concern because the lesions have no potential to become malignant. Lesions are often removed for cosmetic purposes; however, concern arises when there is a sudden eruption of numerous SK lesions over a short period of time. This is called the *sign of Leser-Trélat* and may signal the patient is developing an internal malignancy.

Epithelial Disorders With Malignant Potential

Some benign conditions have malignant potential in all patients afflicted by them. Three will be discussed here.

Actinic Keratosis

Actinic keratosis is a premalignant condition of sun-exposed skin. The term **actinic** refers to exposure to the sun. **Keratosis** refers to rough, raised area of keratinized epithelium. These skin lesions appear as irregular crusty plaques producing excessive amounts of keratin seen against a mottled background of sun-damaged skin. Men are affected more often than women, probably because of the protection provided by lipstick. The presence of actinic keratosis is considered a risk factor for developing skin cancer (squamous cell carcinoma of the skin). Rate of transformation to squamous cell carcinoma is estimated to be 10% to 20% over 10 years. Removal of actinic keratosis helps reduce the risk of developing skin cancer in that area.

Proliferative Verrucous Leukoplakia

Proliferative verrucous leukoplakia (PVL) is a condition characterized by thick white plaques. It is chronic, persistent, and recurrent. Unlike other leukoplakias, PVL has a high rate of malignant transformation to either squamous cell carcinoma or verrucous carcinoma. When the lesions are initially examined, most have benign features. Changes toward premalignant dysplasia and eventually carcinoma are seen over time. An association with HPV infection, particularly strains 16 and 18, has been implicated in some cases, but many cases are HPV negative. Only 30% of patients with PVL report a history of smoking, much lower than in populations affected by hyperkeratosis (Chapter 2), epithelial dysplasia, and oral cancer. Most cases occur in females, with a female-to-male ratio of approximately 4:1 in adults older than 40 years. The peak incidence occurs in women aged 60 to 70 years.

PVL begins as a flat white plaque, much like any other keratotic plaque, such as frictional keratosis (Fig. 7-32A). Progressively, dramatic multiple keratotic plaques with rough corrugated surfaces and papilloma-like projections or thick white fissuring develop (Fig. 7-32B). The plaques slowly spread; multiple sites may be involved at one time. The gingiva and buccal mucosa are typically included. Due to its progressive behavior, multiple serial biopsies are needed to establish the diagnosis of PVL.

Surgical excision is the current treatment for PVL. Because of the high recurrence rate, multiple surgeries may be necessary. Carbon dioxide laser, radiation, topical bleomycin solution, oral retinoids, beta-carotene, and systemic chemotherapy have all failed to reduce recurrence rates. Laser ablation and topical photodynamic therapy hold some promise in research trials.

Oral Submucous Fibrosis

Oral submucous fibrosis is a precancerous condition seen in individuals who chew a concoction called *betel quid* and its derivatives, *pan masala* and *gutka.* This is an

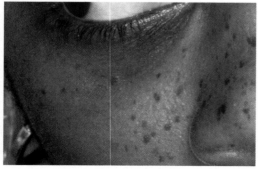

Figure 7–31 **Dermatosis papulosa nigra.** Multiple SKs across the malar skin of an African American patient.

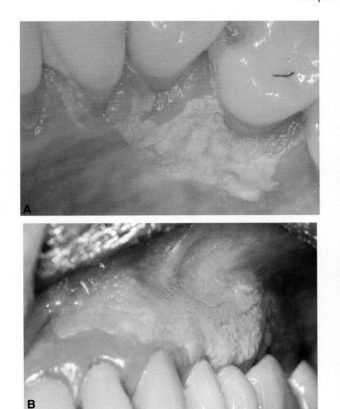

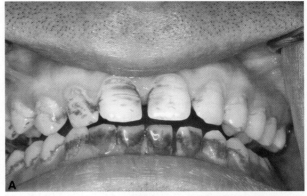

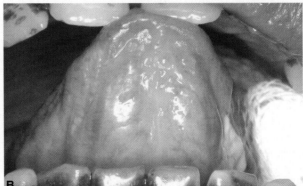

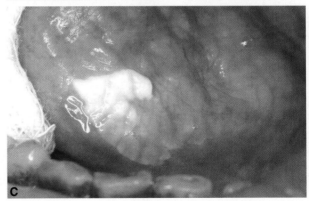

Figure 7–32   Proliferative verrucous leukoplakia.
A. Thick, white plaques with no obvious source of friction showed early stages of dysplasia on biopsy. **B.** Heavy corrugated premalignant lesions of the gingiva and vestibule.

Figure 7–33   A. Betel quid chewer. Tell-tale orange brown stain of teeth in patient who habitually used betel quid. **B.** Oral submucous fibrosis. Same patient with diffuse premalignant white lesions of ventral and lateral tongue. **C.** Same patient with thick white plaque that is well-defined anteriorly and diffuse posteriorly.

addictive habit most commonly used by residents of Southeast Asia and immigrants from this area. This habit leaves a tell-tale orange-brown extrinsic stain on the teeth (Fig. 7-33A). Early lesions may develop after only a short period of use. The buccal mucosa, soft palate, and floor of the mouth become stiff and rigid. This may result in **trismus**, an inability to open the mouth completely. If the tongue is involved, it may eventually become immobile. The tissues appear pale and white (Fig. 7-33B). Eventually, the mucosa develops thick white plaques that are precancerous (Fig. 7-33C). Discontinuing use of betel quid will not result in the mucosa reverting to normal. Patients are at increased risk for development of squamous cell carcinoma and must be followed indefinitely for signs of malignant transformation.

Malignant Epithelial Tumors

The most common malignant epithelial tumor is oral squamous cell carcinoma, discussed previously in this chapter. Other epithelial malignancies inside the oral cavity are very rare; however, several epithelial malignancies occur on the skin of the face that can be readily observed during a dental appointment. Most arise ***de novo*** (from the beginning; anew), but others can arise from pre-existing benign lesions.

Basal Cell Carcinoma

Basal cell carcinoma (BCC) is a malignancy that commonly affects the skin of the face and neck, but not the oral cavity. It is characterized by proliferation of abnormal cells in the basal layer of the epithelium as a result of chronic overexposure to ultraviolet (UV) radiation from sunlight or tanning bed exposure. Mutations of genes in the basal cells occur, resulting in malignant transformation, unregulated growth, and invasion into the underlying connective tissues. Generally, BCC is seen in fair-skinned individuals older than 40 years. However, the mean age has been decreasing in recent years, possibly due to the increased popularity of artificial UV light for tanning the skin. BCC may also occur in patients with nevoid basal cell carcinoma syndrome (Gorlin syndrome, see Chapter 6), where the mutation is inherited rather than caused by UV light.

BCCs most often present as a slow-growing exophytic mass, usually with raised rolled borders and fine blood vessels on the surface (Fig. 7-34A). Early lesions may resemble "pimples" which patients tend to pick until they enlarge and fail to resolve (Fig. 7-34B). The center of the lesion becomes depressed and ulcerated as the mass grows and expands (Fig. 7-34C). Some BCCs become pigmented due to the presence of benign melanocytes in the basal layer.

BCCs can invade deep into the underlying tissues but they are not known to metastasize. If left untreated, they may expand into vital structures and destroy large amounts of skin and subcutaneous tissues. If lesions are properly treated, recurrence is not expected. Proper treatment includes a process called *Mohs surgery*, in which the tumor is removed and examined immediately under the microscope while the patient is still present. If microscopic tumor is still present at the margins of the excised tissue, more tissue is removed until all margins are free of tumor.

Field cancerization principles apply to basal cell carcinoma. The cumulative sun damage may leave other areas of the skin at risk for developing new tumors. Continued monitoring and regular dermatologic examination are important.

Squamous Cell Carcinoma of the Skin

Squamous cell carcinoma (SCC) of the skin is less common than basal cell carcinoma. Light-colored skin, exposure to UV light, immunosuppression, therapeutic radiation, and several hereditary syndromes predispose patients to develop premalignant actinic keratoses, discussed earlier in this chapter. Untreated

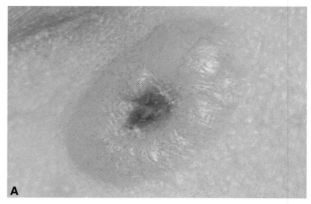

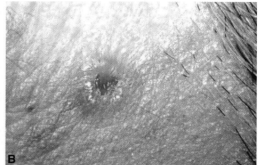

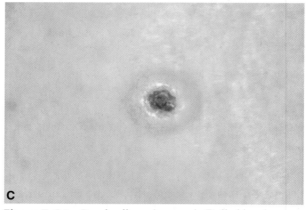

Figure 7–34 Basal cell carcinoma. A. Rolled borders show fine blood vessels; endophytic ulcerated center. **B.** Patient thought he cut himself shaving but lesion did not heal and became indurated. **C.** Long-standing tumor with well-defined rolled margin.

actinic keratosis may develop into a SCC of the skin (Fig. 7-35A).

SCC of the skin begins as a firm, skin-colored or erythematous nodule on the face, ear, neck, or nose (Fig. 7-35B). Because SCC can invade deeply, it can cause damage and disfigurement. Unlike basal cell carcinomas, SCC can metastasize. Treatment is complete surgical excision. Patients have a high risk of

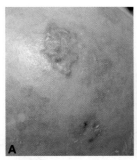
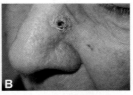

Figure 7–35   Squamous cell carcinoma of facial skin.
A. Diffuse red, crusted lesions of sun-exposed skin.
B. Deeply invasive, crusted tumor of lateral nose; patient
thought it was a "pimple" and picked at it.

recurrence or developing a second tumor because of
field cancerization. Close monitoring of individuals
with a history of excessive sun exposure and SCC of
the skin is indicated.

Melanoma

Melanoma is a malignant neoplasm that arises from
melanocytes. Melanocytes are pigment-producing
cells that are normally located within the basal layer of
stratified squamous epithelium. Most deaths from skin
cancer are from melanoma. Because all melanomas are
malignant, the term "malignant melanoma" is redundant and should be discouraged. Melanoma may occur
both on the skin surface (Fig. 7-36A and B) and on the
oral mucosa. Damage from UV light is considered to
be a major etiologic factor in the development of
melanoma of the skin; however, the etiology of intraoral melanoma is not completely understood. Genetic
alterations that are either inherited or acquired may
play a significant role in their development.

Twenty-five percent of all melanomas are located
on the skin of the head and neck of Caucasian adults
older than age 30. The appearance of skin melanomas
can vary from flat to nodular.

Using the A-B-C-D-E guidelines will help distinguish melanoma from melanocytic nevi or seborrheic
keratosis of the skin.

> **A** – **Asymmetrical shape**: irregular, not symmet-
> rical in shape
> **B** – **Border**: irregular border that is difficult to
> define
> **C** – **Color**: variegated - more than one color (blue,
> black, brown, tan, etc.) or uneven distribution of
> color
> **D** – **Diameter**: greater than 6 mm in diameter (size
> of a pencil eraser)
> **E** – **Evolution**: pigmented lesion has gone through
> recent changes in color and or size

Melanomas may occur in the oral cavity; however,
they are more common in the nasal cavity where they
present with unilateral nasal obstruction and epistaxis.
The gingiva/alveolar ridge and hard palate are the
most common intraoral locations (Fig. 7-37). Lesions
begin as a flat macule with an irregular border but
progress to develop into an exophytic mass. Lesions
may become ulcerated and erythematous. Mucosal
melanomas have a far more aggressive behavior when
compared to skin melanomas and are more likely to
metastasize.

Treatment of skin melanomas is wide surgical excision. Malignant melanocytes are generally resistant to
radiation. The treatment for intraoral melanoma is
surgery, with radiation reserved for advanced cases.
Palliative chemotherapy is used. There is a TNM classification system for melanoma. Survival rates for skin
(dermal) melanoma range from 95 percent for Stage I
to 10 percent for Stage IV, a number that reinforces

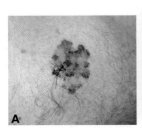
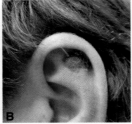

Figure 7–36   Melanoma of facial skin. A. Large,
asymmetric variegated lesion with irregular borders of
sun-exposed skin. **B.** Melanoma of ear in a young patient
who spent long hours in the sun.

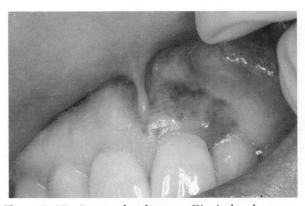

Figure 7–37   Intraoral melanoma. Gingival melanoma.

the need for early detection. The prognosis for intra-oral melanoma is very poor, with only 10% to 15% of patients surviving beyond 5 years.

SALIVARY GLAND NEOPLASIA

Salivary gland neoplasia is exclusively found in the oral cavity and tissues of the head and neck. Understanding their clinical features is essential because many salivary gland tumors are discovered during a dental visit. Most salivary gland tumors are benign; however, some can be malignant. Therefore, early diagnosis may help save a patient's life.

Salivary gland neoplasms can occur wherever there is salivary gland tissue. Considering the large number of minor salivary glands within the oral mucosa, this includes almost the entire oral cavity, with the exception of the gingiva and anterior hard palate. Normal glands are composed of a variety of duct cells, saliva-producing *acinar cells*, and specialized *myoepithelial cells*, which contract and help expel saliva from the gland. This variety of cells helps explain the large number of both benign and malignant salivary gland tumors that arise from them. More than 34 different types of salivary gland tumors exist but only the most common are discussed here (Table 7-5).

Benign Salivary Gland Tumors

Pleomorphic Adenoma

Pleomorphic adenoma is the most common salivary gland tumor. *Pleo* means "many" and *-morphic* means "form." Pleomorphic refers to the microscopic appearance of these tumors rather than their clinical appearance.

The most common location for pleomorphic adenoma is the parotid gland, where it produces a very slow-growing firm and painless mass (Fig. 7-38) that may sometimes be superimposed over the angle of the mandible (Fig. 7-39). Upon palpation, these tumors have the consistency of a raw potato. They are usually well encapsulated; however, the facial nerve is often

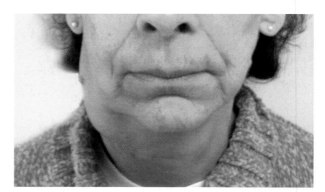

Figure 7–38   Pleomorphic adenoma. Mass of lower lobe of parotid gland.

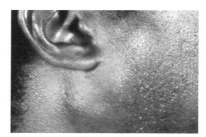

Figure 7–39   Pleomorphic adenoma of parotid. Firm, freely movable mass at angle of the mandible.

Table 7.5	Common Salivary Gland Neoplasms	
	Neoplasm	**Most Common Locations**
Benign	Pleomorphic adenoma	Posterior palate
	Warthin tumor	Parotid
	Canalicular adenoma	Minor glands; upper lip
	Basal cell adenoma	Parotid
	Salivary duct papillomas	Minor glands
Malignant	Mucoepidermoid carcinoma	Posterior palate
	Adenoid cystic carcinoma	Palate and major glands
	Polymorphous low-grade adenocarcinoma	Minor glands most commonly the palate; rare in major glands
	Acinic cell adenocarcinoma	Parotid
	Carcinoma ex-pleomorphic adenoma	Posterior palate

located in close proximity to the tumor, increasing the risk for facial nerve damage during surgery. If the entire capsule is not removed at surgery, the risk of recurrence increases.

Pleomorphic adenomas that occur on the posterior hard palate in minor glands are smooth-surfaced and mucosal colored (Fig. 7-40A) but may become ulcerated from repeated trauma (Fig. 7-40B). Another common location is the submandibular gland (Fig. 7-41), where swelling occurs in the cervical area.

Warthin Tumor

Warthin tumor is almost exclusively found in the parotid gland, where it shares many clinical features with pleomorphic adenoma. However, a distinguishing clinical feature is that Warthin tumor is seen almost exclusively in smokers. Historically, there was a male-to-female ratio of 10:1; however, as the number of women smokers has increased, the male-to-female ratio has dropped to 2:1. Another interesting feature of this tumor is that it can occur bilaterally at different

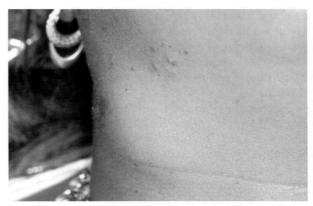

Figure 7–41   Pleomorphic adenoma: submandibular gland. Firm mass of right submandibular gland causing cervical swelling.

times (**metachronous** rather than **synchronous**). Treatment is conservative surgical excision with care to spare the facial nerve.

Canalicular Adenoma

Canalicular adenoma is seen almost exclusively in minor salivary glands, strongly favoring the upper lip of older adults. The tumor assumes its name from its microscopic appearance, which shows ductal structures that mimic a network of canals. It appears as a slow-growing painless mass that can mimic a mucocele, which is rare on the upper lip. Like Warthin tumor, they can occur at multiple sites. Treatment is conservative surgical excision and there is a low rate of recurrence.

Surgery is the treatment of choice for benign salivary gland tumors. Most develop a capsule, which helps with their surgical removal; however, risk of damage to the facial nerve is increased when the surgery occurs in the parotid gland.

Malignant Salivary Gland Tumors

Malignant salivary gland tumors are termed adenocarcinomas, though the prefix *adeno-* often is routinely dropped. Surgery is the standard of care; radiation and chemotherapy are reserved for poorly differentiated tumors and those that have spread to lymph nodes or metastasized to distant sites. Patients often develop significant morbidity and xerostomia as a result of treatment.

Mucoepidermoid Carcinoma

Mucoepidermoid carcinoma is the most common malignant salivary gland neoplasm. It derives its name from the mixture of neoplastic mucous acinar cells and

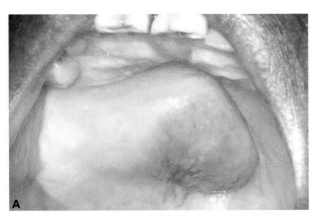

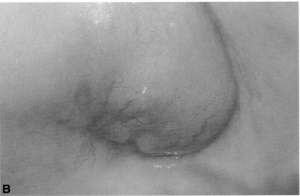

Figure 7–40   Pleomorphic adenoma of palate. A. Firm exophytic mass of the posterior palate. **B.** Close-up view shows small ulcerations.

epidermoid ductal cells. The most common type is the low-grade variant that is slow growing and follows a relatively benign clinical course, rarely causing death. High-grade mucoepidermoid carcinomas tend to grow more quickly and metastasize, reducing the chance of survival.

Mucoepidermoid carcinoma may occur at any age and is the most common salivary gland malignancy among children. The most frequent site is the parotid, where the low-grade type shares clinical characteristics with pleomorphic adenoma and Warthin tumor. However, high-grade tumors may invade the facial nerve and cause facial nerve pain and paralysis. When the tumor develops in minor glands, it may resemble a mucocele. The abundance of neoplastic mucous cells produce mucin that gives the tumor a fluctuant, bluish appearance (Fig. 7-42). If it is ignored, the tumor may enlarge, necessitating a more extensive surgery to remove it. Treatment depends on tumor grade. Low-grade tumors are conservatively excised and have low risk of recurrence. High-grade tumors may require presurgical and postsurgical radiation and neck dissection to remove any lymph nodes that contain spreading tumor cells.

On rare occasions, mucoepidermoid carcinoma may develop within the body and ramus of the mandible, causing signs that mimic an odontogenic tumor (Chapter 8). Some believe they develop from salivary gland tissue that became entrapped during embryogenesis. Others propose that the neoplastic mucous cells form from remnants of odontogenic epithelium. The true answer is unknown.

Polymorphous Low-Grade Adenocarcinoma

Polymorphous low-grade adenocarcinoma (PLGA) is the second most common malignancy of salivary glands. It is most frequently seen in the minor salivary glands, predominantly in the palate where it causes a painless swelling often near the junction of the hard and soft palate (Fig. 7-43). It may be mucosal-colored or have a bluish tint. As with other palatal masses, it may become ulcerated because of local trauma. It is rarely seen in the major glands. As the name implies (low-grade), the tumor has a favorable prognosis.

Adenoid Cystic Carcinoma

Adenoid cystic carcinoma occurs in both the minor salivary glands of the posterior hard palate and major salivary glands (Fig. 7-44). It is unusual among salivary gland neoplasms in that pain is an early sign. This is because this tumor is **neurotropic**, meaning it tends to invade peripheral nerve. It rarely occurs in individuals younger than age 20 and tends to predominate among females. The tumors tend to recur later in life rather than sooner, unlike other malignancies. Unlike other salivary gland malignancies, the 5-year survival is relatively high and the 10-year survival rate is very low, with few patients surviving beyond 20 years due to widespread metastasis. Adenoid cystic carcinoma has a tendency to metastasize to the brain.

Acinic Cell Carcinoma

Acinic cell carcinoma is derived from the saliva-producing serous acinar cells of the parotid gland. Along with mucoepidermoid carcinoma, it is one of the few salivary gland tumors seen in children. It presents as an asymptomatic slow-growing mass that may be present for many months before the patient seeks treatment. It is considered to be a low-grade malignancy with a favorable prognosis.

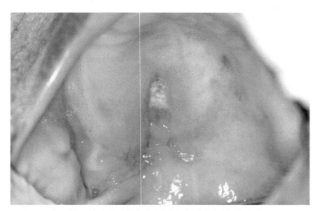

Figure 7–42   Mucoepidermoid carcinoma. Ulcerated exophytic mass of palate; patient reports denture no longer fits.

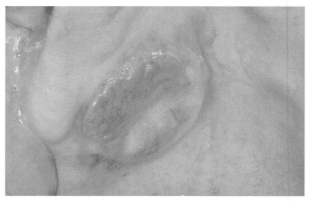

Figure 7–43   Polymorphous low-grade adenocarcinoma. Ulcerated exophytic mass of palate; patient reports denture no longer fits.

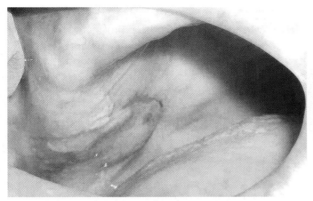

Figure 7–44 Adenoid cystic carcinoma. Painful swelling of palatal mucosa extending to alveolar ridge.

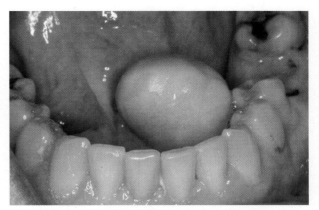

Figure 7–45 Lipoma. Well-encapsulated exophytic soft mucosal colored-to-yellow mass of floor of mouth.

Carcinoma Ex-Pleomorphic Adenoma

Carcinoma ex-pleomorphic adenoma is the malignant form of pleomorphic adenoma. It forms in an existing pleomorphic adenoma or in a patient whose pleomorphic adenoma was previously removed. In either case, sudden rapid growth of a previously stable salivary gland mass presents the clinical clue that the tumor is malignant.

SOFT TISSUE NEOPLASIA

Soft tissue has a specific connotation in pathology. Although many tissues are "soft," including epithelium, glands, and muscle, this term is reserved for nonepithelial tissue derived embryologically from mesoderm and neuroectoderm. This includes fibrous connective tissue, blood and lymphatic vessels, adipose tissue, skeletal and smooth muscle, peripheral nerves and their supporting tissues. Benign tumors of soft tissues are identified by using the tissue name and adding -oma. Malignancies of the nonepithelial soft tissues are termed sarcomas.

Adipose Tissue

Lipoma is benign tumor of fat, or adipose, tissue and one of the most common tumors in the body. Most occur in the arms, legs, and trunk of adults but rarely in children. Intraoral lipoma is far less common than extraoral lipoma. The etiology is unknown and they are not associated with any syndromes or genetic abnormalities.

Intraoral lipoma is often yellow in color, reflecting the natural yellow color of mature fat. However, if a layer of fibrous connective tissue lies between the tumor and the surface mucosa it may appear the color of normal mucosa (Fig. 7-45). The most common location is the buccal mucosa. Others occur as mobile submucosal masses on the tongue, floor of mouth, and lips. As is typical of benign tumors, they are well-circumscribed, often encapsulated, and when removed surgically they tend to come out in a solid mass. They rarely recur.

Liposarcomas of the head and neck area are typically well-differentiated and carry an excellent 5-year survival rate, unlike liposarcomas that occur in deep body cavities that have a low survival rate. Once removed, liposarcomas of the head area must be closely followed for recurrence.

Connective Tissue Proper

Myofibromas arise from myofibroblasts, a common connective tissue cell. This cell has features of both fibroblasts and smooth muscle cells. Myofibromas are most common in the tongue, lips, and buccal mucosa. Typically, they are firm, slow-growing submucosal nodules or exophytic masses. Although patients are frequently asymptomatic, the lesions may be tender or painful. Treatment for oral myofibromas is conservative excision. The recurrence rate is low and spontaneous regression (lesion resolves on its own) has been reported.

Fibrosarcoma in the head and oral cavity accounts for less than 10 percent of all fibrosarcoma cases in the body. They tend to be slow-growing nasal and sinus masses in children and young adults. Obstructive symptoms and pain are frequent complaints. After surgical therapy, tumors often recur. The 5-year survival rate is approximately 50 percent.

Nerve and Nerve Sheath Tumors

Tissue that surrounds and supports peripheral nerves (nerve sheath) can produce a number of neoplasms such as schwannoma, neurofibroma, and granular cell tumor.

Schwannoma, also called neurilemoma, is a benign neoplasm arising from the myelin-producing Schwann cells that surround and support peripheral nerves. Myelin is an insulating material that forms the myelin sheath to protect the nerve axon and help with nerve impulse conduction. Up to 50 percent of all schwannomas occur in the head, neck, and oral cavity, with the tongue being the most common location. They tend to occur as a single tumor that grows slowly to reach up to 1 cm. Schwannomas are not painful because they do not affect the nerve axon; however, if they surround a nerve, they may push the nerve out of its normal position, causing tenderness. Most schwannomas are easily removed without damaging the nearby nerve.

Granular cell tumor tends to favor the oral cavity. Its name is derived from the unusual microscopic appearance of large pink cells with grainy-looking cytoplasm. The origin of these granular cells was the subject of much debate over the years until special tests became available that showed similarities between the granular cells and Schwann cells. The most common location is the dorsal tongue, where it appears as a single asymptomatic sessile submucosal mass that averages less than 1 cm in size (Fig. 7-46). Other locations include the buccal mucosa, labial mucosa, and the skin. Surgical excision is the treatment and they rarely recur.

Neurofibroma is the most common benign neoplasm of the peripheral nervous system. They arise from both Schwann cells and neurofibroblasts, cells that produce collagen to support the nerve. They are slow-growing, painless lesions of the skin and mucosal surfaces that appear in young adulthood. On the skin, their texture is soft and spongy but in the oral cavity they may be firm, similar to a pencil eraser. They tend to be small (Fig. 7-47A), but lesions greater than 1 cm have been reported. Neurofibromas are treated by simple excision and rarely recur. Lesions that develop along the inferior alveolar nerve are detected radiographically (Fig. 7-47B). Neurofibromatosis Types 1 and 2 are two hereditary conditions caused by genetic mutations that produce hundreds of neurofibromas.

Neurofibrosarcoma, also called malignant peripheral nerve sheath tumor (MPNST), is a malignancy that arises in a neurofibroma and has only a 15% to 20% 5-year survival rate. Patients typically develop MPNST during their 50s. When lesions occur, they appear as asymptomatic masses that grow quickly. They cause pain only after they have invaded adjacent

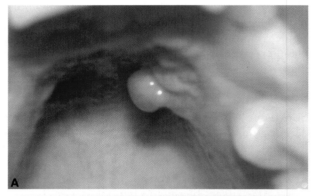

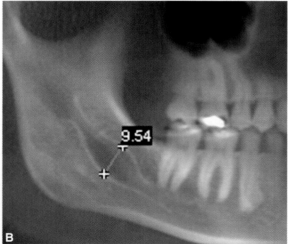

Figure 7–47 Neurofibroma. A. Neurofibroma of the palate. Painless exophytic soft mucosal-colored mass of palatal mucosa. **B.** X-ray of the mandible. Tender enlargement of mandibular canal.

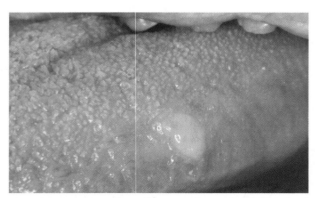

Figure 7–46 Granular cell tumor of tongue. Well-defined painless soft yellow mass of left dorsolateral tongue.

tissue. Early diagnosis may improve a patient's chance of survival. Treatment is radical surgery.

Neoplasms of Blood and Lymphatic Vessels

Vascular channels or blood vessels are a special form of connective tissue that carry blood and lymph. The Greek word for vessel is *angeion*; the Latin word for vessel is *vasculo*. When the vessel carries blood, the prefix *heme-* is used; when the vessel carries lymphatic fluid, the prefix *lymph-* is used. These terms are used in naming tumors that develop from these vessels and can be seen in Table 7-6.

Lymphangioma

Lymphangioma is a benign congenital tumor present at or shortly after birth and is comprised of a slowly enlarging proliferation of lymphatic vessels. Most pathologists believe they are actually *hamartomas*, a developmental disorder. They occur mainly in the head and neck, and are seen in dental patients.

Lymphangiomas that occur in the cervical (neck) area are termed *cystic hygroma*. They appear as fluctuant enlargements of the lower face or neck that generally occupy a great amount of space and may extend inferiorly to the chest cavity or superiorly to the oral cavity. Large lesions may cause upper respiratory problems and infections that may be life-threatening.

Smaller intraoral lymphangiomas are more common and frequently occur on the dorsal tongue. Small blister-like exophytic fluctuant nodules appear in a circumscribed mass. They represent dilated lymphatic channels filled with lymphatic fluid, giving the lesion the appearance of "bubble-wrap" (Fig. 7-48A). Occasionally, blood will leak into the space, creating a red/blue appearance (Fig. 7-48B) that leads to the erroneous diagnosis of a hemangioma (discussed next). Occasionally, superficial lymphangiomas develop in adulthood. These most likely represent small, occult lesions that were present at birth. The lesions were not clinically apparent until trauma and inflammation caused lymphatic fluid to build up in them.

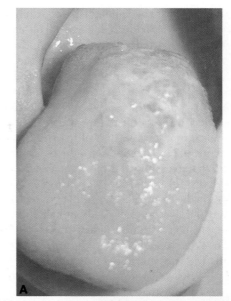

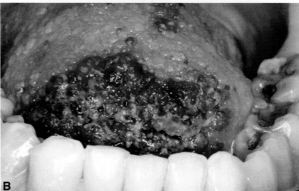

Figure 7–48 **A.** Lymphangioma tongue. Present since early childhood; multiple soft red-to-mucosal colored papules on the mid-dorsum filled with fluid. **B.** "Bubble-wrap" appearance with secondary extravasation of blood into the lesion.

Hemangioma

Hemangiomas are benign congenital tumors, seen shortly after birth, that are composed of a large tangle of blood vessels. They are caused by a proliferation

Table 7.6	Blood Vessel Pathology Nomenclature			
	Latin	**Example**	**Greek**	**Example**
Blood Vessel	Vasculo-	Vasculitis: inflammation of a blood vessel	Angio-	Angiosarcoma: malignancy of blood vessels
Blood	Sangui-	Sanguinous: bloody	Heme- (from iron of hemoglobin)	Hemangioma: benign tumor of blood vessels

of endothelial cells, specialized cells that line normal blood vessels. As the endothelial cells proliferate, vessels form and eventually fill with blood. This gives hemangiomas their characteristic blue/red appearance. If the tumor is composed of tiny blood vessels, it is a *capillary hemangioma*. If the vessels have a large diameter, it is a *cavernous hemangioma*. There may be no difference in the clinical appearance.

The most common location of hemangiomas is the head and neck. They begin as a light blue/red macule of the skin that may show the appearance of small bright red blood vessels at the periphery (Fig. 7-49A). The lesions gradually enlarge as the child ages but then may resolve (involute) by age 5 or 6. About half of the tumors completely resolve with no residual effects, others show scarring or skin color changes in the area where the hemangioma was present. Some may remain throughout life (Fig. 7-49B). Most are superficial and form under skin; however, they may also occur deep within organs or tissues, including bone (Fig. 7-49C).

Other than obvious cosmetic problems, hemangiomas may result in ulceration, local hemorrhage, and obstruction of vital structures caused by their enlargement. They can be life-threatening if a vital structure is involved. Medications that cause *sclerosis* (obliteration) of the vessels may be injected into the tumors to help to shrink their size; however, the tumor itself is benign and is not life-threatening.

Clinical Implications

Another condition called **vascular anomaly** or **vascular malformation** is often confused clinically with hemangioma. Unlike hemangiomas, they are caused by abnormalities in the structure of the vessels and are not due to a proliferation of endothelial cells. **Port wine stain** is a form of vascular malformation that develops along the path of the trigeminal nerve. If the first (ocular) division of the trigeminal nerve is affected, the patient may have a condition called **Sturge-Weber syndrome**. If the second or third divisions of the trigeminal nerve are affected, the patient may exhibit raised red/blue gingival lesions.

Angiosarcoma

Angiosarcoma is a malignancy of blood vessels, specifically of the endothelial cells that line blood and lymphatic vessels. The skin of the head and neck area is one of the favored sites. Patients tend to be elderly

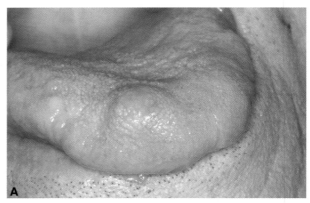

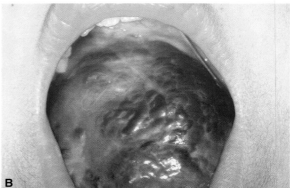

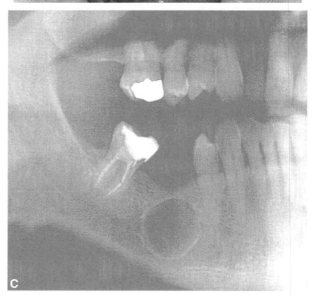

Figure 7–49 **Hemangioma. A.** Adult male with lifelong soft blue mass that blanches upon gentle pressure. **B.** Extensive diffuse congenital blue lesion in child. **C.** Well-defined radiolucency associated with inferior alveolar canal; blood was aspirated.

and present with a "bruise" of the scalp or forehead that does not heal, and eventually enlarges into a tumor mass. Angiosarcoma has a very poor prognosis, with a less than 20 percent 5-year survival rate.

Kaposi's Sarcoma

Kaposi's sarcoma (KS) is a type of angiosarcoma that is associated with an oncogenic virus called human herpes virus 8 (HHV8). This virus infects endothelial cells and causes them to proliferate, forming tiny vascular channels. The vessels are just large enough for red blood cells to pass through single-file, giving the skin a red/blue appearance. Tumors begin as flat, painless macular lesions that grow slowly into nodules, seen mainly on the skin. Intraorally, they appear in areas exposed to trauma, such as the hard palate (Fig. 7-50) and gingiva. KS differs significantly from other angiosarcomas in that it is very low-grade and is rarely life-threatening. Once diagnosed, many lesions are not treated.

Kaposi's sarcoma was virtually unknown before the onset of HIV/AIDS in the 1980s. Before then, the so-called classical form of KS was seen in elderly men in Mediterranean and Slavic countries. Endemic KS affecting internal organs was seen in children in Africa. Some forms of endemic KS are **indolent** (cause few or no symptoms), but others can cause significant **morbidity** (illness) and even **mortality** (death) when vital organs are affected.

Kaposi's sarcoma typically seen in the United States and other developed countries is associated with immune suppression. Since the advent of highly active antiretroviral therapy (HAART), the incidence of KS among HIV-positive patients has declined. However, KS unrelated to HIV/AIDS is not rare among organ transplant patients who receive drugs that cause immunosuppression to prevent organ rejection. Lesions may develop soon after the transplant or later at any time, since immunosuppression is long term.

Tumors of Muscle

Two types of muscle are found in the head and neck: 1) voluntary striated skeletal muscle, and 2) involuntary smooth muscle, typically found around arterioles and in the erector pili muscles of the skin. The prefix used to indicate tumors of striated skeletal muscle is *rhabdomyo-*; the prefix used to indicate tumors of smooth muscle is *leiomyo-*.

Rhabdomyoma is a benign tumor of mature striated skeletal muscle cell origin. Intraorally, these are found in or near normal skeletal muscles in adults, mainly in the posterior oropharynx where airway obstruction can be the presenting feature. There are no clinical features that are unique to this tumor, and its diagnosis is usually a surprise to the surgeon and the pathologist. Treatment is surgical excision.

Rhabdomyosarcoma is a malignant tumor of striated skeletal muscle. Although a rare form can occur in adults older than age 45, this is primarily a childhood tumor generally seen in children younger than age 10. The head and neck are the most common sites. Many tumors appear as painless asymmetrical swellings in the maxillary sinus or nasal cavity that often arise rapidly over a short period of time. Tumors may invade adjacent bone readily and cause dramatic facial asymmetry. Recent advances in chemotherapy have improved long-term survival, but rhabdomyosarcoma continues to have a poor prognosis.

Leiomyoma is a benign tumor of smooth muscle cells that is most common in the uterus, where it is commonly called *fibroids*. Other common locations are the erector pili muscles of the skin and the smooth muscle layer of the GI tract. Oral leiomyomas may be seen in association with the smooth muscle of blood vessel walls, in which case they are termed *angioleiomyoma* or *vascular leiomyoma*. They present as a painful or tender red/blue submucosal nodule anywhere in the oral cavity. Leiomyomas are treated by surgical excision and rarely recur.

Leiomyosarcoma is a malignant tumor of smooth muscle found in locations where smooth muscle is abundant. In the head and neck, they occur in association with the smooth muscle of blood vessel walls. There are so few cases in the oral cavity that generalizations

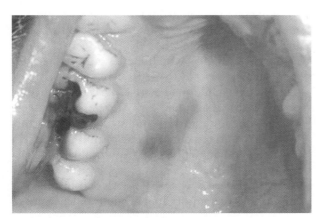

Figure 7–50 Kaposi's sarcoma. Slightly raised blue lesion with ill-defined border on right palate.

about age, location, and clinical features cannot be made. Treatment is surgery, but recurrence and metastasis are not rare. The 5-year survival rate is about 50 percent.

Metastases to Oral Soft Tissues

When cancers metastasize, they tend to favor major organs such as the lung, liver, and brain. Metastases to the soft tissues of the oral cavity may also occur. Tumors from any site in the body can metastasize to the mouth but the most frequent are from the lung, breast, kidney, bone, and colorectum (Table 7-7). Metastasis to the bones of the jaws is discussed in Chapter 8.

Intraorally, the gingiva is a favored intraoral site; greater than 50 percent of soft tissue metastases occur here (Fig. 7-51A). Other intraoral sites include the hard and soft palate, the tongue (Fig. 7-51B), and lips (Fig. 7-51C). Clinically, lesions appear in several forms that mimic common inflammatory and reactive lesions that are common to the oral region, such as pyogenic granuloma, gingival hyperplasia, or traumatic granuloma.

Clinical Implications

Most patients who present with intraoral metastases have already been diagnosed with cancer. However, approximately 30 percent of oral metastases are the first sign of cancer spread. The prognosis is often poor for neoplasms that have spread to the oral cavity.

NEOPLASTIC DISORDERS OF BLOOD CELLS AND BONE MARROW

Classification of neoplasms of blood cells and bone marrow origin is complex due to the wide variety of blood and bone marrow cells. Benign neoplastic conditions of blood and bone marrow are not commonly reported; therefore, they are not discussed here. However, leukemia and lymphoma are two common classes of blood cell and bone marrow malignancy that are important for the dental team.

Leukemia

Leukemia is a malignancy of white blood cells (leukocytes). Leukemia is actually a group of malignancies rather than one condition. Leukemias are unusual in that they rarely form a solid mass commonly thought

Table 7.7	Origin of Metastatic Tumors Found in the Oral Soft Tissues	
Males		**Females**
Lung: 31%		Breast: 24%
Kidney: 14%		Genital organs (uterus, ovaries, cervix, fallopian tubes): 14.8%
Skin: 12%		
Liver: 7.5%		Kidney: 12%
Colorectum: 5.2%		Lung: 9.4%
Bone: 5.2%		Bone: 9.4%
Testis: 4.5%		Skin: 6.8%
Esophagus: 4.5%		Colorectum: 6.8%
Stomach: 3.7%		Rare tumors:16.8%
Rare tumors: 12.4%		

Retrieved July 29, 2012 from http://emedicine.medscape.com/article/1079102-overview#a0199

of as a "tumor"; rather, the neoplastic cells are found within circulating blood, bone marrow, and spleen. Malignant leukocytes are overproduced by the bone marrow and crowd out normal bone marrow cells. Signs and symptoms can vary among types of leukemia, but all represent deficiency in bone marrow function. Leukemias have been associated with exposure to radiation and workplace chemicals. Many represent a genetic abnormality that may be inherited or occur as a *mutation* (see Chapter 6).

Discussion of the entire classification of leukemias is beyond the scope of this text; however, the four major types are briefly described here.

- *Acute lymphoblastic leukemia* (ALL) is a common type of leukemia in which the bone marrow overproduces lymphocyte precursor (stem) cells called *lymphoblasts*. People with ALL experience sudden symptoms caused by malfunctioning erythrocytes and platelets as well as leukocytes. ALL is most common in childhood with a peak incidence at 2 to 5 years of age, and a second peak in old age. Chemotherapy, radiation, and stem cell transplants must be instituted quickly. The overall cure rate in children is about 80 percent. Adults older than age 65 respond less well.
- *Chronic lymphocytic leukemia* (CLL) is of B-lymphocyte origin. It is seen most often in adults older than age 55. It sometimes occurs in younger adults, but is rare in children. Approximately 50 percent of patients

a progressive treatment-resistant phase lasting 1 to 2 years.

- *Acute myelogenous leukemia (AML)* occurs more commonly in adults than in children. It is a cancer of the myeloid (**myelogenous**) line of blood cells that begins quickly with rapid production of abnormal white blood cells. These accumulate in the bone marrow and interfere with the production of other normal blood cells. Patients quickly develop fatigue and fever, and may present with bleeding gums and bruising related to *thrombocytopenia* (decreased platelets for clotting). Rapid proliferation of tumor cells causes enlargement of the spleen and liver. The 5-year-survival rate is 18% to 25%.
- *Chronic myelogenous leukemia* (CML) affects adults in their 50s and 60s and a very small number of children. It is characterized by increased proliferation in the bone marrow of *granulocytic cells (neutrophils, eosinophils, and basophils)* and their immature precursors. The clinical manifestations are nonspecific and include fatigue, weight loss, and decreased exercise tolerance. Chemotherapy is very effective and the 5-year survival rate is 90 percent.

Oral manifestations of leukemia may vary depending on the type, but some of the most common findings are spontaneous bleeding of the gingiva due to loss of normal thrombocytes; mucosal ulceration due to loss of normal defense cells that maintain mucosal integrity; and infections, such as candidiasis, due to loss of normal defense cells that fight infection. Patients may also demonstrate lowered resistance to normal oral flora, leading to gingivitis and periodontitis. Additionally, once the bone marrow becomes filled with neoplastic leukocytes, the excess cells enter the circulation and travel to other body sites. If they reach the gingiva, gingival enlargement occurs. Nodular enlargement of the palate (Fig. 7-52A), tongue (Fig. 7-52B), and other oral tissues may occur. Occasionally, lesions develop within the mandible and present as jaw infection.

Treatment of leukemia depends on the type of cells that have become malignant, but most involve some form of chemotherapy. Other treatments include **bone marrow** or **stem cell transplant**, which involves removing all marrow cells and replacing them with healthy cells from another individual.

Lymphoma

Lymphoma is similar to leukemia in that it is actually a group of malignancies involving leukocytes, usually T-lymphocytes or B-lymphocytes. Lymphomas, like

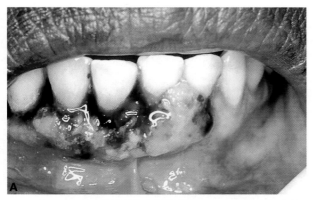
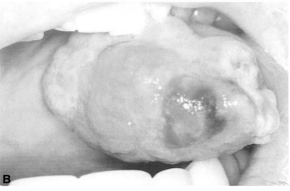
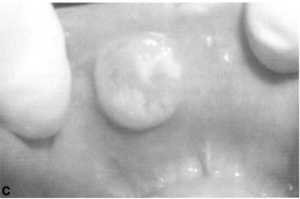

Figure 7–51 Metastasis to oral soft tissue: A. Breast. Gingival enlargement in patient with history of breast carcinoma thought to be in remission. **B.** Exophytic blue-red mass with surface ulcer of the tongue in patient with history of renal cell carcinoma. **C.** Exophytic mass on upper lip in patient with history of lung carcinoma.

are asymptomatic at first. It is not unusual for CLL to be discovered incidentally after a blood cell count is performed for another reason. The initial course is relatively benign and patients are not treated with chemotherapy until they become symptomatic. The 5-year survival rate is 75 percent, but is followed by

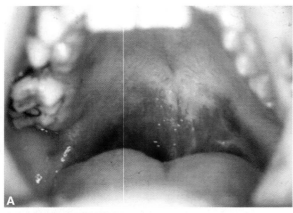

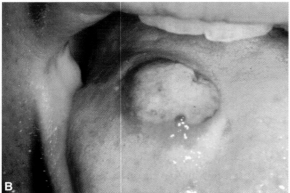

Figure 7–52 Leukemia. A. Diffuse nodular changes to palate in patient with AML. **B.** Exophytic ulcerated mass on dorsal tongue in patient with AML.

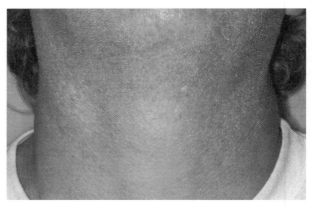

Figure 7–53 Hodgkin's lymphoma. Slight enlargement of right neck is firm and fixed to underlying musculature.

leukemias, are named according to the cell line that has become malignant. Unlike leukemia, lymphomas are solid tumors that develop within lymph nodes instead of bone marrow. Extranodal lymphomas occur in the oral cavity where lymphoid tissue is found, such as tonsils and lymphoid aggregates of the tongue, floor of mouth, and oropharynx.

Hodgkin's and non-Hodgkin's are two broad categories of lymphoma. Each has many subtypes that have different signs, symptoms, treatment, and prognosis, making generalizations difficult.

■ **Hodgkin's lymphoma.** Hodgkin's lymphoma is a group of four different lymphomas that are characterized by the neoplastic proliferation of Reed-Sternberg cells, a type of B-cell. It occurs in two peaks, between 15 to 30 years of age or 50 to 55 years of age. The first presenting symptom is nonpainful lymph nodes that slowly enlarge. The cervical lymph nodes are commonly involved (Fig. 7-53). Early Hodgkin's lymphoma of the cervical nodes can often

be detected during a routine head and neck examination. Patients may experience fever, weight loss, and other nonspecific symptoms. Early detection is critical because treatment of Hodgkin's lymphoma in early stages is highly successful.

■ **Non-Hodgkin's lymphoma.** Non-Hodgkin's lymphoma is a broad classification of lymphoma that includes more than 25 different tumors. The classification system of lymphomas has changed several times, reflecting an increasing and evolving knowledge about the etiology, pathogenesis, treatment, and prognosis of these tumors. Most occur within lymph nodes, but extranodal disease is not uncommon. Patients with Sjögren syndrome, immune deficiency disorders and certain viral infections, such as Epstein-Barr virus and HHV-8, are at higher risk of developing lymphoma.

Non-Hodgkin's lymphoma predominantly affects adults. Patients usually become aware of a nontender enlargement of the lymph nodes, which gradually become firm and fixed to the underlying tissues. The tumor will spread to other lymph nodes if left untreated. Intraoral lymphomas present as gingiva swellings (Fig. 7-54A) palatal masses (Fig. 7-54B) or lingual tonsil masses that are nontender, often erythematous, and ulcerated (Fig. 7-54C). Lymphomas may begin within the jaws, where they will show an ill-defined radiolucency that may mimic periapical or periodontal disease. Occasionally, teeth will show resorption (Fig. 7-54D). Once the tumor has achieved significant size, the bone will expand. If an early lesion is mistaken for an abscessed tooth and the tooth is extracted, the tumor will grow into the oral cavity through the non-healing socket (Fig. 7-54E), mimicking *epulis granulomatosum* (see Chapter 2).

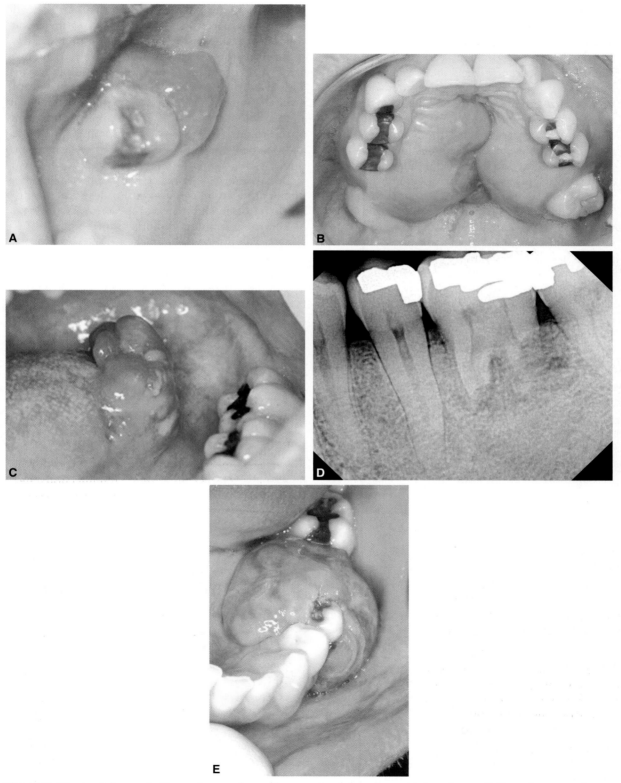

Figure 7–54 Lymphoma. A. Pyogenic granuloma-like mass in adult patient with lymphoma. **B.** Lymphoma causing bilateral enlargement of the hard palate with surface ulceration. **C.** Lymphoma arising in lingual tonsil. **D.** Lymphoma arising within bone causing resorption of molar roots. **E.** Tooth in D was extracted; mass grew out of extraction site.

■ **Burkitt's lymphoma.** Burkitt's lymphoma primarily affects young children and adolescents in two main forms: endemic and sporadic. *Endemic Burkitt's* is believed to be caused by Epstein-Barr virus. It was first identified in African children and termed "African Burkitt's," though children in other countries have been reported to have the disease. Patients develop relatively painless intraosseous maxillary lesions that cause gross facial deformity, tooth mobility, and premature exfoliation of deciduous teeth. *Sporadic Burkitt's* is believed to be caused by a chromosomal abnormality. It was first identified in American children and is therefore termed "American Burkitt's." These children develop abdominal tumors with only rare jaw involvement. Immunosuppressed patients such as HIV-positive patients or transplantation patients have also been reported to develop Burkitt's lymphoma. Regardless of form, the radiographic features include ill-defined radiolucent bone destruction that may be preceded by loss of lamina dura. Treatment includes aggressive chemotherapy and recurrence is possible.

Plasmacytoma and Multiple Myeloma

Plasmacytoma and multiple myeloma are two related malignancies of plasma cells. Plasma cells are responsible for producing antibodies. *Plasmacytoma* is a solitary (single) tumor of malignant plasma cells that is most commonly seen in adult females older than age 40. The marrow spaces of the spine are the most common location, though many cases have been reported in the jaws (Fig. 7-55). The tumor causes a single unilocular radiolucency with jaw expansion. Occasionally, the tumor is found outside the marrow spaces (*extramedullary*). Treatment consists of surgical excision and radiation therapy.

Plasmacytoma patients who are observed over many years often go on to develop multiple lesions. This condition is called *multiple myeloma*. Multiple myeloma is rarely diagnosed before age 40. Bone pain and pathologic fracture may be the presenting signs of the tumor. The classic radiographic appearance is "punched out" or "coin" lesions/radiolucencies (Fig. 7-56).

Because normal plasma cells are responsible for antibody production, patients with widespread multiple myeloma often suffer from repeated infections due to abnormal immunoglobulins (antibodies). These abnormal immunoglobulins can be detected in the urine in the form of *Bence-Jones proteins*. Also, other abnormal proteins called *amyloid* are deposited in the soft tissues. If the tongue is affected, macroglossia may result.

Treatment is mainly aggressive chemotherapy, but long-term survival is less than 20 percent. Bisphosphonate therapy has been shown to be helpful in strengthening the bone and reducing fractures. Patients being treated with bisphosphonates are at increased risk for developing *bisphosphonate osteonecrosis* (Chapter 2).

Langerhans Cell Histiocytosis

Langerhans cells are found in the skin and mucous membranes, lymph nodes, and bone marrow, where they act as part of the immune system that helps destroy foreign antigens. *Langerhans cell histiocytosis* is

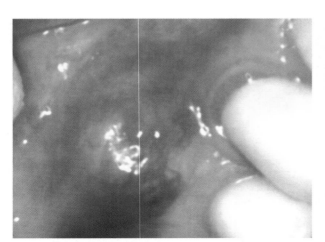

Figure 7-55 **Plasmacytoma.** Enlargement within maxillary vestibule with loss of underlying bone.

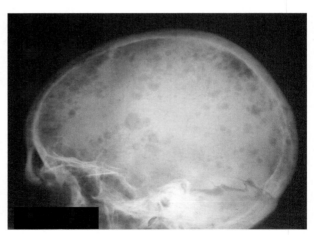

Figure 7-56 **Multiple myeloma x-ray.** "Punched-out" radiolucencies associated with bone destruction.

a neoplastic process that is characterized by proliferation of abnormal Langerhans cells in their normal anatomic locations.

Two basic forms are named based on how widespread lesions are. The *chronic localized form* is confined to one bone (*monostotic*) and is referred to as *eosinophilic granuloma*. This form is seen mainly in adults as localized bone destruction (Fig. 7-57A and B). Frequently, the Langerhans cells of the overlying mucosa are also affected, resulting in severe ulcerative mucositis. Early lesions resemble localized periodontitis that does not respond to conventional periodontal therapy. Treatment of eosinophilic granuloma usually involves curettage of bone lesions, radiation, or local injections of corticosteroids.

The *chronic disseminated form* is named Hand-Schüller-Christian disease after the three doctors who first described it. This form is seen mainly in children younger than 15 years of age who develop multiple lesions that involve the skin, mucosa, bone, deep visceral organs, and/or lymph nodes. Lesions can be found in multiple bones (*polyostotic*). When the jaws are affected, radiographs show teeth that appear to be "floating" in bone that is destroyed around them. The overlying soft tissues will appear ulcerated as in eosinophilic granuloma.

The chronic disseminated form is more difficult to treat than the localized form. Patients may require chemotherapy. Prognosis is better for individuals whose diagnosis is made at an older age. Younger patients tend not to do as well; however, death from this disease rarely occurs.

The *acute disseminated form* is called Letterer-Siwe disease and is seen in neonates. The disease is rapidly progressive and lethal. Patients generally do not reach age 2.

Critical Thinking Questions

Case 7-1:   Your 55-year-old patient informs you he has just been diagnosed with chronic myelogenous leukemia (CML). His presenting signs and symptoms included fatigue, weight loss, and decreased exercise tolerance. He is just starting chemotherapy and wants his teeth cleaned.

• • •

What are some oral manifestations of leukemia you might encounter during his visit?

How does leukemia affect the patient's ability to fight infection? What impact will this have on his oral health in terms of caries? Periodontal disease?

What is his long-term outlook? How will this impact his future dental care?

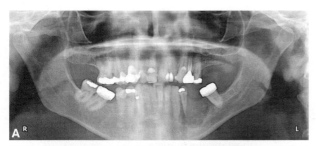
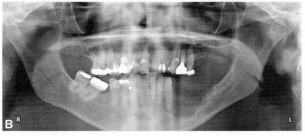

Figure 7–57   Langerhans cell histiocytosis. A. Premolar and first molar were lost to what appeared to be "periodontal disease." **B.** Following extraction of second molar, the tissue submitted showed Langerhans cell histiocytosis.

Case 7-2:   Your 60-year-old male patient has smoked three packs of cigarettes a day for approximately 40 years and regularly consumes beer on the weekends. You find nothing abnormal after a thorough head and neck and intraoral examination. He asks you, "What does an early oral cancer look like? What are my chances for developing oral cancer, since I smoke and drink?" He also asks if oral cancer can be inherited.

• • •

How do you answer his questions?

What will you tell him about the risk factors for oral cancer?

What information can you provide him about smoking and drinking habits?

Case 7-3: A 64-year-old female comes in for a routine dental examination. She spends a great deal of time outdoors gardening, sailing, and playing golf. You observe dryness, white-colored sun damage, and an indistinct vermillion border to her lower lip. One area appears crusted but it is nontender and not hard or indurated. When you palpate her neck, no firm lymph nodes are found.

• • •

What do you suspect is happening to her lip?

What can you tell the patient about sun exposure to the skin and lips?

What can you do to actively involve her in the care and protection of her lips?

How can this current lesion be treated? What is the long-term outlook for these types of lesions?

Case 7-4: Your 65-year-old patient has recently undergone extensive radiation therapy for squamous cell carcinoma on the posterior lateral tongue. He reports his doctor may have to do some surgery to remove the small tumor that is left. He quit smoking after his diagnosis.

• • •

What are some potential radiation side effects this patient may experience in the oral cavity?

How might these complications affect the patient's quality of life? Oral health?

Is this patient at risk for developing additional intraoral cancers? Why?

Case 7-5: An 18-year-old male presents to your office for routine treatment. On routine head and neck examination, you easily detect several prominent non-painful cervical lymph nodes. He reports that they have been present for several months and he believes they are slowly increasing in size. On questioning he states he has lost some weight, had bouts with fatigue, and, on occasion, a low-grade fever. Based on your findings and his history, answer the following questions.

• • •

What benign and malignant neoplastic process might be responsible for the cervical lymph node enlargement?

What is your course of action for this patient?

What does his prognosis depend on?

Review Questions

1. **Oncogenes cause transformation of normal cells and**
    A. cause cell death.
    B. prevent cells from growing on their own.
    C. are capable of repairing damaged DNA.
    D. are capable of causing a neoplasm.

2. **Neoplastic and reactive processes**
    A. differ in that reactive processes generally resolve when the originating stimulus is removed.
    B. both produce damage to the cell's DNA that results in gene alterations.
    C. are similar in that they both progress to tumorigenesis.
    D. both require ongoing stimulus for continued cell growth.

3. **Metastasis of tumors**
    A. is synonymous with infiltration.
    B. occurs regularly with both benign and malignant neoplasms.
    C. with rare exception, is associated with malignant tumors.
    D. results in a neoplasm that does not resemble the original tumor.

4. **What percent of all oral cancers are squamous cell carcinomas?**
    A. 5 percent
    B. 25 percent
    C. 60 percent
    D. 90 percent

5. **As a general pathology term, *dysplasia* means**
   - A. caused by friction.
   - B. loss of normal maturation of cells and tissues.
   - C. precancerous.
   - D. caused by sunlight.

6. **Of the locations listed below, which one is the most common intraoral site for squamous cell carcinoma?**
   - A. hard palate.
   - B. floor of the mouth.
   - C. gingiva.
   - D. lateral tongue.

7. **Which intraoral neoplasm is characterized by a thick, wart-like surface texture and is seen most often in smokeless tobacco users?**
   - A. Myofibroma
   - B. Rhabdomyosarcoma
   - C. Verrucous carcinoma
   - D. Hemangioma

8. **Therapeutic radiation-induced bone death**
   - A. is known as osteoradionecrosis.
   - B. heals completely over time.
   - C. is due to radiation-induced xerostomia.
   - D. can be prevented by the use of sialogogues.

9. **Cumulative sun exposure may leave large areas of skin of a person with skin cancer at risk for developing new skin cancers. This phenomenon is known as**
   - A. programmed cell death.
   - B. Mohs phenomenon.
   - C. micro-invasion potential.
   - D. field cancerization.

10. **Which one of the following is the most common salivary gland tumor?**
    - A. Mucoepidermoid carcinoma
    - B. Polymorphous low-grade adenocarcinoma
    - C. Pleomorphic adenoma
    - D. Warthin tumor

11. **Which one of the following is a benign neoplasm arising from the myelin-producing cells that surround and support peripheral nerves?**
    - A. Neurofibrosarcoma
    - B. Schwannoma
    - C. Myofibroma
    - D. Hemangioma

12. **Which one of the following is a malignant tumor of striated skeletal muscle?**
    - A. Leiomyoma
    - B. Leiomyosarcoma
    - C. Rhabdomyoma
    - D. Rhabdomyosarcoma

13. **Leukemia patients may present with bleeding gums and bruising. This is related to**
    - A. excess production of red blood cells in the spleen.
    - B. decreased platelets for clotting (thrombocytopenia).
    - C. onset of fatigue, weight loss, and decreased exercise tolerance.
    - D. a relative increase in thrombocytes.

14. **Which one of the following is a malignancy of plasma cells that may show multiple "punched out" radiolucencies in bone?**
    - A. Burkitt's lymphoma
    - B. Multiple myeloma
    - C. Plasmacytoma
    - D. Hodgkin's lymphoma

15. **Radiographs of a 5-year-old child with Langerhans cell histiocytosis show teeth that appear to be "floating" in the jaws. What name is given to the chronic disseminated form of this disease?**
    - A. Eosinophilic granuloma
    - B. Hand-Schüller-Christian disease
    - C. Letterer-Siwe disease
    - D. Bence-Jones disease

16. **Which one of the following terms is used to describe abnormal cells that show changes that are considered cancerous?**

    A. Anaplastic
    B. Well-differentiated
    C. Hyperchromatic
    D. Metastatic

17. **A white lesion that does not wipe off and cannot be attributed to any specific source or cause is known as**

    A. carcinoma.
    B. leukoplakia.
    C. erythroplakia.
    D. carcinoma-in-situ.

18. **Epithelial disorders with malignant potential include all of the following EXCEPT**

    A. dermatosis papulosa nigra.
    B. proliferative verrucous leukoplakia.
    C. actinic keratosis.
    D. oral submucous fibrosis.

19. **Which one of the following is true of basal cell carcinomas?**

    A. They occur 90 percent of the time in the oral cavity.
    B. They do not commonly metastasize.
    C. They do not invade or expand into vital structures.
    D. They are considered to be premalignant.

20. **All of the following are considered benign soft tissue neoplasms EXCEPT**

    A. myofibroma.
    B. lipoma.
    C. schwannoma.
    D. fibrosarcoma.

REFERENCES

Books

Ellis, GL, Auclair, PL: Tumors of salivary gland. Armed Forces Institute of Pathology Atlas of Tumor Pathology. Washington, DC, 2008.
Neville, B, Damm, DD, Allen, CM, Bouquot, J: Oral and Maxillofacial Pathology, ed. 3. Elsevier, St. Louis, 2009.
Neville, B, Damm, D, White, D: Color Atlas of Clinical Oral Pathology, ed. 2. Williams and Wilkins, Baltimore, 1999.

Regezi, J, Scuibba, J, Jordan, R: Oral Pathology: Clinical Pathologic Correlations, ed. 4. Saunders, Philadelphia, 2007.
Robbins, SL, Kumar, V, Abbas, AK, Cotran, RS, et al: Pathologic Basis of Disease, ed. 10. Saunders Elsevier, Philadelphia, 2010.
Rubin, E, Reisner, H: Essential Pathology, ed. 5. Lippincott, Williams and Wilkins, Philadelphia, 2008.

Journal Articles

Abla, O, Egeler, RM, Weitzman, S: Langerhans cell histiocytosis: Current concepts and treatments. Cancer Treatment Review 36:354–359, 2010.
Aziz, SR: Coming to America: Betel nut and oral submucous fibrosis. Journal of the American Dental Association 141:423–428, 2010.
Berk, LB, Shivnani, AT, Small, W: Pathophysiology and management of radiation-induced xerostomia. Journal of Supportive Oncology 3:191–200, 2005.
Ferner, RE: Neurofibromatosis 1 and neurofibromatosis 2: A twenty-first century perspective. Lancet Neurology 6:340–351, 2007.
Geller, AC, Annas, GD: Epidemiology of melanoma and non-melanoma skin cancer. Seminars in Oncology Nursing 19:2–11, 2003.
Geraminejad, P, Memar, O, Aronson, I, Rady, PL, et al: Kaposi's sarcoma and other manifestations of human herpes virus 8. Journal of the American Academy of Dermatology 47:641–655, 2002.
Jose, BO, Koerner, P, Spanos, WJ, Paris, KJ, et al: Hodgkin's lymphoma in adults - Clinical features. Journal of the Kentucky Medical Association 103:5–7, 2005.
Philipsen, HP, Reichart, PA: The development and fate of epithelial residues after completion of human odontogenesis with special reference to the origins of epithelial odontogenic neoplasms, hamartomas and cysts. Oral Biosciences and Medicine1:171–179, 2004.
Pulte, D, Brenner, H: Changes in survival in head and neck cancers in the late 20th and early 21st century: A period analysis. Oncologist 15(9):994–1001, 2010.
Rosenthal, DI, Trotti, A: Strategies for managing radiation-induced mucositis in head and neck cancer. Seminars in Radiation Oncology 19:29–34, 2009.
Simard, EP, Engels, EA: Cancer as a cause of death among people with AIDS in the United States. Clinical Infectious Diseases 51(8):957–962, 2010.
Smith, MA, Seibel, NL, Altekruse, SF, Ries, LA, et al: Outcomes for children and adolescents with cancer: Challenges for the twenty-first century. Journal of Clinical Oncology 28:2625–2634, 2010.

Online Resources

Oral Cancer Foundation. Retrieved July 2012 from http://oralcancerfoundation.org/
Rahat, S, Azfar, MD, James, WD, Gross, PR: Proliferative verrucous leukoplakia: Treatment and medication. Retrieved January 2012 from http://emedicine.medscape.com/article/1081559

Neoplasms of the Bones of the Mandible and Maxilla

Neoplasms of the Bones of the Maxilla and Mandible

Odontogenic Neoplasms

Ameloblastoma

Calcifying Epithelial Odontogenic Tumor

Squamous Odontogenic Tumor

Odontogenic Myxoma

Odontoma

Adenomatoid Odontogenic Tumor

Ameloblastic Fibroma and Ameloblastic
  Fibro-odontoma

Cementoblastoma

Keratinizing Cystic Odontogenic Tumor

Neoplasms of Bone Tissue

Osteoma

Ossifying Fibroma

Osteoblastoma

Osteosarcoma

Metastasis of Other Tumors to Bone

Neoplasms of Cartilage

🌑 Learning Outcomes

At the end of this chapter, the student will be able to:

8.1. Define all key terms in the chapter.

8.2. Explain the difference between an odontogenic neoplasm and a nonodontogenic neoplasm.

8.3. Give examples of odontogenic tumors that occur mainly in adults and those that occur mainly in children.

8.4. Identify on a radiograph the key features of odontogenic neoplasms. Explain why some tumors appear multilocular.

8.5. Describe two odontogenic tumors that can mimic periodontitis radiographically.

8.6. Explain why compound and complex odontomas have different radiographic features.

8.7. Explain why peripheral odontogenic tumors have a different prognosis than central odontogenic tumors.

8.8. Recognize the key radiographic features of osteoma versus osteosarcoma.

8.9. Give examples of malignant tumors of the body that are known to metastasize to the jaws.

NEOPLASMS OF THE BONES OF THE MAXILLA AND MANDIBLE

Many different neoplasms (tumors) arise within the maxilla and mandible. **Primary jaw tumors** are those that originate in the jaw bones. They are either **odontogenic** (arising from tooth-forming tissues) or **non-odontogenic** (not arising from tooth-forming tissues). Many other neoplasms may arise in this location, but this chapter focuses on odontogenic tumors and tumors of bone and cartilage tissue. Tumors that develop in distant sites and metastasize to the jaws will also be briefly discussed.

Many primary jaw tumors are found incidentally on radiographs or other types of imaging. Early symptoms may include pain, bone expansion and swelling, numbness, drifting of teeth, and changes in occlusion. Most jaw tumors require surgical management. Benign tumors tend to be encapsulated, making surgical removal less of a challenge than those with no capsule. Often, infiltrating tumors with a high rate of recurrence may require **resection** (removal) of a section of the jaw followed by reconstruction to replace the lost tissue. Occasionally, teeth will need to be removed and replaced with dental prosthetics and/or implants.

ODONTOGENIC NEOPLASMS

Odontogenic neoplasms arise from remnants of the developing tooth germ that undergo neoplastic transformation. (See Chapter 7 for a discussion of neoplastic transformation.) A review of the histologic development of teeth will provide insight into the complex structure of the developing tooth. Figure 8-1 indicates the portion of the developing tooth germ from which each odontogenic neoplasm is believed to arise.

With rare exceptions, odontogenic tumors are found in the tooth-bearing areas of the jaws. Odontogenic tumors closely approximate teeth but they do not always affect the health of adjacent teeth. Teeth remain vital, though they may be displaced. Odontogenic tumors are either *central* or *peripheral*. Most odontogenic tumors are **central**, meaning they develop within bone of the mandible or maxilla. Some odontogenic tumors are **peripheral**, meaning they develop outside the bone cortex in overlying soft tissues. Overall, peripheral odontogenic tumors are less aggressive and more easily treated than central odontogenic tumors.

Classification of odontogenic tumors can be based on tissue of embryologic origin (see Fig. 8-1), age (Table 8-1), or radiographic appearance (see Table 8-1). However, the most clinically useful classification is by age and radiographic appearance. Often these are used together in formulating a differential diagnosis or a list of possible tumors. For example, a radiolucent lesion in a pediatric patient could be cystic ameloblastoma, ameloblastic fibroma, or keratinizing cystic odontogenic tumor.

There are many odontogenic tumors; only the most common ones are discussed in this chapter. Odontogenic tumors seen more commonly in adults are discussed first.

Ameloblastoma

The most common benign odontogenic tumor is *ameloblastoma*. It is characterized by the proliferation

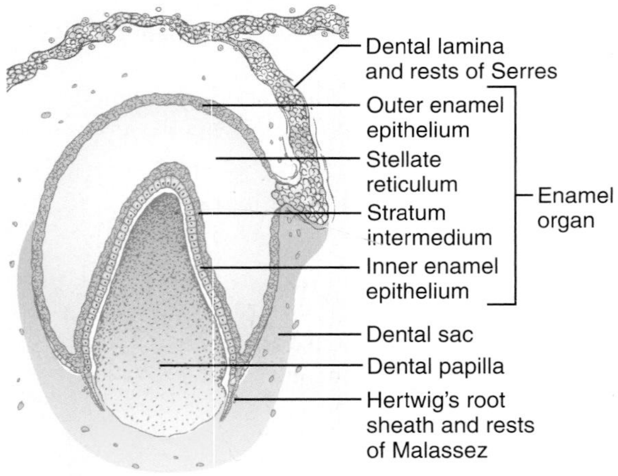

Neoplasm	Tooth Germ Layer
Ameloblastoma	Enamel organ
Adenomatoid odontogenic tumor	Dental lamina
Squamous odontogenic tumor	Rests of Malassez
Ameloblastic fibroma/fibro-odontoma	Inner enamel epithelium and dental papilla
CEOT	Dental lamina
KCOT	Dental lamina
CCOT	Dental lamina
Odontogenic myxoma	Dental papilla
Odontoma	All layers
Cementoblastoma	Dental sac
Peripheral odontogenic neoplasms	Rests of Serres or basal layer of oral epithelium

Figure 8–1 **Odontogenic tumors are derived from cells of the tooth germ.**

Table 8.1	Classification Schemes for Odontogenic Tumors	

Classification Based on Age

Adult	Pediatric	Any Age
Multicystic solid ameloblastoma	Cystic ameloblastoma	Keratinizing cystic odontogenic tumor (KCOT)
Calcifying epithelial odontogenic tumor (CEOT)	Ameloblastic fibroma	Calcifying cystic odontogenic tumor (CCOT)
Squamous odontogenic tumor	Ameloblastic fibro-odontoma	
Odontogenic myxoma	Adenomatoid odontogenic tumor	
Ameloblastic carcinoma	Cementoblastoma	
	Compound or complex odontoma	

Classification Based on Radiographic Appearance

Radiolucent (RL)	Radiopaque (RP)	Mixed RL/RP
Multicystic solid ameloblastoma	Complex odontoma	Compound odontoma
Ameloblastic fibroma	Cementoblastoma	Ameloblastic fibro-odontoma
Squamous odontogenic tumor		Adenomatoid odontogenic tumor
Odontogenic myxoma		CCOT
Ameloblastic carcinoma		KCOT
KCOT		

of cells resembling three of the four layers of cells constituting the enamel organ: outer enamel epithelium, stellate reticulum, and inner enamel epithelium, which forms the ameloblasts. Because no dental hard tissues form, ameloblastomas are radiolucent.

There are three types of ameloblastoma: multicystic solid, cystic intraosseous, and peripheral. Each has a different clinical and radiographic presentation, treatment, and prognosis.

Multicystic Solid Ameloblastoma

Multicystic solid ameloblastoma, sometimes called *conventional ameloblastoma*, is the most worrisome of the three types due to its aggressive and recurrent nature. It is rarely seen in patients under age 20 or over age 40. The pathogenesis of ameloblastomas remains controversial. Ameloblastomas may occur in any location within the jaws but are most common in the posterior mandible. The classic radiographic appearance is a multilocular "soap-bubble" appearance (Fig. 8-2A). Early lesions may appear unilocular (Fig. 8-2B). Patients present with a painless swelling of the jaw, which can grow to dramatic proportions if left untreated (Fig. 8-2C). As the tumor expands, it can destroy or thin the buccal and/or lingual cortex, producing an "egg shell" consistency (Fig. 8-2D). Ameloblastomas do not form capsules even though they are benign tumors. This allows them to insidiously infiltrate bone, complicating surgical removal. Microscopic remnants of tumor left behind after surgery can lead to recurrence years later.

Treatment is complete surgical excision. This may necessitate removal of large amounts of bone depending on tumor size. Reconstruction with bone grafting may be necessary. Recurrence is a serious risk and patients must be followed throughout their lives.

When malignant transformation of ameloblastoma occurs, the malignant tumor is called *ameloblastic carcinoma*. Most patients who experience ameloblastic

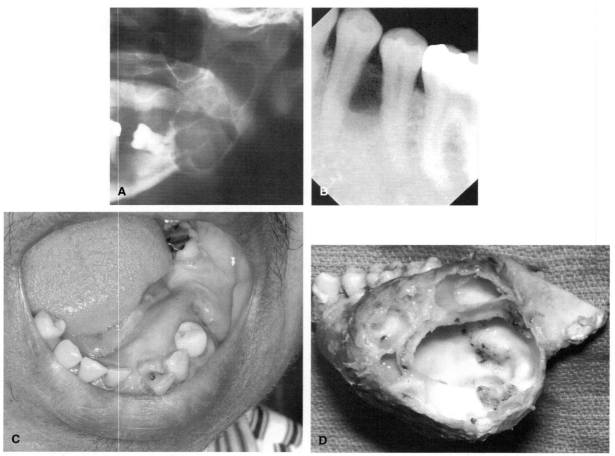

Figure 8–2 Multicystic ameloblastoma. A. Multilocular radiolucency in the posterior mandible that extends into the ramus and TMJ. **B.** Early ameloblastoma with unilocular appearance. **C.** Clinical appearance of painless enlargement of the left mandible and malpositioning of teeth. **D.** Ameloblastoma: Gross specimen. Ameloblastoma of the mandible with lingual bone removed; bony walls produce multilocular radiographic appearance.

carcinoma have had a previous long-term history of ameloblastoma, usually with multiple recurrences.

Benign ameloblastomas have been found in extraoral sites. Many believe these are metastatic lesions from the jaws; however, this activity is unusual for benign tumors.

Peripheral Ameloblastoma

Peripheral ameloblastomas originate within the gingival soft tissues of adults. Patients present with a painless, firm nodular swelling of the gingiva, most often in the mandibular premolar area, that has a smooth or papillary surface (Fig. 8-3A). There is no bone involvement and radiographs appear normal (Fig. 8-3B). Occasionally, multicystic solid ameloblastomas perforate the cortex and cause gingival swelling. These are *not* considered peripheral tumors because the point

of origin is within bone. Unlike multicystic solid ameloblastoma, peripheral ameloblastomas are not aggressive, are easily treated with conservative local excision, and pose little risk for recurrence. Peripheral ameloblastomas must be differentiated from intraosseous ameloblastomas because treatment and prognosis differs significantly.

Calcifying Epithelial Odontogenic Tumor

Calcifying epithelial odontogenic tumor (CEOT) is a benign tumor composed of cells that resemble stratum intermedium of the enamel organ. Cells resembling ameloblasts are not seen. CEOT is comparable to ameloblastoma in age, location, and treatment. CEOT presents as a painless, slow-growing mass of the jaw (Fig. 8-4A). Radiographic appearance is that of a unilocular or multilocular radiolucency with a well-defined

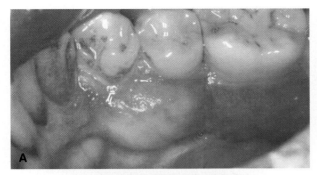

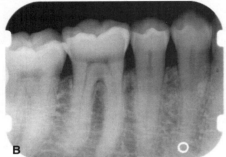

Figure 8–3 Peripheral ameloblastoma. A. Firm nodular mass on lingual surface of mandible; underlying bone was intact. **B.** Periapical radiograph shows no evidence of intrabony lesion.

but noncorticated border (Fig. 8-4B), containing scattered radiopacities. Significant expansion and a "honeycombed" (Fig. 8-4C) appearance may be present. The scattered radiopacities help differentiate it from ameloblastoma. Treatment involves wide surgical excision and close clinical follow up for recurrence.

Squamous Odontogenic Tumor

Squamous odontogenic tumor (SOT) arises from the Rests of Malassez within the periodontal ligament space. It occurs at any age but is more common in adults. SOTs present as painless swellings of gingiva, which may result in displaced and mobile teeth. Radiographic appearance is that of localized radiolucent loss of alveolar bone and lamina dura along the periodontal ligament space. Treatment is conservative curettage. SOTs tend not to recur.

Odontogenic Myxoma

Odontogenic myxoma is a benign neoplasm that arises from the mesenchymal portion of the tooth germ. Microscopically, it resembles tissues of the dental papilla. It presents as a mild jaw swelling (Fig. 8-5A) with either a unilocular (Fig. 8-5B) or multilocular

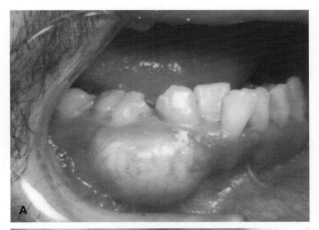

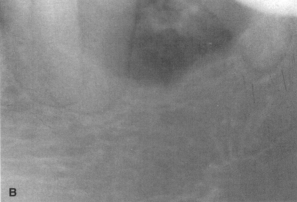

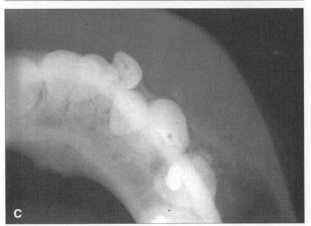

Figure 8–4 Calcifying epithelial odontogenic tumor (CEOT). A. Swelling of the jaw and malpositioning of teeth. **B.** CEOT periapical radiograph. Well-defined but noncorticated lesion with central radiopaque material. **C.** CEOT occlusal radiograph. CEOT has perforated the cortex; note radiopacities within tumor.

radiographic appearance. Myxomas frequently develop along the lateral aspect of teeth where early lesions can mimic periodontal bone loss (Fig. 8-5C). The tumor is not encapsulated and has a gelatinous consistency. This allows easy infiltration of the marrow spaces, making complete removal very difficult and recurrence common.

> ### Clinical Implications
> Squamous odontogenic tumor and odontogenic myxoma should be suspected when there is a non-inflamed isolated periodontal defect in an otherwise healthy adult mouth.

Odontogenic tumors seen predominantly in the pediatric population are discussed next.

Odontoma

Controversy exists as to whether *odontomas* represent neoplasms or developmental **hamartomas**. If they are considered a neoplasm, then they are the most common odontogenic neoplasm, exceeding the number of all other odontogenic neoplasms combined. They present as well-defined masses composed of a combination of all tooth-forming and hard dental tissues. The two basic types of odontomas are described next.

Compound Odontoma

Compound odontoma is a well-defined encapsulated mass of tiny "toothlets," miniature teeth, often 4 to 8 mm in length, with identifiable crowns and roots. Compound odontomas may be seen anywhere in the jaws but favor areas where deciduous teeth are or have been located. They may impede the eruption of permanent teeth, which is how they are often first recognized. Radiographs show a radiolucent follicular sac-like structure (Fig. 8-6A) filled with identifiable toothlets (Fig. 8-6B). Treatment is surgical removal and they do not recur.

Complex Odontoma

Complex odontoma is a well-defined, encapsulated, disorganized, jumbled mass of mature tooth tissues with no identifiable toothlets (Fig. 8-7A). Radiographically, it appears as a radiodense structure with a radiolucent rim that may be misinterpreted as a more ominous tumor (Fig. 8-7B). The diagnosis is often not apparent until it is removed and examined microscopically. Once removed, they do not recur.

Occasionally, a compound odontoma may occur in conjunction with a complex odontoma. When this happens, the term *compound/complex odontoma* is used (Fig. 8-8).

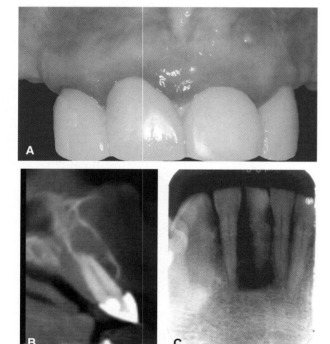

Figure 8–5   Odontogenic myxoma. A. Swelling between maxillary central incisors. **B.** Myxoma lateral slice radiograph. Same case as 4A. Radiolucent lesion pushing cortex toward facial surface. **C.** Myxoma periapical. Destruction of bone by odontogenic myxoma mimics periodontal bone loss.

> ### Clinical Implications
> Because odontomas are essentially "impacted teeth," they are vulnerable to the same problems as other impacted or unerupted teeth. For example, dentigerous cysts may develop within the follicular sacs surrounding odontomas. Surgical removal not only allows eruption of blocked teeth but prevents further associated pathologic changes.

Cystic Ameloblastoma

Cystic ameloblastoma (formerly termed *unicystic ameloblastoma*) occurs in individuals under age 20, much

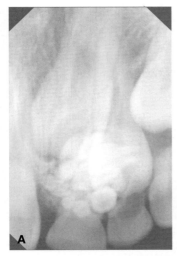

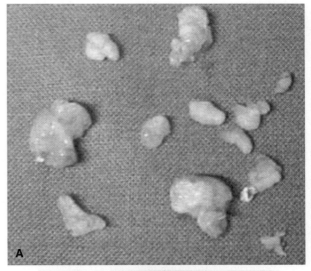

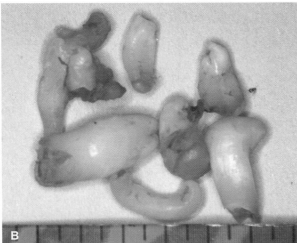

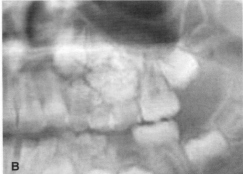

Figure 8–7   Complex odontoma. A. Fragments of calcified tooth material with no identifiable toothlets. **B.** Complex odontoma radiograph. Radiopaque mass with no identifiable toothlets.

Figure 8–6   Compound odontoma. A. Compound odontoma impeding eruption of maxillary incisors; toothlets are clearly visible. **B.** Toothlets from compound odontoma; crowns and roots recognizable.

younger that those with multicystic solid ameloblastoma. It appears unilocular on radiographs (Fig. 8-9) and may be associated with an unerupted tooth and mimic a dentigerous cyst. Dentigerous cysts usually do not cause jaw expansion. Cystic ameloblastomas often cause significant jaw expansion. These lesions are not encapsulated but tend to be well-defined. Cystic ameloblastomas incompletely removed by curettage tend to recur. Complete surgical excision and examination for evidence of small tumor islands is needed to reduce the risk of recurrence.

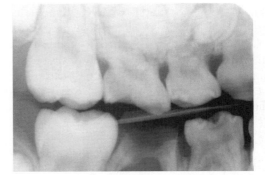

Figure 8–8   Compound/complex odontoma. Radiopaque mass with toothlets plus solid component apical to primary molars.

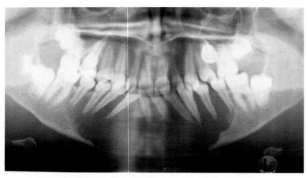

Figure 8–9   Cystic ameloblastoma. Teeth drifting within large unilocular ameloblastoma in 12-year-old patient.

Clinical Implications

For both multicystic and cystic ameloblastoma, recurrences are more difficult to treat. Patients lose additional jaw structure and teeth with each surgery. Aggressive initial surgical intervention is often the best opportunity to cure these lesions.

Adenomatoid Odontogenic Tumor

Adenomatoid odontogenic tumor (AOT) is a benign tumor seen in adolescents. It has a female predominance. It is most common around unerupted or impacted teeth, most often the maxillary canines. Radiographically, it appears as a well-defined, well-corticated, unilocular, pericoronal radiolucency in association with an unerupted tooth (Fig. 8-10). The radiolucency often extends far below the cemento-enamel junction (CEJ). Scattered small foci of calcifying hard tissue called "snowflake" calcifications may be seen radiographically within the radiolucency. Extension of the tumor apically from the CEJ and the presence of calcifications can help differentiate AOTs from dentigerous cysts. Patients rarely complain of pain but they may notice swelling of the jaw where the tumor is located. Sometimes the tooth will "erupt through the tumor," leaving the tumor situated at the apex of the tooth. This mimics periapical pathology, but the tooth will be vital and asymptomatic. Because AOT is so well-encapsulated, it can easily be removed from the bone. Recurrence is rare. Malignant transformation has not been reported.

Clinical Implications

The typical case scenario of AOT is an adolescent girl with an impacted maxillary canine tooth. A nonpainful, well-defined, mixed radiolucent/radiopaque lesion is present surrounding the crown and extending down along the root surface below the CEJ.

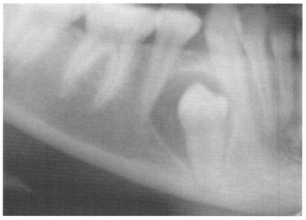

Figure 8–10   Adenomatoid odontogenic tumor. Unerupted premolar with unilocular radiolucency containing small calcified flecks.

Ameloblastic Fibroma and Ameloblastic Fibro-odontoma

Ameloblastic fibroma is rarely seen in patients older than age 20. Because the tumor is derived from a combination of enamel organ cells (ameloblasts) and dental papilla cells (mesenchyme), the possibility of tooth tissue formation exists. If no tooth tissue forms, the term *ameloblastic fibroma* (AF) is used. AF is an asymptomatic radiolucent lesion that can vary in size from a small lesion found incidentally on routine radiographs to a large jaw swelling most often seen in the posterior mandible (Fig. 8-11). It is a well-defined, encapsulated lesion that may be readily removed from the bone; however, the risk of incomplete removal and recurrence exists. The very rare malignant *ameloblastic fibrosarcoma* has been seen in patients whose AFs have recurred multiple times.

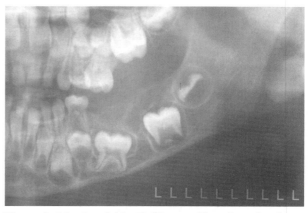

Figure 8–11   Ameloblastic fibroma. Eruption of molars is impeded by radiolucent ameloblastic fibroma in a child.

Ameloblastic fibro-odontoma (AFO) forms when an AF forms tooth tissue. AFO shares many clinical features with AF, except that the lesion will appear mixed radiolucent/radiopaque. The degree of radiopacity depends on the amounts of enamel and dentin that are formed and how well they calcify (Fig. 8-12). Therefore, lesions may show either faint radiopacity or large radiodense areas within the encapsulated tumor. AFOs appear more "mature" than AFs, with hard tissue formation. For this reason, they have less tendency to recur and malignant transformation is more rare.

Clinical Implications

There are major clinical differences between ameloblastoma and ameloblastic fibroma. Ameloblastoma is an aggressive recurrent lesion that often requires major surgery and close clinical follow up throughout the patient's life span. AFs and AFOs in general require more conservative surgical treatment and recurrence is not common.

Cementoblastoma

Cementoblastoma is a benign neoplasm of cementum. It presents in patients younger than age 30 as a solid, radiopaque mass found most frequently around the apex of a tooth. The neoplasm is most frequently associated with the mandibular first molars (Fig. 8-13A). Deciduous

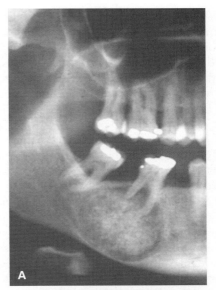

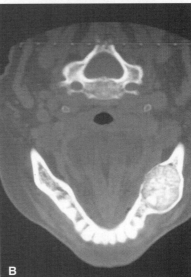

Figure 8–13   Cementoblastoma. A. Well-defined mixed radiolucent/radiopaque mass attached to the roots of mandibular first molar. **B.** Cementoblastoma CT scan. CT scan showing expansion of mandible with cementoblastoma.

and other permanent teeth may be involved. Cementoblastomas may be aggressive and cause jaw expansion with accompanying pain (Fig. 8-13B). Treatment is complicated as the tumor adheres directly to the tooth root, making extraction of the tooth and tumor excision very difficult. Recurrence is common.

Two developmental odontogenic cysts have recently been reclassified as odontogenic neoplasms because their biologic behavior is more consistent with that of a neoplasm. They can be found in any age group and are presented here.

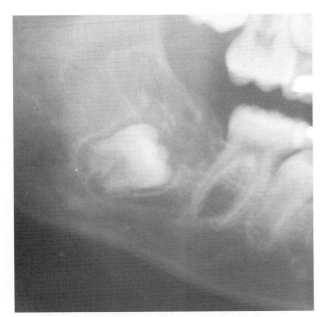

Figure 8–12   Ameloblastic fibro-odontoma. Eruption of second molar impeded by mixed radiolucent/radiopaque ameloblastic fibro-odontoma.

Keratinizing Cystic Odontogenic Tumor

Keratinizing cystic odontogenic tumor (KCOT) has been more commonly called *odontogenic keratocyst* (OKC). It is called "keratinizing" because the cystic spaces or lumen fill with desquamated keratin from an epithelial lining. It is known for its aggressive and recurrent behavior. Patients with the diagnosis of KCOT require a lifetime of close clinical observation for recurrence. KCOT is a feature of nevoid basal cell carcinoma syndrome (Gorlin syndrome) discussed in Chapter 6. Early diagnosis can help reduce associated morbidity associated with the syndrome.

KCOT typically will not cause jaw expansion but may insidiously destroy large amounts of trabecular bone, leaving the patient vulnerable to jaw fracture. Figure 8-14A shows one KCOT that caused expansion because it was in thinner bone of the anterior mandible. Radiographically KCOT appears as a unilocular (Fig. 8-14B) or multilocular radiolucency (Fig. 8-14C) seen around the crown of an impacted tooth, at the apices of vital teeth, in the maxillary sinus, or elsewhere in the jaws. Complete removal is difficult because of residual "daughter cysts," which may be left behind after surgery and lead to recurrence.

Calcifying Cystic Odontogenic Tumor

Calcifying cystic odontogenic tumor (CCOT) is also called *calcifying odontogenic cyst* (COC) or *Gorlin cyst*. This tumor can occur anywhere in either jaw as a painless swelling that may reach a large size. CCOT may cause root divergence but rarely root resorption. It has a unilocular radiolucent appearance with varying numbers of calcified epithelial "ghost cells" that tend to fill up the cystic spaces of the tumor (Fig. 8-15). Treatment is surgical **enucleation**. Unlike KCOT, it rarely recurs.

NEOPLASMS OF BONE

In addition to odontogenic tumors of the jaws, neoplasms of the bone itself can develop. Neoplasms of bone often cause expansion. This is detectable by the patient who presents to the dental office with a chief complaint of swelling. Expansion of bone may also occur when tumors from other parts of the body metastasize to the jaws.

Osteoma

Osteomas are benign tumors composed of mature bone tissue. They are rarely seen outside the bones of the head and neck. They may resemble torus palatinus and torus mandibularis; however, tori are development

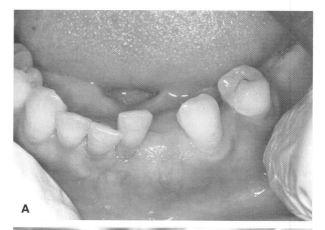

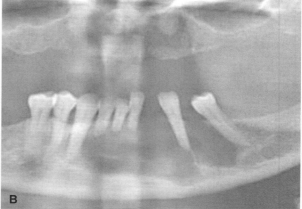

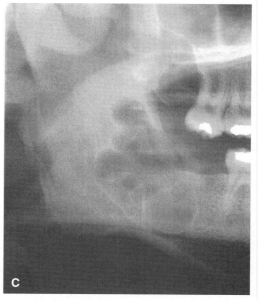

Figure 8–14   Keratinizing cystic odontogenic tumor (KCOT)/odontogenic keratocyst. A. Movement of teeth and swelling of jaw with KCOT. **B.** Large unilocular radiolucency and resorption of tooth roots. **C.** Multilocular radiolucent lesion originally thought to be an ameloblastoma. Biopsy showed KCOT.

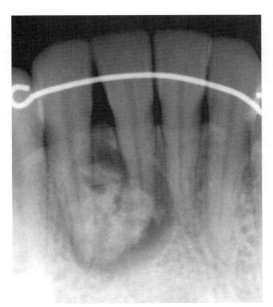

Figure 8–15   Calcifying cystic odontogenic tumor (calcifying odontogenic cyst). Well-defined mixed radiolucent/radiopaque mass of anterior mandible.

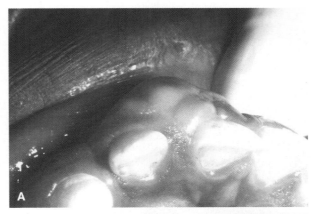

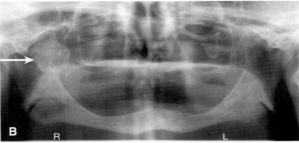

Figure 8–16   Osteoma. A. Developing osteoma causing hard swelling of anterior maxilla. **B.** Osteoma in area of the temporomandibular joint (arrow).

abnormalities that grow as the patient grows, whereas osteomas develop autonomously later in life.

Osteomas arise on the surface of the bone and can be detected by palpation. Most are small but some can become large enough to cause mild facial distortion (Fig. 8-16A). They rarely cause difficulties for the patient unless they impinge on the temporomandibular joint (TMJ) or occur within the sinuses. Radiographically, osteoma appears as well-circumscribed radiopacities (Fig. 8-16B). If they are large enough to include bone marrow, the central portions may appear radiolucent.

Gardner's syndrome is a hereditary autosomal dominant condition of significance to dentistry because it often presents with dental and jaw abnormalities, including multiple osteomas. A serious consequence for patients with this syndrome includes development of polyps of the colon that eventually undergo malignant transformation. See Chapter 6 for more details on Gardner's syndrome.

Ossifying Fibroma

Ossifying fibroma is a benign neoplasm comprised of bone and cementum-like material. Although the term *cemento-ossifying fibroma* is still used, the more accepted term is ossifying fibroma because there is no true cementum in this tumor. Ossifying fibroma occurs mainly in young adults but can be seen at any age. It is found most commonly in the premolar area of the mandible. In the early stages of development, fibrous transformation

of normal bone gives the tumor a radiolucent appearance. As the tumor grows, the fibrous tissue undergoes calcification. This causes a well-defined, unilocular mixed radiolucent/radiopaque appearance with a distinctly corticated rim (Fig. 8-17A). The tumor is aggressive but causes painless expansion of the jaw with accompanying facial asymmetry. Teeth may be moved but are rarely resorbed (Fig. 8-17B). Small tumors tend to "shell out" at surgery because they have a well-defined capsule. If the tumor is large, a portion of the mandible or maxilla may have to be removed *en bloc*, causing a large surgical defect. Bone grafting may be needed to replace the missing section of jaw.

Clinical Implications

The term *central* implies that the neoplasm occurs within the bone rather than "peripheral" on the soft tissues that cover the bone. A peripheral ossifying fibroma is a non-neoplastic benign reactive disorder that occurs on the gingiva and is unrelated to central ossifying fibroma. They should not be confused. See Chapter 2 for a discussion of peripheral ossifying fibroma.

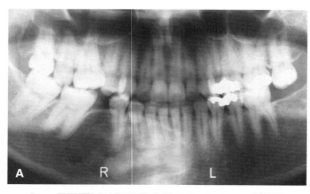

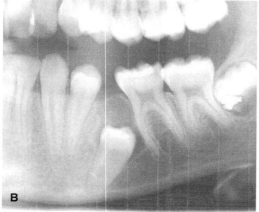

Figure 8–17 **Ossifying fibroma of bone. A.** Well-defined mixed radiolucent radiopaque mass of the anterior mandible. **B.** Small COF impeding eruption of premolar; radiopaque component not fully developed.

Osteoblastoma

Osteoblastoma is a benign tumor that differs from osteoma in that the neoplastic bone tissue is immature and weak rather than mature and hard. Osteoblastoma can occur in any bone, including the mandible and the maxilla, and can reach a size of up to 4 cm (1.57 in.). Most jaw osteoblastomas occur before age 30. Tumor osteoblasts produce bone of poor quality that appears radiographically as a mixed radiolucent radiopaque mass destroying normal adjacent bone. Due to infiltration of peripheral nerve fibers, they tend to be painful, unlike osteomas. The tumors do not metastasize or reduce life expectancy; however, they require surgery, which may cause morbidity. Once surgically removed, recurrence is rare.

Osteosarcoma

Osteosarcoma is cancer of bone tissue. Osteoblasts undergo malignant transformation and show the features

of *anaplasia*, discussed in Chapter 7. Anaplastic osteoblasts lose their ability to form normal bone and instead produce immature abnormal nonfunctional bone. The tumor osteoid fails to calcify completely. Osteosarcomas range from radiolucent to mixed radiolucent/radiopaque appearance depending on the amount of the abnormal bone that undergoes calcification.

In the jaws, osteosarcoma tends to peak between 30 and 35 years of age. Osteosarcoma of the jaws is less frequent than osteosarcoma of the long bones, which peaks between 10 and 20 years of age.

Swelling and pain are the most common symptoms (Fig. 8-18A). Because the new abnormal bone is weak, the patient is vulnerable to jaw fracture. If the tumor begins in the alveolar bone, there is loss of the radiographic lamina dura accompanied by tooth mobility (Fig. 8-18B). The apices of the teeth may be resorbed at an angle, causing a "spiked" appearance. The tumor bone may appear **sclerotic** and blend in with the adjacent normal bone, making it difficult to view the borders of the tumor radiographically (Fig. 8-18C). Therefore, advanced imaging is necessary to determine the true dimensions of the tumor (Fig. 8-18D). A "sunburst" appearance may be seen radiographically at the periphery of the bone in approximately 25 percent of cases. This is due to alternating bands of calcification within the abnormal bone. Treatment and prognosis depend on the degree of anaplasia of the tumor cells, the size of the tumor, and the extent of spread. Chemotherapy often precedes extensive and sometimes radical surgery. Osteosarcomas of the jaws can metastasize but more commonly they recur locally and threaten vital structures. **Local recurrence** may occur despite the best surgical procedures. Removal of the entire mandible or maxilla may be required to control this neoplasm. Depending on the size of the tumor and the success of the surgery, the 5-year survival rate ranges from 30% to 75%.

Clinical Implications

Early osteosarcoma of the jaws may destroy alveolar bone and mimic periodontitis; however, in periodontitis the loss of lamina dura will initially appear at the alveolar crest rather than the lateral socket wall (PDL space) or apices as seen in osteosarcoma. Pain and tissue expansion/swelling seen in osteosarcoma are not characteristic of periodontitis.

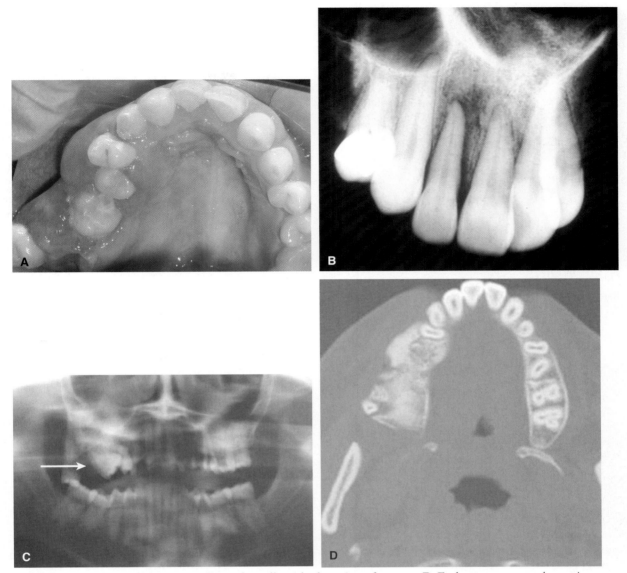

Figure 8–18 **Osteosarcoma. A.** Swelling of maxilla with ulceration of mucosa. **B.** Early osteosarcoma destroying lamina dura of lateral incisor. **C.** Same patient as A. Tumor in the right maxilla (arrow). **D.** CT of same patient that shows extent of the tumor.

Metastasis of Other Tumors to Bone

Carcinomas from distant sites may favor metastasis to bone, including the maxilla and mandible. The most common tumors to metastasize to the jaws are adenocarcinomas from the breast, prostate, thyroid, gastrointestinal (GI) tract, and lung, as well as carcinomas from the kidney and lung (Table 8-2). Sarcomas other than osteosarcoma rarely metastasize to bone. In most cases, patients present with a previous history of carcinoma. Occasionally, metastasis of cancer to the jaws is occasionally identified and diagnosed before the discovery of the **primary tumor**.

Signs and symptoms vary widely depending on the location of the metastasis. Patients may complain of swelling, loose teeth, and pain or numbness if the tumor impacts the mandibular nerve. Radiographs typically show ill-defined radiolucent alterations of the bone, sometimes described as "moth eaten" (Fig. 8-19). Occasionally **dystrophic calcifications** may be seen in breast and prostate cancer metastases. When the

Table 8.2	Origin of Metastases to the Bone of the Jaws	
Men	**Women**	
Lung: 25%	Breast: 36.6%	
Kidney: 10.8%	Genital organs (uterus, ovaries, cervix, fallopian tubes): 9.5%	
Liver: 8.6%		
Prostate :7.5%	Kidney: 8.5%	
Bone: 7.5%	Colorectum: 7.1%	
Adrenal gland: 5.3%	Bone: 6.7%	
Colorectum: 4.7%	Adrenal gland: 5.8%	
Testis: 4.4%	Thyroid: 5.4%	
Esophagus: 3.6%	Rare tumors: 20.4%	
Stomach: 2.5%		
Bladder: 2.5%		
Rare tumors: 17.0%		

Source: http://emedicine.medscape.com/article/1079102-overview#a0199, July 2012.

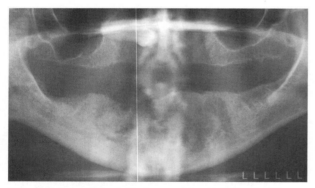

Figure 8–19   Metastatic tumor. Poorly defined diffuse mixed radiolucent/radiopaque expansile mass in patient with metastatic carcinoma to the mandible.

lesions are biopsied, the microscopic features of the original tumor are seen. It is a misnomer to call carcinomas that metastasize to the jaws "bone cancer."

NEOPLASMS OF CARTILAGE

Chondroma is a benign tumor composed of mature cartilage produced by normal-appearing chondrocytes. Chondromas are found in body locations where normal cartilage is typically found, including the ribs, fingers, legs,

nasal septum, and occasionally the TMJ. They require surgical removal and rarely recur. Multiple chondromas are characteristic of several syndromes for which the patient should be assessed.

Chondrosarcoma is cancer of cartilage composed of anaplastic chondroblasts producing immature cartilage that fails to calcify properly. Chondrosarcomas may be found in the anterior maxilla, nasal cartilage, sinuses, TMJ, and laryngeal cartilage of adults. Jaw tumors cause bone expansion with loosening and resorption of teeth, but patients rarely complain of pain. Radiographic images show a poorly defined radiolucency with scattered radiopacities that may enlarge as the tumor progresses. Prognosis depends on surgical removal because chemotherapy and radiotherapy are not always effective. Five-year survival rates are greater than 60 percent but the rates decrease in later years due to propensity for recurrence.

Critical Thinking Questions

Case 8-1:   Your 14-year-old female patient presents to your office with failure of eruption of tooth #6. Her jaw is slightly swollen in the area. A radiograph shows that the tooth is impacted. The well-defined, well-corticated radiolucent lesion surrounding it shows some fine radiopaque flecks.

• • •

Which two odontogenic tumors should be considered in this case?

What features will differentiate your two choices?

How will the final diagnosis be reached?

Case 8-2:   Your 26-year-old male patient presents for routine care and new bitewings before he enlists in the Marines. He complains that he thinks his wisdom tooth is erupting because he feels a swelling. On his bitewing, you note a radiolucent lesion distal to this second molar. A subsequent panoramic radiograph shows a large multilocular radiolucent lesion extending to the lower third of the ramus. The third molar is not present.

• • •

Name two possible odontogenic neoplasms this may represent.

Because the swelling is not being caused by a third molar, how do you explain the patient's symptoms?

Your patient states he does not want to "do anything about it now" because he is about to leave for training. He proudly tells you he is planning on trying out for the boxing team on the base.

What precautions should you relate to the patient?

After the dentist examines the patient, he relents and decides to seek care for his swelling.

What will be the first step in determining what this lesion is?

Case 8-3: Your 64-year-old female patient presents for routine care. Her medical history includes past history of breast cancer for which she received radiation and chemotherapy. She has been disease-free for 13 months. During scaling, you notice that tooth #29 and tooth #30 have +1 mobility. Radiographs show a diffuse loss of bone density at the apices of the teeth. They respond positively to percussion tests. There is no tenderness or swelling in the area.

• • •

There is a possibility that this lesion represents a metastasis of her breast cancer. How can that be determined? What steps will be taken to investigate this lesion?

How will this impact your treatment plan?

What types of cancer arise from bone in the jaw? What types of cancer commonly metastasize to the jaw?

Review Questions

1. **Which one of the following is true of odontogenic neoplasms?**
   A. They include osteomas and osteosarcoma of the jaws.
   B. They arise from remnants of the developing tooth germ.
   C. They include those that develop in a distant site and metastasize to the jaws.
   D. They are always malignant.

2. **Most odontogenic tumors are central. This means they**
   A. originate in the soft tissues covering the jaws.
   B. closely approximate the center of the ramus.
   C. are made up of mandibular or maxillary bone.
   D. develop within the bone of the jaws.

3. **Of the neoplasms listed below, which one is the most common benign odontogenic tumor?**
   A. Ameloblastoma
   B. Ameloblastic carcinoma
   C. Calcifying epithelial odontogenic tumor
   D. Odontogenic myxoma

4. **All of the following are true about multicystic solid ameloblastoma EXCEPT**
   A. the posterior mandible is the most common location.
   B. it is the most worrisome type of ameloblastoma.
   C. recurrence is rare.
   D. it is the "conventional" or most common form of ameloblastoma.

5. **Which one of the following is true of peripheral ameloblastomas?**

   A. They originate within the soft tissues of the gingiva in adults.
   B. They are aggressive and require wide surgical excision.
   C. They are known to frequently recur after treatment.
   D. They have a tendency to metastasize to the lung.

6. **Under which one of the following circumstances can squamous odontogenic tumor and odontogenic myxoma be suspected?**

   A. If the patient is under 12 years of age.
   B. When there is a non-inflamed isolated periodontal defect in an otherwise healthy mouth.
   C. When an encapsulated mass of tiny "toothlets" is present.
   D. When there is a well-defined radiolucency with "snowflake" calcifications.

7. **Compound odontomas**

   A. are well-defined encapsulated masses of tiny "toothlets."
   B. may occur as both benign and malignant neoplasms.
   C. are well-defined, encapsulated, disorganized, jumbled masses of mature tooth tissues.
   D. are not considered odontogenic.

8. **Which one of the following odontogenic tumors often occurs around the crown of an unerupted maxillary canine in an adolescent female?**

   A. Cystic ameloblastoma
   B. Adenomatoid odontogenic tumor
   C. Squamous odontogenic tumor
   D. Odontogenic myxoma

9. **Which one of the following is a benign radiopaque lesion that may be found around the apex of a tooth in a patient younger than 30?**

   A. Ameloblastic fibro-odontoma
   B. Ameloblastoma
   C. Odontogenic myxoma
   D. Cementoblastoma

10. **Odontogenic keratocyst has recently been reclassified as an odontogenic neoplasm. The new name is**

    A. calcifying cystic odontogenic tumor.
    B. keratinizing cystic odontogenic tumor.
    C. ameloblastic cystic fibro-odontoma.
    D. cystic odontogenic myxoma.

11. **What benign tumor is composed of mature bone and may resemble a torus?**

    A. Osteoblastoma
    B. Osteosarcoma
    C. Osteoma
    D. Chondroma

12. **Multiple osteomas of the jaws are seen in what syndrome?**

    A. Gardner's syndrome
    B. Nevoid basal cell carcinoma syndrome
    C. Chondroblastic osteosarcoma syndrome
    D. Ameloblastic cell syndrome

13. **All of the following are true about osteosarcoma EXCEPT**

    A. occurrence of jaw tumors tends to peak between 30 and 35 years of age.
    B. there is a direct link with tobacco and alcohol use.
    C. it is a cancer of bone with osteoblasts undergoing malignant transformation.
    D. swelling and pain are the most common symptoms.

14. **A "sunburst" appearance is seen radiographically in approximately 25 percent of cases of which one of the following neoplasms?**

    A. Osteosarcoma
    B. Osteoma
    C. Ameloblastoma
    D. Compound odontoma

15. **Which one of the following tumors may metastasize to the mandible?**

    A. Breast cancer
    B. Prostate cancer
    C. Lung cancer
    D. All of the above

REFERENCES

Books

Neville, BW, Damm, DD, Allen, CA, Bouquot, JE: Oral and Maxillofacial Pathology, ed. 3. Saunders Elsevier, St. Louis, 2009.

Robbins, SL, Kumar, V, Abbas, AK, Cotran, RS, et al: Pathologic Basis of Disease, ed. 10. Saunders Elsevier, Philadelphia, 2010.

Journal Articles

Arndt, CA, Rose, PS, Folpe, AL, Laack, NN: Common musculoskeletal tumors of childhood and adolescence. Mayo Clinic Proceedings 87(5):475–487, May 2012.

Boffano, P, Roccia, F, Campisi, P, Gallesio, C: Review of 43 osteomas of the craniomaxillofacial region. Journal of Oral Maxillofacial Surgery 70(5):1093–1095, May 2012.

Boxberger, NR, Brannon, RB, Fowler, CB: Ameloblastic fibroodontoma: A clinicopathologic study of 12 cases. Journal of Clinical Pediatric Dentistry 35(4):397–403, Summer 2011.

D'Silva, NJ, Summerilin, DJ, Cordell, KG et al: Metastatic tumors in the jaws: A retrospective of 114 cases. Journal of the American Dental Association1 37:1667–1672, 2006.

Morgan, PR: Odontogenic tumors: A review. Periodontology 2000 57(1):160–176, October 2011.

Triantafillidou, K, Venetis, G, Karakinaris, G, Iordanidis, F: Ossifying fibroma of the jaws: A clinical study of 14 cases and review of the literature. Oral Surgery, Oral Medicine, Oral Pathology, Oral Radiology and Endodontology 114(2):193–199, August 2012.

Chapter 9

Systemic Pathology and Oral Manifestations of Systemic Diseases

Learning Outcomes

At the end of this chapter, the student will be able to:

9.1. Illustrate by examples how a Review of Systems can impact the dental hygiene appointment.

9.2. Describe systemic and oral manifestations of endocrine gland dysfunction, including endocrinopathies of the pituitary, adrenal, pancreas, thyroid, and parathyroid glands.

9.3. Contrast the difference in oral and systemic manifestations of endocrinopathies when onset occurs in adulthood versus childhood.

9.4. Discuss oral and systemic manifestations of diabetes mellitus, and relate how this disorder impacts patients and dental treatment.

9.5. Compare the hemoglobinopathies including their etiologies, clinical features, laboratory findings, and dental appointment management considerations.

Continued

9.6. Describe the types and causes of anemia, and laboratory tests used in evaluation of red blood cells.

9.7. Discuss the different types of bleeding disorders and their impact on dental care.

9.8. Describe systemic and oral manifestations of gastrointestinal tract dysfunction, including the main difference between inflammatory bowel disease and Crohn's disease.

9.9. Explain how jaundice develops and its significance.

9.10. Discuss how connective tissue disorders affect dental treatment.

9.11. Compare systemic and oral features of hyper-vitamin states and vitamin deficiencies.

9.12. Explain how vitamin C and vitamin D deficiencies impact the oral hard and soft tissues.

ORAL MANIFESTATIONS OF SYSTEMIC DISEASE

An important part of every dental visit is the gathering of information on a patient's general health. Completing the medical history includes a Review of Systems. This involves questioning patients or parents about diseases of body systems such as the respiratory, cardiovascular, digestive, and neuromuscular systems. Regardless of the chief dental complaint, a thorough health history is necessary to safely provide appropriate treatment.

Systemic diseases can remain undetected until signs appear in the oral cavity and become apparent. Dental hygienists are in an ideal position to recognize the oral signs of systemic disease, leading to their diagnosis.

Some signs and symptoms of underlying systemic disease that present in the oral cavity can be disease-specific, whereas others are nonspecific. Knowledge of systemic diseases and their oral signs and symptoms is important not only in disease recognition and detection but in understanding implications for patient management and treatment. Discovery of undetected medical conditions also allows for timely referral of patients to a physician for evaluation and treatment. This chapter discusses the **pathophysiology** of selected systems along with their oral manifestations and clinical implications for patients and dental hygiene practice.

OVERVIEW OF THE ENDOCRINE SYSTEM AND ENDOCRINOPATHIES

The endocrine system consists of a group of organs that use extracellular molecules called **hormones** that act in a coordinated manner to communicate with other body systems (Fig. 9-1). The endocrine system acts to control metabolism, growth, and a variety of tissue functions by secreting hormones directly into the bloodstream for transport to target organs. Cells in the target organs

respond by signaling the secreting gland when sufficient hormone has been received, causing secretion to stop.

Most hormone secretion is controlled by a physiological *negative feedback inhibition loop*. For example, the hypothalamus secretes thyroid-releasing hormone (TRH) that directs the anterior pituitary gland to secrete thyroid-stimulating hormone (TSH). TSH stimulates thyroid cells to secrete T3 and T4, two common thyroid hormones. These hormones produce their designated effects on the body, including heat regulation. When temperature is adequately regulated, normal levels of T3 and T4 signal the pituitary gland that enough thyroid hormone has been produced. The pituitary gland responds by slowing or stopping the production of TRH. A similar negative feedback loop is seen with other pituitary hormones.

Endocrine disorders may occur as a result of underproduction or overproduction of hormones. This may be due to endocrine gland dysfunction, an abnormal interaction between the hormone and its target organ, or disease preventing the hormone from being metabolized. Endocrine diseases discussed in this chapter include those of the pituitary, thyroid, parathyroid, adrenal glands, and pancreas.

Pituitary Gland

The pituitary gland consists of anterior and posterior lobes. The anterior lobe secretes growth hormone (GH), adrenocorticotrophic hormone (ACTH), melanocyte-stimulating hormone (MSH), thyroid-stimulating hormone (TSH), prolactin, follicle-stimulating hormone (FSH), and luteinizing hormone (LH). A summary of pituitary hormones, their effects on target organs, and diseases is provided in Table 9-1. Not all diseases associated with alterations of pituitary hormones have oral manifestations of immediate concern to dental hygiene

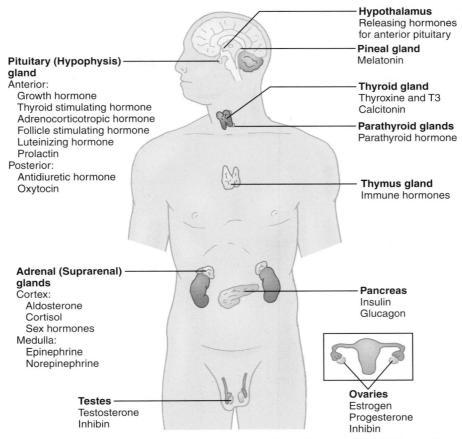

Figure 9–1   The endocrine system and its glands. (From Tamparo, CD: Diseases of the Human Body, ed. 5. F.A. Davis, Philadelphia, 2011, p 284.)

Table 9.1	Pituitary Hormones			
	Hormone	**Target Organs**	**Hormone Effects**	**Diseases**
Anterior Pituitary	Growth hormone (GH)	Mainly liver, bones, muscles	Overall growth and protein, fat and glucose homeostasis	Excessive GH - Gigantism - Acromegaly Deficiency of GH - Dwarfism
	Adrenocorticotrophic hormone (ACTH)	Adrenal gland (cortex)	Stimulates the production of glucocorticoids	Excess ACTH - Cushing's syndrome Deficiency of ACTH - Addison's disease
	Melanocyte stimulating hormone (MSH)	Melanin-producing cells, usually present in the skin	Stimulates the production of melanin, causing darkening of the skin	Seen in Addison's disease

Continued

Table 9.1	Pituitary Hormones—cont'd			
	Hormone	**Target Organs**	**Hormone Effects**	**Diseases**
	Thyroid stimulating hormone (TSH)	Thyroid gland	Regulates thyroid function	Excess TSH -Graves' Disease Deficiency of TSH -Hashimoto's Disease
	Follicular stimulating hormone (FSH)	Reproductive organs	Regulates the development, growth, pubertal maturation, and reproductive processes	Deficiency of LH - Hypogonadism (lack of development of sex organ)
	Luteinizing hormone (LH)	Reproductive organs	Stimulates the secretion of testosterone	Deficiency of LH - Hypogonadism (lack of development of sex organ)
Posterior Pituitary	Antidiuretic hormone/ Vasopressin (ADH)	Kidney	Conservation of water	Excess ADH - Low blood levels of sodium Deficiency of ADH - Diabetes insipidus
	Oxytocin	Uterine muscles, mammary glands	Uterine contraction, lactation in females	

practice. Following is a brief discussion of selected disorders that may be encountered.

Hyperpituitarism

Hyperpituitarism most often refers to an excess production of hormones originating from the anterior lobe of the pituitary gland. The most common cause is pituitary adenoma, a benign neoplasm that overproduces hormones. Other causes include hyperplasia of the gland or other pituitary and nonpituitary tumors. Disease manifestations depend on the type of pituitary cells affected. For example, overproduction of growth hormone from the anterior pituitary during childhood results in *gigantism*, or *acromegaly* after the individual has achieved their growth potential.

Gigantism

Elevation of growth hormone levels in children before they reach their normal growth potential results in *gigantism*. Children with gigantism are extremely tall for their age because the disorder occurs before the bone (epiphyseal) growth plates are closed. They have abnormal height, long arms and legs, large hands, and disproportionate body size. In the oral cavity, oral structures appear morphologically normal but abnormally large. Enlargement of the jaws and generalized macrodontia are oral features commonly observed in gigantism.

Acromegaly

Elevation of growth hormone after the closure of bone (epiphyseal) growth plates results in *acromegaly*. Adults with this condition exhibit generalized enlargement of bones of the skeleton and soft tissues. Gradually enlarging hands, feet, and head are common features. Bone and soft tissue growth in the face creates coarse features with an increasing lower facial height, enlargement and protrusion of the mandible, enlarged tongue, and widening of interproximal spaces between normal sized teeth. Excess growth hormone production is a serious condition that contributes to many other systemic problems including hypertension, diabetes mellitus, osteoporosis, arthritis, and congestive heart failure.

Blood tests revealing elevated growth hormone levels are required to confirm the diagnosis of gigantism or acromegaly. Appropriate treatment of the underlying cause is required. Early detection is vital to prevent serious complications, which can ultimately result in death.

Hypopituitarism

Hypopituitarism is defined as reduction in production of one or more pituitary hormones due to pathology affecting the pituitary gland. Symptoms depend on which hormone is missing or deficient. The condition most often involves the hypothalamus and/or anterior pituitary. The hypothalamus produces growth hormone-releasing hormone, which stimulates the anterior pituitary to release growth hormone. *Pituitary dwarfism* is due to either a reduction in growth hormone production or a lack of tissue response to the hormone. Anatomical structures continue to develop in normal proportions but are significantly smaller than normal. Individuals with this condition have short stature, normal body proportions, and may appear younger than their actual age. The maxilla, mandible, and teeth are all smaller than normal and delayed tooth eruption and shedding of the primary teeth may be observed.

The condition is detected when growth and development lag far behind normal rates by age. Deficiency in growth hormone production may present with associated serious systemic complications depending on the underlying cause. Growth hormone replacement therapy can be used in children before the bone growth plates have closed.

Thyroid Gland

The thyroid gland is located in the neck anterior to the larynx. It is butterfly-shaped with two lobes joined by an isthmus in the midline. The thyroid gland is responsible for the secretion of triiodothyronine (T3) and thyroxin (T4), hormones responsible for the regulation of metabolism. The thyroid gland is stimulated by thyroid-stimulating hormone (TSH), secreted by the anterior pituitary gland, which is under the influence of the thyroid-releasing hormone (TRH) produced by the hypothalamus. Thyroid gland disorders result from either excessive T3 and T4 production (hyperthyroidism) or a deficiency in T3 and T4 production (hypothyroidism).

Hyperthyroidism: Graves' Disease

Hyperthyroidism, or overactive thyroid, is a disorder caused by unregulated production of thyroid hormones (T3 and T4). This may occur as a result of hyperplasia of thyroid tissue, benign or malignant thyroid tumors, or overproduction of TSH by the pituitary gland. Clinical effects caused by excess of thyroid hormones in the blood are known as *thyrotoxicosis*. Clinical manifestations may include tremor, anxiety, intolerance to heat and sweating, insomnia, tachycardia, increased susceptibility to heart failure, heart murmur, hypertension, and increased appetite accompanied by weight loss. The dangers of untreated hyperthyroidism include heart dysfunction and high metabolic rate, which may be fatal.

Head and neck manifestations of thyrotoxicosis include increased susceptibility to caries and periodontal disease, enlargement of **extraglandular** thyroid tissue on the lateral posterior tongue, osteoporosis of the jaws, burning oral pain, and accelerated dental eruption in young patients. Enlargement of the thyroid gland, called goiter (Fig. 9-2), may occur in the presence or absence of clinical signs and symptoms of disease.

The autoimmune condition (see Chapter 4) known as **Graves' disease** is a common cause of hyperthyroidism. In this disease, autoantibodies directed at the thyroid cause a continuous stimulation of the gland, leading to overproduction of T4. Graves' disease affects mainly women aged 20 to 40 years. Clinical features include excessive sweating, warm skin, palmar erythema, fine tremors, **alopecia** (hair thinning and loss), weight loss despite an increased appetite, and sagging of eyelids. Patients with Graves' disease may also have a wide-staring gaze called **exophthalmos** (Fig. 9-3) in which the eyeballs protrude forward and bulge out of the orbits due to swelling of tissues behind the eyes. Patients may complain of burning pain in the mouth. They also may concurrently have Sjögren's syndrome, which causes dry mouth. The thyroid may be enlarged and more noticeable when the patient is in a supine position in the dental

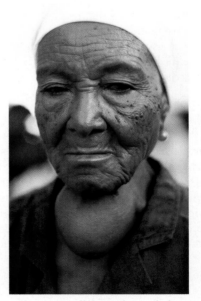

Figure 9–2 Goiter. Swelling in the neck due to goiter. (From Tamparo, CD: Diseases of the Human Body, ed. 5. F.A. Davis, Philadelphia, 2011, p 290.)

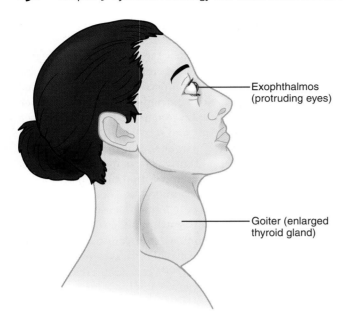

Exophthalmos (protruding eyes)

Goiter (enlarged thyroid gland)

Figure 9–3 Exophthalmos. Bulging of eyes in patient with Graves' disease.

chair, though severely enlarged thyroids may be visible when the patient is sitting upright or standing. Anxiety, restlessness, tachycardia, palpitations, and hypertension are common. Pretibial myxedema, characterized by thickening of the skin and pitting edema of the lower legs, may also be present in Graves' disease.

The diagnosis of Graves' disease is confirmed by physical examination, blood tests, and radioactive iodine uptake rates. Clinical manifestations of Graves' disease such as hypertension, **tachycardia**, palpitations, and anxiety are treated using beta-blockers. Many patients with Graves' disease also develop other autoimmune disorders such as systemic lupus erythematosus, type 1 diabetes, or Addison's disease (discussed later in this chapter).

Clinical Implications

Untreated thyrotoxicosis can lead to a life-threatening condition known as *thyroid storm*. This is characterized by a sudden and excessive release of thyroid hormones, resulting in a hypermetabolic state. Thyroid storm is usually brought on by stress, infection, or trauma and can lead to shock, sudden heart failure, and pulmonary edema. When treating patients with Graves' disease, it is important to minimize anxiety by scheduling short appointments and instituting effective pain control measures. Use of epinephrine may be contraindicated in patients with uncontrolled hyperthyroidism due to cardiac complications.

Hypothyroidism

Hypothyroidism, or underactive thyroid, is a condition frequently encountered on the medical history review of systems. It involves inadequate levels of thyroid hormones T3 and T4. The most common cause of hypothyroidism is an autoimmune condition known as Hashimoto's thyroiditis. Immune-mediated destruction of the thyroid gland leads to inadequate production of thyroid hormones and eventual thyroid failure. Hashimoto's thyroiditis tends to occur in females usually between 45 to 65 years of age. There is a strong genetic predisposition and an increased susceptibility to other autoimmune diseases such as Sjögren's syndrome, lupus erythematosus, and type 1 diabetes mellitus.

Cretinism is hypothyroidism that develops in infancy or early childhood. It is characterized by impaired development of the central nervous and skeletal systems, severe intellectual disability, and short stature. Abnormal facial features include an overdeveloped maxilla, underdeveloped mandible, and a large protruding tongue (macroglossia). Delayed eruption of primary and permanent teeth is common.

Hypothyroidism in older children or adults varies with age of onset and is known as *myxedema*. This manifests as a gradual slowing of physical activity, generalized fatigue and weakness, mental sluggishness, unintentional weight gain, intolerance to cold, bradycardia, decreased sweating, and constipation. Oral manifestations in those who have not been treated include enlarged tongue and thick lips, xerostomia, and osteoporosis of the jaws.

Both forms of hypothyroidism are diagnosed by measuring free thyroid hormone levels in the blood. Management involves supplementation with synthetic hormones. Early detection is critical to implementing treatment, mitigating permanent disability, and facilitating recovery where possible.

Parathyroid Glands

The parathyroid glands are found attached (*para*, meaning alongside) to each lobe of the thyroid gland, hence the name *parathyroid*. However, despite the name, their function is unrelated to thyroid function. These glands help synthesize parathyroid hormone (PTH), which plays an important role in the regulation of serum calcium and bone health. When serum calcium levels decrease, release of PTH from the parathyroid glands occurs. PTH acts to elevate the serum calcium by:

- Mobilizing calcium from bone
- Enhancing adsorption of calcium from the small intestine
- Decreasing calcium loss in the urine

Diseases of the parathyroid glands are clinically evident when PTH levels are abnormally increased or decreased. This may be due to insufficient parathyroid hormone production related to disease states, parathyroid tumors, or loss of the parathyroid glands after thyroid surgery.

Hyperparathyroidism

Hyperparathyroidism is caused by abnormal increased synthesis and secretion of PTH. It may be primary or secondary. *Primary hyperparathyroidism* involves overproduction of PTH due to a benign or malignant tumor or non-neoplastic hyperplasia of the parathyroid gland. Primary hyperparathyroidism most often occurs in adults, predominantly women. *Secondary hyperparathyroidism* is often a consequence of prolonged decreased calcium levels (*hypocalcemia*) that leads to the continuous stimulation of the parathyroid glands to compensate for the low calcium levels. The most common cause of secondary hyperparathyroidism is *chronic renal failure*. Because the kidneys play an important role in calcium metabolism, renal failure can lead to impaired active vitamin D production. Vitamin D is essential for calcium absorption in the gut. Reduced absorption of calcium from the gut and decreased reabsorption of calcium within the renal tubules leads to a lower serum calcium level. Lower serum calcium levels send a feedback message to the parathyroid glands to remove calcium from bones, making up for calcium lost from the kidneys.

The classic signs and symptoms of primary hyperparathyroidism are referred to as "stones, bones, and groans." *Stones* refers to kidney stones. Individuals have increased risk of developing renal (kidney) stones due to elevated serum calcium levels (*hypercalcemia*) caused by excess parathyroid hormone. This can result in kidney failure. *Bones* refers to bone-related pathology. Bone and/or root resorption causes a "ground-glass" radiographic appearance similar to that seen in fibrous dysplasia. Additionally, loss of the lamina dura can be seen in dental radiographs (Fig. 9-4). In chronic cases, especially with secondary hyperparathyroidism, unilocular or multilocular radiolucencies may be seen (Fig 9-5A), sometimes accompanied by jaw swelling (Fig. 9-5B). These lesions are known as "brown

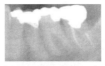

Figure 9–4   Hyperparathyroidism. Loss of lamina dura in a patient with hyperparathyroidism.

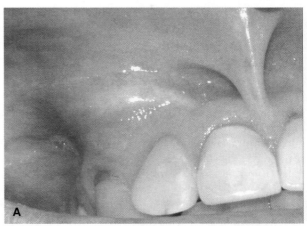

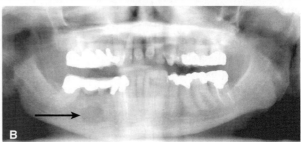

Figure 9–5   Brown tumor of hyperparathyroidism.
A. Swelling of maxilla in patient with brown tumor of hyperparathyroidism. **B.** Radiograph showing brown tumor in right mandible.

tumors" of hyperparathyroidism. Accumulation of red blood cell end products, such as hemosiderin, gives the tumors a red-brown appearance upon excision, hence the name "brown tumor." These are similar microscopically to central giant cell granulomas (see Chapter 2). *Groans* refers to abdominal discomfort due to indigestion, constipation, gastrointestinal ulcers, nausea, and vomiting.

Diagnosis of hyperparathyroidism is based on finding elevated PTH and calcium levels in the blood. Surgical removal of parathyroid glands in order to reduce PTH levels is the main treatment. Management of secondary hyperparathyroidism requires elimination of the cause of the hypocalcemia. For example, in chronic renal failure, vitamin D supplements and dietary control are provided to prevent hypercalcemia. A kidney transplant may restore the calcium homeostasis in some cases.

Clinical Implications

Hyperparathyroidism may go undiagnosed until loss of lamina dura and bony changes are noted on routine dental radiographs or biopsy shows findings suggestive of "brown tumor."

Hypoparathyroidism

Hypoparathyroidism is an uncommon condition characterized by decreased levels of PTH. The most common cause is *iatrogenic* loss of parathyroid tissue following thyroid surgery. Other causes include congenital absence of the parathyroid glands and autoimmune destruction of the gland. Hypoparathyroidism leads to a reduction in blood calcium level (hypocalcemia). Clinical manifestations of hypoparathyroidism vary depending on the severity of hypocalcemia. Calcium ions play a crucial role in neuromuscular activity. Potentially fatal complications may result. Patients may complain of numbness and tingling sensations of the lips and fingers, muscular spasms of the distal extremities or the respiratory tract, and seizures. When hypoparathyroidism occurs during early childhood development, dental abnormalities such as enamel hypoplasia and defective root formation may be seen.

Diagnosis of hypoparathyroidism is based on blood tests showing decreased PTH levels. Management includes restoring calcium levels to normal through a diet rich in calcium and vitamin D, and with dietary supplements.

Adrenal Glands

The adrenal glands are located on the superior pole of each kidney (*ad* = near; *renal* = kidney). They are composed of a cortex and medulla. The cortex is divided into three distinct zones: zona glomerulosa, zona fasciculata, and zona reticularis. Zona glomerulosa is involved in production of mineralocorticoids, mainly aldosterone, which plays a role in the regulation of blood pressure. Zona fasciculata is under the control of the adrenocorticotropic hormone (ACTH) and produces glucocorticoids such as cortisol. Zona reticularis produces sex steroid androgens such as testosterone. The adrenal medulla is responsible for production of the catecholamines epinephrine (adrenaline) and norepinephrine (noradrenaline). Epinephrine and norepinephrine hormone release is part of the body's "fight-or-flight" response.

Diseases of the adrenal gland result from either increased or decreased hormone secretion by the glands. Diseases involving *cortisol* are featured in this section because they have significant clinical implications for general and oral health. A comparison of the features of Cushing's syndrome and Addison's disease are shown in Fig. 9-6.

Cushing's Syndrome

Cushing's syndrome, or "hypercortisolism," is a hormonal disorder characterized by prolonged elevated levels of cortisol in the body. This disorder has a variety of causes. It most commonly results from medical use of glucocorticoids, such as prednisone, to treat autoimmune and inflammatory disorders including asthma, rheumatoid arthritis, and systemic lupus erythematosus. Benign tumors of the pituitary may also secrete ACTH, which stimulates the adrenal glands to produce excess cortisol.

Patients with Cushing's syndrome have distinctive clinical features including rounding of the face ("moon facies"), accumulation of fat in the supraclavicular region of the neck ("buffalo hump"), obesity of the trunk of the body with muscle wasting in the upper and lower limbs ("moon on stick" appearance), as well as bruises and purplish striae (stretch marks) in areas of skin fragility. Affected individuals also have an increased risk of osteoporosis, menstrual irregularities, and mood disturbances including depression. Because glucocorticoids induce release of glycogen from the liver, **hyperglycemia** may result.

Diagnosis of Cushing's syndrome is made based on physical examination and using the 24-hour urine collection test for free cortisol excretion. Endogenous

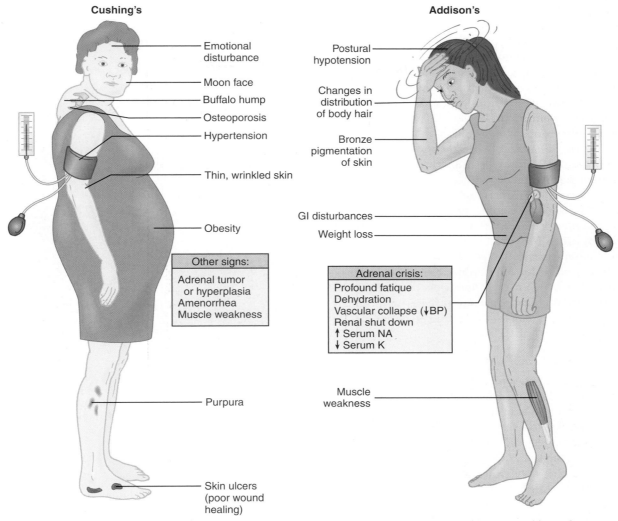

Figure 9–6   Comparison of Cushing's syndrome and Addison's disease. Comparison of adrenocortical hyperfunction (Cushing's syndrome, left) and hypofunction (Addison's disease, right).

forms of Cushing's syndrome are treated by surgical removal of the adrenal glands or pituitary adenoma secreting ACTH. Cushing's syndrome caused by medications is harder to manage. This is because the patients may have other medical conditions that may necessitate continued use of corticosteroids.

Clinical Implications

Patients with Cushing's syndrome are more prone to infection due to immune suppression. Oral candidiasis, viral infections such as recurrent herpes labialis, herpes zoster, as well as periodontal disease are common. When planning invasive procedures for patients on long-term corticosteroid

therapy, it is important to consult with the patient's physician. Additional corticosteroid supplementation may be required to prevent adrenal insufficiency and potentially fatal complications.

Addison's Disease

Addison's disease, or hypocortisolism, is a condition of adrenal insufficiency in which the adrenal glands do not produce sufficient steroid hormones. This may be caused by damage to or disease of the adrenal glands such as lymphoma, hemorrhage, infection, metastatic cancer, or autoimmune disease. Addison's disease is more common in Caucasians than in other ethnicities and there is a slight female predilection. Insufficient cortisol production presents as generalized fatigue and weakness, weight loss, nausea, and vomiting. Patients may also experience hypoglycemia as a result of cortisol deficiency. In stressful conditions such as infection, trauma, or surgery, acute adrenal crisis may occur, which leads to cardiovascular collapse and death. Addison's disease is diagnosed by performing the ACTH stimulation test, which confirms a lack of cortisol production following an intravenous administration of ACTH.

Hyperpigmentation of the skin and oral mucosa are characteristic features of primary Addison's disease. Hyperpigmentation occurs because melanocyte stimulating hormone (MSH) is chemically related to ACTH. The two share the same precursor molecule, pro-opiomelanocortin (POMC). Excess ACTH accompanied by excess MSH results in the hyperpigmentation. In Addison's disease, the skin all over the body may gradually darken or develop a bronze coloration. Hyperpigmented areas that may be homogenous or blotchy also may occur as brown patches or macules on the gingiva, tongue, or vermillion of the lip (Fig. 9-7A and B).

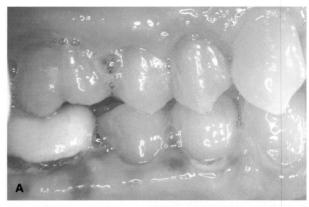

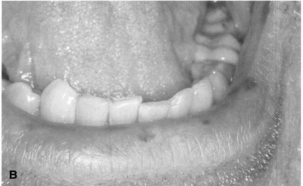

Figure 9–7 **Addison's disease pigmentation. A.** Gingiva; diffuse hyperpigmentation of the gingiva. **B.** Lips of patient with Addison's disease.

> ### Clinical Implications
>
> Onset of Addison's disease is subtle and may not be noticed unless the patient is observed over time. Changes in oral mucosal pigmentation, over multiple dental visits, arouses suspicion of Addison's disease, especially in individuals with little tendency for racial pigmentation. Acute adrenal crisis, a life-threatening event due to insufficient cortisol, may result from stress during medical or dental treatment. This disorder requires prompt recognition and diagnosis.

The Pancreas and Diabetes Mellitus

The pancreas is the endocrine organ responsible for controlling release of insulin. **Insulin** is a hormone produced by beta cells of the islet of Langerhans in response to elevated blood glucose. Insulin is central to regulating carbohydrate and fat metabolism in the body. The pancreas also is an exocrine gland producing pancreatic juices that aid with digestion.

Diabetes Mellitus

Diabetes mellitus (DM) is the most common disease of pancreatic dysfunction. DM is of great interest to oral health-care providers because it can lead to numerous systemic complications such as cardiovascular abnormalities, **neuropathies**, renal failure, and immunosuppression (Fig. 9-8). Diabetes is a disorder of metabolism associated with abnormally high levels of glucose (sugar) in the blood. Hyperglycemia may result from destruction or dysfunction of beta cells in the islets of Langerhans in the pancreas, which produce insulin. The function of insulin is to facilitate transport of glucose from the blood into the cells. Insufficient insulin production causes glucose to accumulate in the blood (hyperglycemia). Cells then have no glucose for energy production and must resort to metabolizing fat for energy. Fat metabolism produces *ketones*, which accumulate in the body fluids. Increase in ketones in the blood is a hallmark of uncontrolled diabetes. Ketones cause decreased pH, dehydration, and electrolyte imbalance, a condition known as **diabetic ketoacidosis** (Table 9-2). Individuals with ketoacidosis may have a distinctive aroma to their breath. The odor has been described as sweet like fruit or resembling acetone in nail polish remover.

Diabetes mellitus can be classified as type 1 or 2. *Type 1 diabetes mellitus*, also known as insulin-dependent diabetes mellitus, is an autoimmune disorder of the

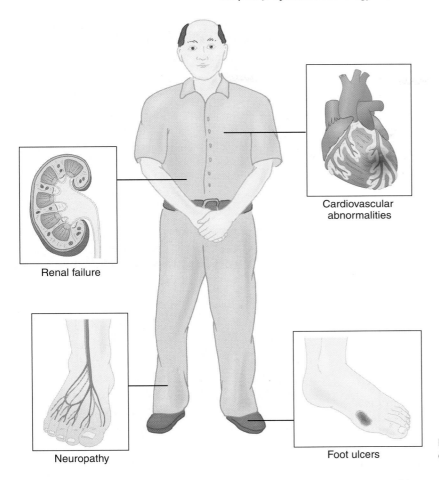

Cardiovascular abnormalities

Renal failure

Neuropathy

Foot ulcers

Figure 9–8   Long-term complications of diabetes.

Table 9.2	**Complications of Uncontrolled Diabetes**	
	Diabetic Ketoacidosis	**Hypoglycemia**
Onset	Gradual	Often sudden
History	Often acute infection in a diabetic or insufficient insulin intake History of diabetes may be absent	Recent insulin injection, inadequate meal, or excessive exercise after insulin
Musculoskeletal	Muscle wasting or weight loss	Weakness Tremor Muscle twitching
Gastrointestinal	Abdominal pains or cramps, sometimes acute Nausea and vomiting	Nausea and vomiting
Central nervous system	Headache Double or blurred vision Irritability	Confusion, delirium, or seizures
Cardiovascular	Tachycardia Orthostatic hypotension	Variable

Continued

Table 9.2	Complications of Uncontrolled Diabetes—cont'd	
	Diabetic Ketoacidosis	**Hypoglycemia**
Skin	Flushed, dry	Diaphoretic, pale
Respiratory	Air hunger Acetone odor of breath Dyspnea	Variable Increased respiratory rate
Laboratory values	Elevated blood glucose (> 200 mg/dl) Glucose and ketones in blood and urine	Subnormal blood glucose (0–50 mg/dl) Absence of glucose and ketones in urine unless bladder is full

From Taber's Cyclopedic Medical Dictionary, ed. 21. F.A. Davis, Philadelphia, 2009, p 631.

pancreas with an unknown cause. Autoantibodies (see Chapter 4) are directed against the beta cells in the islets of Langerhans. This results in insufficient or absent insulin production. Type 1 diabetes mellitus most commonly occurs before age 25 and there is no gender predilection. Individuals with a family history of type 1 diabetes mellitus or other autoimmune disorders have an increased risk of developing diabetes.

Type 2 diabetes mellitus, also known as noninsulin-dependent diabetes mellitus, is the most common form of diabetes. It is characterized by insufficient insulin production in relation to what is known as *insulin resistance*. Insulin resistance is a condition in which cells of the body ignore or become resistant to the effects of insulin. The cells do not respond adequately to normal levels of insulin. A number of etiologic factors play a role in the development of insulin resistance including genetics, obesity, sedentary lifestyle, poor eating habits, and age. Recently increasing rates of obesity in younger individuals have been associated with rising rates of type 2 diabetes.

Patients with diabetes mellitus may present with generalized fatigue and lethargy, increased appetite (**polyphagia**) with weight loss, frequent urination (**polyuria**), and increased thirst (**polydipsia**). They may also experience xerostomia, changes in vision, tingling and numbness of fingers and toes, and burning sensation of the tongue and lips (Table 9-3).

The oral manifestations of diabetes mellitus depend on the extent of blood glucose control. Common oral manifestations of poor glucose control include increased risk of bacterial and fungal infections such as oral candidiasis. Patients may experience burning mouth, impaired wound healing, xerostomia, and parotid gland enlargement. Xerostomia increases the risk for dental caries, candidiasis (Fig. 9-9), traumatic or aphthous ulcers, and cheilitis, also called perlèche (Fig. 9-10). Diabetes mellitus is considered a major risk factor for periodontal disease because of decreased resistance to bacterial infection.

Table 9.3	Signs and Symptoms of Diabetes Mellitus
Signs	**Symptoms**
Acanthosis nigricans	Polydipsia (feeling of thirst)
Ketone breath	Polyuria (frequent urination)
Gingivitis	Polyphagia (feeling of hunger)
Periodontitis	Tender gingiva and bleeding on brushing
Oral candidiasis	
Delayed wound healing	Weight loss despite increased appetite
	Malaise (lack of energy)
	Xerostomia
	Loss of strength
	Recurrent infections
	Blurred vision
	Peripheral neuropathy (numbness and tingling of the hands and feet) including burning oral pain

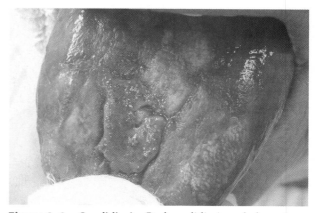

Figure 9–9 Candidiasis. Oral candidiasis and ulceration in a diabetic patient.

The primary goal in managing diabetes mellitus is to maintain a steady, normal blood glucose level. Lifestyle modifications such as diet, weight control, and exercise, along with hypoglycemic medications, are used to help control blood levels of glucose. Type 1 diabetes mellitus patients require insulin injections. Depending on the severity of the disease, patients with type 2 diabetes may also require injections.

Acanthosis Nigricans

Acanthosis nigricans is a skin or mucosal disorder that may be inherited or related to underlying medical problems, most commonly endocrine disorders. The most common cause of acanthosis nigricans is insulin-resistant type 2 diabetes mellitus. The disorder may also be observed in patients using hormonal medications such as oral contraceptives or human growth hormone. Some cancers of the gastrointestinal or genitourinary tracts produce hormones that may cause acanthosis nigricans. The patient may be unaware of the internal malignancy until the skin or mucosal lesions develop.

Acanthosis nigricans is characterized by asymptomatic dark, thick, velvety skin in body folds and creases (Fig. 9-11) in the flexural areas such as in the armpits, groin, neck folds, and over the joints of the fingers and toes. Less commonly the oral mucosa, lips, palms, or soles of the feet may be affected. Large zones of increasing benign papillary eruptions termed *papillomatosis* may present on the lips and palate. Patients with acanthosis nigricans should be screened for diabetes and/or internal malignancy. The lesions often fade or resolve when the cause is found and treated.

ANEMIA

Anemia is not a disease but a sign of underlying disease. It is the most common disorder of blood. Anemia is defined as a reduction in circulating red blood cells (RBCs) or a deficiency of hemoglobin in the blood. Both of these produce reduced oxygen-carrying capacity of blood. Anemia may be due to excessive blood loss or excessive RBC hemolysis (destruction). It may occur as a result of conditions such as renal failure; liver disease; chronic infection or malignancy; deficiency of iron, folic acid, or vitamin B12; and diseases of hemoglobin (Table 9-4). Patients with reduced oxygen-carrying capacity suffer from fatigue and loss of energy, headaches, dizziness, pallor of the skin, and other symptoms depending on the etiology of the anemia.

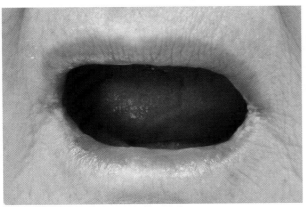

Figure 9–10   **Perlèche.** Red, dry cracked areas of commissures.

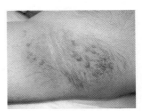

Figure 9–11   **Acanthosis nigricans.** Hyperpigmentation of flexural surface of arm. (From Barankin, B: Derm Notes. F.A. Davis, Philadelphia, 2006, p 52.)

Table 9.4	Causes of Anemia
Causes of Anemia	**Examples**
Chronic blood loss	Stomach ulcers, bleeding due to malignant tumor
Chronic disease	Renal failure, liver disease, systemic lupus erythematosus, sarcoidosis, tuberculosis
Destruction of red blood cells	External causes: prosthetic heart valves inducing damage to the RBCs, enlarged spleen, direct toxic effect from parasites or poisonous venom Internal causes: thalassemia, sickle cell anemia
Nutrient deficiencies	Iron deficiency anemia, folate deficiency anemia, pernicious anemia/vitamin B12 anemia

Anemia is diagnosed by laboratory analysis of a blood sample. (See Table 9-5 for a list of some RBC indices.) RBCs and their oxygen-carrying protein **hemoglobin** are measured. The percentage of RBCs in blood is called the **hematocrit.** Low hematocrit means fewer red blood cells than normal to carry needed oxygen. Hemoglobin is the component in RBCs responsible for oxygen-carbon dioxide exchange. Low hemoglobin means there is an insufficient amount of this protein to transport oxygen and carbon dioxide. Tissues starved for oxygen cause the heart and lungs to compensate by working harder.

Clinical Implications

Skin of anemic patients often appears pale and, in severe cases, intraoral examination may reveal pale oral mucosa. Elective dental procedures should be postponed if the oral mucosa appears pale and/or the patient complains of shortness of breath (**dyspnea**), dizziness, fatigue, muscular weakness, and tingling of extremities.

Diseases of Hemoglobin (Hemoglobinopathies)

Hemoglobinopathies are diseases of hemoglobin. Hemoglobin in RBCs consists of two parts: *heme* and *globin*. The heme part is composed of iron molecules, while the globin part has four polypeptide chains: two alpha and two beta chains. RBCs have a specific shape that helps them carry out the chemical exchange of oxygen-carbon dioxide. They are biconcave disks producing increased surface area for the gas exchanges. Babies are born with fetal hemoglobin and gradually develop the adult form. Both acquired and inherited disorders may cause defective hemoglobin production or function. Three disorders of hemoglobin are presented in this section.

Thalassemia Major and Minor

Thalassemias are a group of inherited blood disorders that feature defective production of hemoglobin. Beta thalassemia is the most common type and is characterized by reduced or absent production of beta globin chains. Beta thalassemia has two forms: minor and major. Individuals with thalassemia minor have one normal beta-chain gene and one beta thalassemia gene. They have mild anemia with slightly low hemoglobin levels and a normal blood iron level.

Table 9.5	Red Blood Cell Indices	
Measurements	**Units**	**Definition**
Hematocrit	%	The ratio of packed red cells to total blood volume
Red cell count	gm/dL	Concentration of hemoglobin in the blood
Mean cell volume	No. x 10^6/ μL	Number of red blood cells present
Mean cell hemoglobin	Femtoliter (fL)	The average size of a red blood cell
Mean cell hemoglobin concentration	Picograms (pg)	The average amount of hemoglobin per red blood cell
Red cell distribution width		The average concentration of hemoglobin per red blood cell

Individuals with thalassemia major (Cooley's anemia) have two genes for beta thalassemia (no normal beta-chain gene). This is a serious condition and eventually causes a striking deficiency in the production of hemoglobin. At birth, a baby with thalassemia major seems normal due to adequate fetal hemoglobin, which does not have beta chains. Anemia begins to develop within the first months after birth when fetal hemoglobin is replaced by markedly defective adult hemoglobin. Observed clinical features include growth retardation, hepatosplenomegaly, and bone marrow hyperplasia as the body attempts to produce more cells.

Bone marrow hyperplasia causes characteristic facial features known as "chipmunk facies" with enlargement of the maxilla and/or mandible and frontal bossing. An altered trabecular pattern in bone is present on dental radiographs with coarse trabecular pattern and enlargement of marrow spaces. "Hair on end" appearance is a common radiographic finding on a skull radiograph (Fig. 9-12). Abnormal tooth and root morphology may be observed along with delayed tooth eruption.

Patients with thalassemia major are dependent on conventional treatment with blood transfusions. Treatment is currently palliative, but gene therapy holds promise for the future.

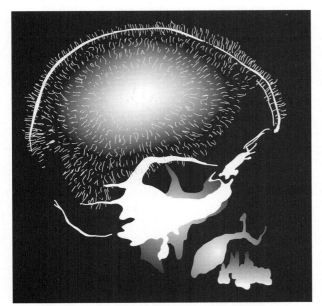

Figure 9–12 "Hair on end" sign indicates reactive bone growth in the thalassemia and sickle cell anemia.

Sickle Cell Disorder

Sickle cell disorder, or *sickle cell anemia*, is an inherited disorder of hemoglobin synthesis caused by a mutation in the beta globin chain of hemoglobin. If two mutated genes are inherited, the individual will develop sickle cell disorder. If one mutated gene is inherited, then the individual has *sickle cell trait*, a mild form of the disease.

RBCs in this disorder can undergo changes in shape from flexible biconcave disks to a less flexible sickle shape. Sickling of RBCs is promoted by conditions associated with low oxygen levels including infections, fever and dehydration, bleeding, exposure to cold, or alcohol abuse. The sickle shape (Fig. 9-13) and decreased flexibility of the abnormal RBCs can obstruct capillaries, restricting blood flow to tissues and organs. This results in ischemia, pain, and necrosis. Sickled cells are recognized as abnormal and destroyed by the spleen. The bone marrow often cannot keep up with new blood cell production and anemia results. *Sickle cell crisis* occurs when sufficient oxygen cannot reach affected tissues. The sites most often affected by the blocking or stacking action of sickled cells are the lungs, liver, bone, muscles, brain, spleen, eyes, and kidneys.

Delayed growth, development, and tooth eruption are seen in children with sickle cell anemia. Other oral manifestations include pale oral mucosa, loss of the papillae on the dorsum of the tongue, oral ulcers, and angular cheilitis. Red blood cells obstructing blood flow may contribute to pulpal necrosis and osteomyelitis of the jaw. Distinct radiographic features observed include altered trabecular pattern, increased marrow spaces, and "hair on end" pattern on a skull radiograph similar to that seen in thalassemia.

Clinical Implications

Antibiotic prophylaxis is common because infections predispose these individuals to sickle cell crisis. Dental appointments should be short because prolonged stress may also trigger a crisis. Use of local anesthetic without epinephrine may be preferred to reduce the risk of tissue hypoxia.

Iron Deficiency Anemia

Iron deficiency anemia is the most common cause of anemia in the world and is more prevalent in developing countries. In the United States, it is most often seen in infants and children, adolescent girls, and in women

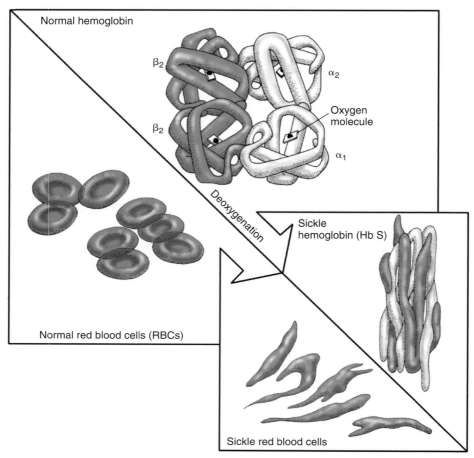

Figure 9–13   Sickle cells. Structure of hemoglobin A and S and their effect on erythrocytes. (From Taber's Cyclopedic Medical Dictionary, ed. 21. F.A. Davis, Philadelphia, 2009, p 119.)

of child-bearing age. The etiology of iron deficiency anemia includes:

- Lack of iron intake in diet
- Impaired absorption of iron
- Increased demand of iron by the body
- Excessive acute or chronic blood loss

Deficiency of iron in the diet is common in the elderly where it may be associated with poor dental health or decreased consumption of iron-rich foods such as meats and vegetables. Patients with gastrointestinal (GI) malabsorption may develop chronic diarrhea leading to poor iron absorption. Increased body demand for iron is seen during pregnancy. Deficiency is common in young children during growth spurts and around puberty. In premenopausal women, heavy menstrual bleeding may lead to iron deficiency due to excessive blood loss. In males, iron deficiency may be related to chronic blood loss due to gastric problems such as ulcers or other unknown conditions including malignancy.

Oral manifestations of iron deficiency anemia include:

- Atrophic glossitis seen as a smooth, glossy tongue (Fig. 9-14)
- Oral candidiasis and angular cheilitis (cracking at commissures, see Fig. 9-10)
- Burning sensation on tongue
- Pallor of oral mucosa

Treatment of iron deficiency anemia involves dietary iron supplements. In individuals with GI malabsorption, iron may be administered via nasal spray or by injections. Signs and symptoms of iron deficiency anemia are usually reversed after iron supplementation.

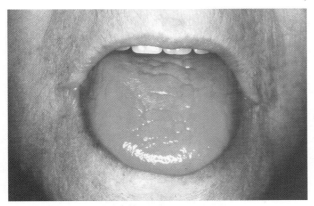

Figure 9–14 **Anemic glossitis.** Loss of filiform papillae and angular cheilitis in patient with anemia.

Plummer-Vinson Syndrome

Plummer-Vinson syndrome presents most often in postmenopausal women. This syndrome has three components: glossitis, dysphagia (difficulty in swallowing), and iron deficiency anemia. The tongue is smooth, shiny, and erythematous, and patients may complain of a burning sensation. Difficulty in swallowing is due to formation of abnormal bands of tissue in the walls of the esophagus. This results in "webbing," which causes esophageal constriction. The condition has been associated with an increased risk of oral and esophageal squamous cell carcinoma; hence, Plummer-Vinson syndrome is considered premalignant and requires close monitoring. Treatment of Plummer-Vinson syndrome involves correcting the iron deficiency with supplements. Elective dental treatment should be delayed in patients with severe anemia until the underlying condition has been treated.

Pernicious Anemia

Pernicious anemia is considered an autoimmune disorder (see Chapter 4 for discussion of autoimmunity) usually associated with atrophic gastritis. In this disorder, the immune system produces antibodies against parietal cells in the stomach. Parietal cells produce a protein called *intrinsic factor*, which is necessary for the absorption of vitamin B12 in the ileum. Vitamin B12 is needed for the production of hemoglobin. In pernicious anemia, parietal cells are destroyed and vitamin B12 is not absorbed. Patients who have undergone gastrointestinal bypass surgery or who are strict vegetarians are at risk for vitamin B12 deficiency and developing pernicious anemia. Early detection of vitamin B12 deficiency is very important because these individuals have an increased risk of developing gastric cancer.

Clinical features of pernicious anemia include dyspnea, fatigue, dizziness, weakness, frequent headaches, and tingling or numbness of fingers and toes. Oral manifestations include tingling and burning of the tongue as well as patchy areas of erythema and atrophy of oral mucosa and tongue (Fig. 9-15). Treatment of pernicious anemia involves regular intramuscular injections or intranasal application of vitamin B12. With proper management, oral lesions of this condition can be reversed.

 Clinical Implication

Referral to a physician for testing of vitamin B12 levels may be indicated for patients with a chief complaint of "burning" tongue.

BLEEDING DISORDERS

Bleeding disorders describes a group of conditions in which there is a problem with clotting of the blood. Common signs include excessive bruising with changes in skin or mucosal coloration due to accumulation of extravasated red blood cells. In oral tissues, this is most commonly seen as a side effect of medications such as aspirin, heparin, or Coumadin. Mucosal hemorrhage is also seen in a variety of other diseases and is not pathognomonic (diagnostic) of any particular disease.

Hemostasis is the stoppage of blood loss from a damaged blood vessel. It initially involves vasoconstriction and formation of a plug of platelets and fibrin clot to seal the damaged area. Clotting factors are

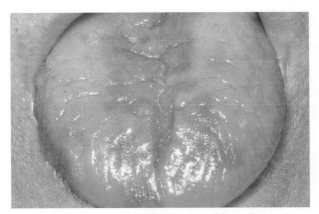

Figure 9–15 **Pernicious anemia.** Painful, tender tongue in patient with pernicious anemia.

chemical and cellular constituents of blood that are responsible for clot formation. At least 12 different factors are known to act in a complex cascade of events leading to formation of a clot. All clotting factors are produced in the liver, except for Factor VIII, made by endothelial cells, and von Willebrand factor, made by endothelial cells, subendothelial connective tissue, and megakaryocytes. The factors are designated by Roman numerals, which indicate the order in which they were discovered rather than their sequence in clot formation (Table 9-6). Lack of any single clotting factor may result in prolonged bleeding and excessive loss of blood that may be life-threatening.

Petechiae are clusters of tiny red-purple spots on a body surface such as the skin or a mucous membrane. They are pinpoint hemorrhages of capillaries (Fig. 9-16A) and measure less than 3 mm in size. **Purpura** describes larger areas of purple or red discoloration caused by bleeding underneath skin or mucous membranes that are greater than 3 to 10 mm in size (Fig. 9-16B). Color varies with age of the lesions with early lesions being red, then purple, and finally turning brown-yellow as they fade. **Ecchymosis** describes larger common bruises or hematomas. Ecchymoses are nonelevated irregular blue-to-purple hemorrhagic spots greater than 1 cm (larger than purpura) in the skin or mucous membrane.

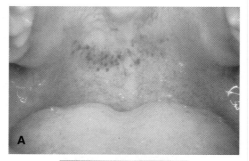

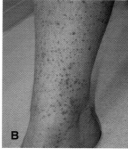

Figure 9–16 **A.** Petechiae; pinpoint submucosal hemorrhage. **B.** Purpura. Purpuric papules on lower leg. (From Barankin, B: Derm Notes. F.A. Davis, Philadelphia, 2006, p 97.)

Polycythemia Vera

Polycythemia vera (PCV) is characterized by an overproduction of red blood cells. In some cases, white blood cells and platelets are also overproduced. PCV increases with age and is more common in the elderly and males. The abnormally increased numbers of blood cells cause increased blood **viscosity** (thickening). Blood flow slows down and this decreased flow, along with abnormalities in platelets, increases the risk of **thrombus** (clot) formation (Fig. 9-17) (plural = *thrombi*) within blood

Table 9.6	Coagulation (Clotting) Factors
Factor Number	**Factor Name**
I	Prothrombin
II	Tissue factor
III	Calcium
IV	Proaccelerin
V	Does not exist
VI	Proconvertin
VII	Antihemophilic factor
VIII	Plasma thromboplastin (Christmas factor)
IX	Stuart factor
XI	Plasma thromboplastin antecedent
XII	Hageman factor
XIII	Fibrin-stabilizing factor
No number	von Willebrand factor
No number	Vitamin K

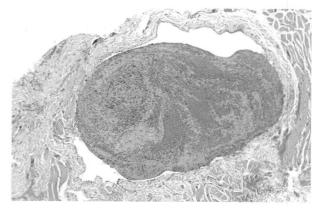

Figure 9–17 **Blood clot.** Thrombus with a vein.

vessels. This means patients with PCV are at higher risk of a heart attack (myocardial infarction) or stroke.

Patients with PCV complain of fatigue, dyspnea, dizziness, and frequent headaches. Shortness of breath with bluish discoloration of the skin (*cyanosis*) and hypertension are common. PCV is treated with *phlebotomy* to maintain normal red blood cell volume in the blood.

Clinical Implications

PCV patients may be on blood thinners (anticoagulants) and require special consideration if dental procedures that induce bleeding are planned. In addition, episodes of thrombosis may alternate with episodes of hemorrhage in this disorder. Gingival bleeding, sometimes spontaneous, can be an oral manifestation of PCV treated with blood-thinning medications. Medical consultation to ensure that the red blood cell counts and clotting are normal is advisable before starting dental treatment.

Hemophilia

Hemophilia, perhaps the best known bleeding disorder, is characterized by deficiency of clotting factors required to stop hemorrhage. However, there are many other types of bleeding disorders associated with specific missing or defective clotting factors. Three bleeding disorders will be discussed in this section: Von Willebrand disease, hemophilia A, and hemophilia B.

Von Willebrand Disease

Von Willebrand disease is the most common inherited bleeding disorder in the United States and can affect both men and women. It may also be acquired as a result of medical conditions. Von Willebrand disease is characterized by deficient or defective von Willebrand clotting factor. This is a protein that causes platelets to adhere to walls of damaged blood vessels. There are several types of this bleeding disorder with manifestations ranging from mild to severe. Patients with milder forms may have symptoms such as nosebleeds, easy bruising tendencies, and prolonged bleeding after injury. In mild cases, the disease may go undetected until the patient suffers serious injury or has surgery. Bleeding gums and prolonged bleeding after dental procedures such as tooth extraction or deep scaling may occur. Aspirin and other nonsteroidal anti-inflammatory drugs are contraindicated in Von Willebrand disease because they make the condition worse.

Hemophilia A

Hemophilia A is an inherited bleeding disorder associated with a lack of clotting factor VIII. It is the most common type of hemophilia. Hemophilia A involves a gene that occurs on the X chromosome and is passed to a son as a sex-linked recessive trait from a mother who carries the gene. Therefore, hemophilia occurs almost exclusively in males. The disease may be mild, moderate, or severe depending on the amount of clotting factor in the blood. The prevalence of hemophilia A in the United States is approximately 1 in 5,000 males and accounts for 80% to 85% of hemophilia.

Hemophilia B

Hemophilia B is an inherited bleeding disorder associated with a lack of clotting factor IX. The disorder is also known as Christmas disease, after the first patient described with this disorder. It is the second most common type of hemophilia. Like hemophilia A, hemophilia B involves a gene that occurs on the X chromosome and is passed to a son as a sex-linked recessive trait from a mother who carries the gene. Hemophilia B almost exclusively occurs in males. Deficiency of factor IX significantly impairs clot formation and control of bleeding. Hemophilia B is less common than hemophilia A, with an estimated prevalence of 1 in 25,000 males. Historically, hemophilia was called "the royal disease" due to increased incidence resulting from intermarriage in European royal families. Recently, genetic testing indicates that hemophilia in European royal family members was hemophilia B.

Clinical features of both hemophilia A and B depend on severity of the condition and levels of clotting factors. Spontaneous bleeding may occur at any time, along with hematomas, ecchymoses in soft tissues and muscles, and bleeding into weight-bearing joints causing **hemarthroses.** Hemarthroses may become a debilitating condition, eventually leading to joint deformity requiring replacement. Excessive bleeding may occur after routine dental and surgical procedures.

In the oral cavity, gingival bleeding may be spontaneous or induced by dental procedures or minor trauma from tooth brushing or flossing. This may cause patients to be afraid of practicing good oral home care or undergoing any type of dental treatment. Hemorrhage into the oral soft tissues and/or temporomandibular joint (TMJ) may form tumor-like masses known as *pseudotumor of hemophilia.*

Medical consultation before rendering dental treatment is vital to prevent episodes of uncontrolled bleeding. Replacement of clotting factors or blood transfusion may be required before dental treatment. Because patients with hemophilia often undergo multiple blood transfusions, their risk of contracting blood-borne diseases such as hepatitis B or C, or HIV infections is increased.

Hereditary Hemorrhagic Telangiectasia

Hereditary hemorrhagic telangiectasia (HHT) is an autosomal dominant inherited disorder of abnormal blood vessel formation. It is also known as Osler-Weber-Rendu disease or syndrome. HHT is characterized by numerous red, vascular lesions usually 1 to 2 mm in size, referred to as **telangiectasias**. These tiny red spots are formed by blood pooling within collections of dilated capillaries under the surface of the mucosa. The lesions blanch (turn white) in response to pressure, unlike hematomas. Telangiectasias may be seen in other disorders but in HHT they are commonly seen in increased numbers on the vermillion zone of the lips (Fig. 9-18), tongue (Fig. 9-19), and buccal and labial mucosa. Lesions may also be found on skin of the hands and feet, within the gastrointestinal and genitourinary tracts, and in the conjunctiva. Excessive blood loss due to rupture of telangiectasias may result in chronic iron deficiency anemia (discussed previously in this chapter). Patients also have an increased risk of developing blood vessel anomalies in the liver, lungs, and brain, which can lead to thrombus formation and thrombotic **emboli**.

History of HHT may include digestive tract bleeding and/or spontaneous nose bleed, also called **epistaxis**. Epistaxis is due to the presence of telangiectasias in the nasal mucosa. Electrocautery or laser ablation may be employed to stop the bleeding. Patients who report episodes of recurrent spontaneous epistaxis and present with telangiectasias in the oral cavity require referral to a physician to rule out HHT.

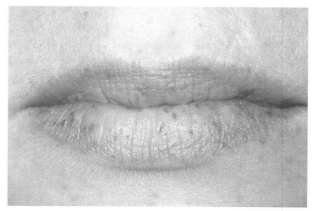

Figure 9–18 Hereditary hemorrhagic telangiectasia (HHT) lips. Patient with HHT shows dilated minute vascular channels.

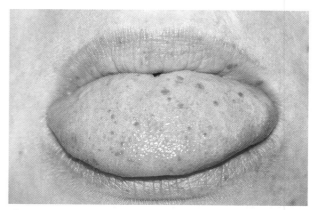

Figure 9–19 Hereditary hemorrhagic telangiectasia (HHT) tongue. Same patient as in Figure 9-18 with lesions on tongue.

Clinical Implications

Mucosal bleeding may occur with manipulation of oral tissues exhibiting telangiectasias. Care must be taken when performing dental procedures. Oral lesions may be the first sign of HHT and lead to the initial medical diagnosis.

GASTROINTESTINAL DISORDERS

The gastrointestinal (GI) tract extends from the mouth to the anus. GI disorders can manifest anywhere along the tract including within the oral cavity. Some oral manifestations may be detected long before the patient experiences other GI signs and symptoms.

Inflammatory Bowel Disease

Inflammatory bowel disease (IBD) is a group of inflammatory diseases of the small intestine and colon. Persistent inflammation causes a variety of symptoms including chronic persistent diarrhea, pain and cramping, and rectal bleeding. The two major types of IBD are Crohn's disease and ulcerative colitis (Table 9-7).

Crohn's Disease

Crohn's disease, also known as regional enteritis, accounts for 50 percent of cases of IBD. The main difference between Crohn's disease and ulcerative colitis is the location of inflammatory changes within the GI tract. Crohn's disease may affect any part of the GI tract from the oral cavity to anus. Ulcerative colitis, on the other hand, primarily affects the large intestine or colon.

Table 9.7	Ulcerative Colitis vs. Crohn's Disease	
Disease features	**Ulcerative colitis**	**Crohn's disease**
Location in gastrointestinal tract	Mainly in the colon and terminal ileum, sometimes the rectum	Part of the small intestines and the colon
Distribution of lesion	Involves the entire portion of the colon	Tends to have multiple localize areas involved, forming 'skip' lesions
Involvement of intestinal mucosa	Usually confined to the superficial mucosa	Tends to involve the entire mucosal layer
Ulcerations	Superficial and broad-based	Deep and knife-like; linear pattern
Perforation of intestinal mucosa	No	Yes, as ulcers tend to be transmural
Constrictions of intestinal mucosa	Rare	Yes
Presence of intestinal pseudopolyps	Numerous pseudopolyps	Seldom
Risk of development of colon cancer	Markedly increased	Moderate
Clinical symptoms	Bloody diarrhea with lower abdominal pain	Mild diarrhea with some abdominal pain

The precise cause of Crohn's disease is unknown. It has been associated with a combination of environmental factors, immune system problems, and genetic factors. Family members of affected individuals are slightly more at risk of developing Crohn's disease. Smokers are more likely to develop Crohn's disease than nonsmokers. Changes in oral mucosa can be found in both Crohn's disease and ulcerative colitis; however, they are more frequently seen in Crohn's disease.

The oral manifestations of Crohn's disease occur in up to 30 percent of patients and may lead to the initial diagnosis. Major aphthous ulcers (Fig. 9-20) (see Chapter 4) and "cobblestone" buccal mucosa (Fig. 9-21) are two of the most common oral manifestations. Their detection in the dental office may be the first clue that a patient has Crohn's disease.

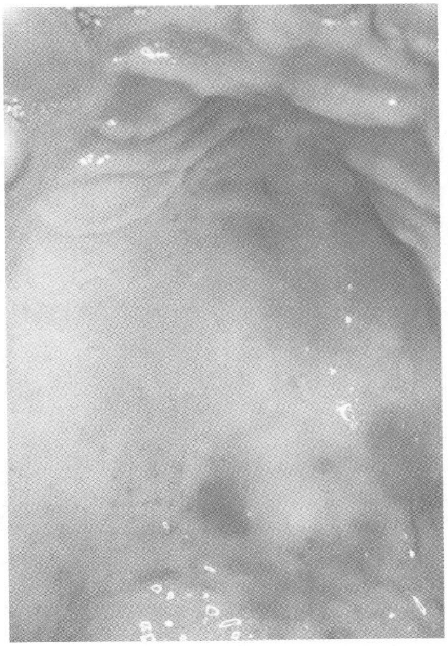

Pyostomatitis Vegetans

Pyostomatitis vegetans is another inflammatory condition seen in patients with Crohn's disease and ulcerative colitis. In the mouth, this condition is characterized by yellowish pustules on the oral mucosa and superficial ulcerations. These yellow pustules have a "snail-track" appearance that may appear on almost any oral mucosal surface (Fig. 9-22). Management of pyostomatitis vegetans depends mainly on the treatment of the underlying GI disorder. Rarely, it occurs as the sole manifestation of the disease.

Figure 9–20 **Palatal ulcers in patient with Crohn's disease.**

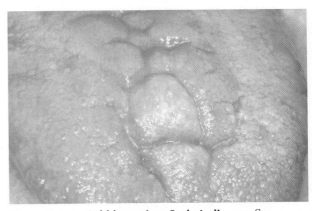

Figure 9–21 **Cobblestoning: Crohn's disease.** Same patient with cobblestone appearance to dorsal tongue.

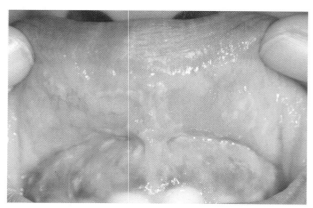

Figure 9–22 Pyostomatitis vegetans. Teenage girl with large number of nonpainful yellow papules.

Jaundice and Hyperbilirubinemia

Jaundice, also called icterus, refers to yellowish coloration of the skin and sclera (white part of the eye) caused by excess bilirubin in the blood (hyperbilirubinemia). Bilirubin is a breakdown product of heme in hemoglobin, a component of red blood cells (RBCs). Bilirubin is formed when old or damaged RBCs are disposed of by the spleen. Bilirubin is normally processed by the liver and eventually excreted in bile and urine. In liver disease, bilirubin may not be processed, allowing it to build up in the bloodstream, pass into tissues, and give the tissues the yellowish coloration associated with jaundice.

Any liver disease may lead to jaundice, including hepatitis A, B and C. Patients with jaundice present with a yellow color to the conjunctiva, skin, oral mucosa, or nail beds. Intensity of the yellow discoloration depends on the amount of excess bilirubin present.

> **Clinical Implications**
>
> Identifying patients with jaundice is important because it may indicate underlying liver disease. Liver diseases often increase bleeding tendencies due to decreased levels of clotting factors produced by the liver. Medical consultation may be indicated when deep scaling or invasive dental procedures are contemplated in patients with known liver disease and/or jaundice.

Neonatal hyperbilirubinemia results in jaundice in newborns and may be caused by hemolytic disease, biliary atresia, and/or blood group and Rh factor incompatibility. Some conditions may occur *in utero* and affect the developing fetus. Bilirubin may be deposited throughout the body, including within developing teeth. Hyperbilirubinemia may produce permanent intrinsic yellow to dark green staining of the primary teeth (see Chapter 5) (Fig. 9-23).

CONNECTIVE TISSUE DISORDERS

Connective tissue diseases are a group of disorders affecting two major components of connective tissue: collagen and elastin. Collagen functions to connect and support tissues and internal organs. It is also present in teeth. Collagen is composed of fibers that contribute to the external and internal structure of cells. It works in conjunction with elastin, the major component of ligaments and skin. Elastin allows tissues to stretch and then return to their original size.

There are more than 200 disorders that impact connective tissues. Many connective tissue diseases are the result of autoimmunity (see Chapter 4). Collagen and elastin may be injured by inflammation and the immune response. Other connective tissue diseases are the result of infection, injury, or genetics. Some have no known cause. Those with oral manifestations are listed in Table 9-8.

Raynaud's Phenomenon and CREST Syndrome

Raynaud's phenomenon is characterized by marked changes of the skin due to vasoconstriction of underlying blood vessels. Distinct red, white, and blue skin changes are observed in the toes and fingers, ears, and nose. The color changes are related to vasodilatation, vasoconstriction, or cyanosis. Two main precipitating events for Raynaud's phenomenon are emotional stress

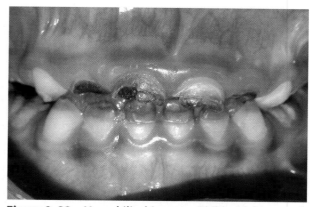

Figure 9–23 Hyperbilirubimemia. Child with history of congenital liver disease shows effects of bilirubin deposition into developing teeth.

Table 9.8	Oral Manifestations of Connective Tissue Disorders	
Connective Tissue Disorder	**Oral Manifestations**
Systemic lupus erythematosus	Malar rash, desquamative gingivitis, RAU
Rheumatoid arthritis	TMJ arthritis
Sjögren's syndrome	Xerostomia, xerophthalmia
Systemic sclerosis	Trismus, dysphagia, xerostomia, xerophthalmia, trigeminal neuralgia
Polymyositis	Dysphagia
Relapsing polychondritis	Nasal deformity, laryngeal hoarseness
Wegener's granulomatosis	"Strawberry" gingivitis
Behçet's disease	Major aphthous ulcers
Temporal arteritis	Temporal headache, intraoral ischemia

and cold temperature. Less common instigators are insufficient blood supply to the extremities due to an underlying systemic condition such as systemic lupus erythematosus, scleroderma, or arteriosclerosis.

Clinical Implications

Removal of triggering factors for this disorder can reverse observed vascular changes. The stress of dental appointments and treatment may be enough to trigger an episode of Raynaud's phenomenon in some patients.

CREST syndrome is a multifactorial disease that includes Raynaud's phenomenon. CREST is characterized by five cardinal clinical signs, the first letter of which constitute the name. Three of the five are required to make a diagnosis:

- Raynaud's phenomenon (Fig. 9-24)
- Calcinosis cutis—tiny calcium deposits under the skin of elbows, knees, and fingers (Fig. 9-25)
- Esophageal dysmotility or reflux and dysphagia

- Sclerodactyly (contractures of the digital joints) (Fig. 9-26)
- Telangiectasia (refer to Figs. 9-18 and 9-19)

CREST has no cure but can be treated with immunosuppressive drugs. Treatments reduce the symptoms of esophageal reflux, pulmonary hypertension, and Raynaud's phenomenon.

Clinical Implications

In the connective tissue disorder systemic sclerosis, tightening of facial skin creates limited mouth opening, making tooth brushing and flossing a challenge (Fig. 9-27). Restricted opening also limits access for dental procedures such as routine prophylaxis. Patients may experience xerostomia with increased risk of dental caries. Most patients also experience acid reflux, resulting in erosion of enamel and dentin.

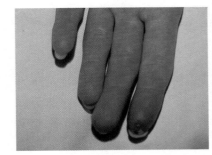

Figure 9–24   Raynaud's phenomenon. Raynaud's phenomenon with blue discoloration to the finger tips. (From Taber's Cyclopedic Medical Dictionary, ed. 21. F.A. Davis, Philadelphia, 2009, p 1978.)

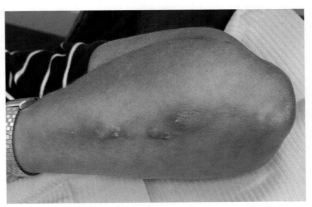

Figure 9–25   Calcinosis cutis. Hard calcium deposits under the skin.

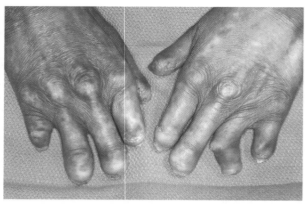

Figure 9–26 Sclerodactyly. Contracture of hands in patient with scleroderma.

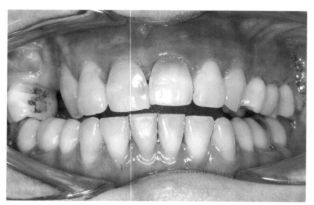

Figure 9–27 Trismus from scleroderma. Patient with limited ability to open her mouth due to contracture of facial skin.

Ehlers-Danlos Syndrome

Ehlers-Danlos syndrome (EDS) is an inherited connective tissue disorder involving production of defective collagen. Various forms of Ehlers-Danlos syndrome are based on specific gene mutations but most patients present with a set of classic features including increased elasticity of the skin, extremely flexible joints, easy bruising due to increased fragility of blood vessel walls, abnormal wound healing, and connective tissue scarring (Fig. 9-28).

Oral manifestations of EDS include high palatal vault and a narrow maxillary arch. Dental crowding may develop, making the teeth difficult to clean. Individuals are more susceptible to periodontal disease at an early age, due to defective collagen weakening periodontal ligament fibers. Increased joint flexibility increases the tendency for dislocation of the jaw. This is a consideration for dental procedures that require prolonged jaw opening.

An important and potentially serious complication of Ehlers-Danlos syndrome is excessive bleeding after an invasive dental procedure. This is a result of increased fragility of blood vessels.

AMYLOIDOSIS

Amyloid refers to proteins produced in the bone marrow that become "folded" into insoluble fibrous forms when they interact with normal body proteins. Abnormal accumulation of amyloid in organs is known as *amyloidosis*. Amyloidosis can be seen in at least 20 diseases affecting various organs including the skin (Fig. 9-29), heart, kidneys, liver, spleen, central nervous system, and gastrointestinal tract. There are three types of amyloidosis: primary, secondary, and hereditary.

Primary systemic amyloidosis is the most common form. It tends to occur in adults older than age 50 and has an unknown etiology. Primary amyloidosis occurs by itself and is not associated with other diseases. Secondary amyloidosis has been associated with other disorders such as multiple myeloma (see Chapter 7), tuberculosis (see Chapter 3), rheumatoid arthritis, and osteomyelitis. Renal dialysis increases the risk of amyloidosis because dialysis cannot remove large proteins from the blood. Treatment of underlying disease may stop or help control this form of amyloidosis. The hereditary (familial) type of amyloidosis primarily affects the liver, nerves, heart, and kidneys.

The most common oral manifestation of amyloidosis is macroglossia. Enlargement of the tongue develops and scalloping occurs along the lateral borders due to imprinting from adjacent teeth along the bite line. Clinically, the tongue may show yellow nodules on the lateral surfaces. Salivary hypofunction may also occur as a result of amyloid deposition within the salivary glands.

Clinical Implications

Suspected amyloid deposition in the tongue or other intraoral site requires medical evaluation for underlying systemic disease. Occasionally, isolated lesions of amyloidosis are found in areas exposed to chronic inflammation. These are not associated with a serious underlying disease.

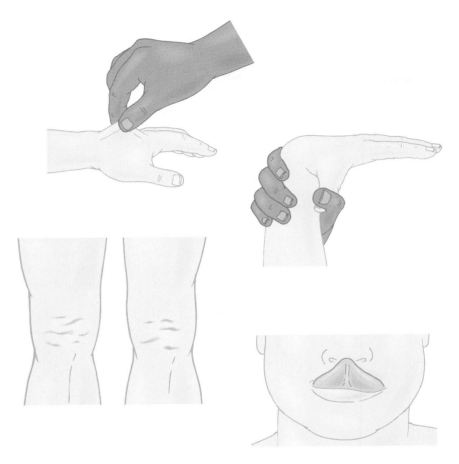

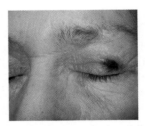

Figure 9–28   Ehlers-Danlos syndrome. Extreme flexibility of joints and skin is a feature of Ehlers-Danlos syndrome.

Figure 9–29   Amyloidosis. Amyloid nodule on left eyelid. (From Barankin, B: Derm Notes. F.A. Davis, Philadelphia, 2006, p 191.)

NUTRITIONAL DISORDERS AND VITAMIN DEFICIENCIES

Nutritional disorders most often involve inadequate intake or absorption of one or more nutrients essential for health. The disorders may also result from intake of food that has poor nutritional value.

Thirteen fat- and water-soluble vitamins and organic substances are essential in minute amounts for normal body growth and activity. These are obtained naturally from plant and animal foods. Dietary vitamin deficiencies are uncommon in the United States. However, deficiencies do occur associated with malnutrition states resulting from gastrointestinal disorders affecting absorption of vitamins, eating disorders, and alcoholism.

Fat-Soluble Vitamins

Fat-soluble vitamins include vitamins A, D, E, and K. Animal sources include fish and fish oil, fortified milk and juices, beef liver, fortified cereals, and eggs; other sources include green leafy vegetables and vegetable oils. Excess consumption of fat-soluble vitamins promotes their storage. This can result in a potentially dangerous situation called *hypervitaminosis*. Deficiency of fat-soluble vitamins also may result from compromised absorption. This may occur as a result of drugs that interfere with absorption from the intestine. Cystic fibrosis is associated with a deficiency of enzymes from the pancreas that interferes with fat absorption in the intestines. Oral manifestations of vitamins A, E, and K deficiency are uncommon.

Vitamin D plays an important role in bone metabolism, maintaining calcium and phosphate levels in the body. Vitamin D is found in fortified milk, cheese, whole eggs, liver, and salmon. Skin synthesizes vitamin D when exposed to sunlight. Deficiency of vitamin D in children produces the condition known as rickets. Adult onset of deficiency of vitamin D is known as osteomalacia.

Rickets is most common in the first year of life. It presents with spine deformities, bowing of legs, prominence of costochondral junctions (called "rachitic rosary"), and protrusion of the sternum (called "pigeon breast" deformity) (Fig. 9-30). Teeth may show enamel pits and hypoplasia, large pulp chambers, and a thin layer of dentin.

Osteomalacia literally means "soft bones." It is a disease of defective bone mineralization. Causes include dietary deficiency of calcium and phosphate due to vitamin D deficiency, gastrointestinal absorption problems, lack of sunlight, gastrectomy, celiac disease, kidney or liver disorder, renal dialysis, and medications that block cellular calcium or phosphorous uptake. The result is accumulation of nonmineralized bone matrix (osteoid) and a decrease in the activity and

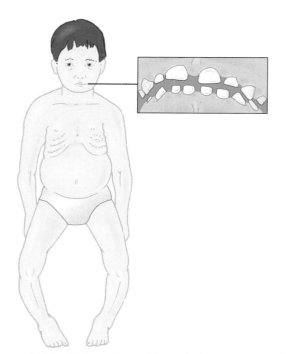

Figure 9–30   Rickets. Enamel hypoplasia, prominent rib joints and sternum, protruding abdomen are features of rickets.

number of osteoclasts and osteoblasts. Clinical signs of osteomalacia include skeletal deformities, bone pain, fractures, and decreased muscle tone with weakness of arms and legs. Alveolar ridge resorption and periodontal bone loss may occur.

Water-Soluble Vitamins

Water-soluble vitamins include vitamin C, all of the B vitamins, and folic acid. These vitamins dissolve in water when they are ingested and excess amounts are excreted in the urine. They cannot be stored and continuous supply is needed daily to prevent deficiency states. The B-complex group is found in a variety of foods: cereal grains, meat, poultry, eggs, fish, milk, legumes, and fresh vegetables. These vitamins are easily destroyed during food storage and preparation, promoting dietary deficiencies. Water-soluble vitamin deficiencies have both systemic and oral manifestations of interest to dentistry.

Vitamin B1 is called thiamine. Thiamine deficiency leads to *beriberi*, a condition that occurs in chronic alcohol abusers or elderly patients who have poor or limited diets. Beriberi is characterized by poor appetite, fatigue, and nausea. It may also present with cardiovascular problems such as heart failure and peripheral edema. Neurological problems including tingling and numbing sensation of the extremities and tip of tongue may occur. Severe cases may result in neurological symptoms such as mental deterioration, coma, and death.

Vitamin B2 is called riboflavin. Deficiency of riboflavin may result in glossitis, angular cheilitis, and generalized erythema of the oral mucosa. Other clinical features include twitching of eyelids and photophobia (sensitivity to light).

Vitamin B3 is called niacin. Niacin deficiency in the diet leads to a condition known as *pellagra*, classically associated with "the four D's": diarrhea, dementia, dermatitis, and death. Oral manifestations include beefy red glossitis and aphthous ulcers. Prolonged niacin deficiency eventually leads to death.

Vitamin B6 is called pyroxidine. Deficiency is rarely due to poor diet but most often related to poor absorption caused by medications such as corticosteroids and certain antibiotics. Vitamin B6 deficiency can be seen in alcoholics and those with poor absorption due to aging. This vitamin is important for neurological health. Signs of deficiency include weakness, dizziness, or episodic seizures. Oral manifestations include glossitis and angular cheilitis.

Vitamin B12 is called cobalamin. Cobalamin has a key role in normal brain and nervous system function as well as blood formation. Cobalamin deficiency is called *pernicious anemia* (previously discussed in this chapter). It is typically associated with autoimmune **gastritis** (see Chapter 4 for discussion of autoimmunity). Intrinsic factor involved in the absorption of vitamin B12 is not produced because the gastric parietal cells are destroyed by autoantibodies. Resultant vitamin B12 deficiency leads to defective red blood cell production and anemia. Gastrointestinal bypass patients and strict vegetarians are at risk for vitamin B12 deficiency. Clinical features of pernicious anemia include dyspnea, fatigue, dizziness, weakness, frequent headaches, and tingling or numbness of fingers and toes. Oral manifestations include tingling and burning tongue, patchy areas of erythema, and atrophy of the oral mucosa and tongue (see Fig. 9-15).

Folic acid (also called folate) is the water-soluble form of vitamin B9. It is needed to synthesize and repair DNA and plays a role in rapid cell division and growth during infancy and pregnancy. Deficiency of folic acid may produce neural tube defects in developing embryos, resulting in developmental conditions such as spina bifida. Clinical signs and symptoms of deficiency include diarrhea, macrocytic anemia, peripheral neuropathy, glossitis, aphthous ulcers, headaches, and behavioral disorders. In deficiency states, impaired DNA repair may predispose to cancer.

Clinical Implications

Patients with oral burning pain, commonly called burning mouth syndrome, should be assessed for possible folic acid and vitamin B12 deficiencies. Relief of oral symptoms is achieved when deficiency states are treated with proper supplementation.

Vitamin C is called ascorbic acid. Ascorbic acid deficiency is known as *scurvy*. It develops in individuals who lack citrus fruits and vegetables in their diets. Vitamin C is involved in collagen synthesis, which is required in the production of normal connective tissue. Deficiency of vitamin C leads to weakened blood vessels, joints, gingiva, periodontal ligaments, and bone. Oral manifestations include generalized swollen spongy gingiva with spontaneous bleeding called *scorbutic gingivitis*. Aphthous ulcers, tooth mobility, and loss of periodontal support also occur. Wound healing is affected and is a treatment consideration, particularly in surgical patients.

Critical Thinking Questions

Case 9-1: Your 12-year-old male patient presents with a long history of painful oral ulcers. His father had similar ulcers as a child. He now shows diffuse small yellow papules along the lips and buccal mucosa that are not painful. He has missed a lot of school lately because his stomach has been bothering him.

• • •

What disease produces this combination of signs and symptoms?

What is the name given to the yellow papules?

How will his disease receive a proper diagnosis? What specialist might be involved in his care?

Case 9-2: Your 45-year-old female patient returns for a routine recall examination. She tells you about a recent missionary trip to Africa where she helped build a school. She worked in an impoverished village that did not have a safe water supply. Since returning home she reports she "has been a little run down." You notice her eyes and skin appear jaundiced.

• • •

Is there a possible relationship between her signs and symptoms and her trip to Africa?

What causes jaundice? What organ systems might be involved?

What questions will you ask on her medical history update?

How will the findings of jaundice affect her dental appointment and treatment?

Case 9-3: A 14-year-old male patient has been coming to see you for about 3 years. Since his last visit (1 year ago) you notice he has suddenly lost a lot of weight. He looks very thin and his mother is concerned. She reports he drinks a lot of water, has a great appetite, but is not gaining weight.

• • •

What disease process might be the cause of his sudden weight loss? Explain how this causes weight loss.

What questions on the medical history are important to evaluate this patient's condition?

What oral manifestations of disease would you look for in this patient?

Case 9-2: Your 63-year-old female patient complains that her tongue "feels like it is on fire." It has felt this way for several months.

• • •

List several different conditions that may cause oral burning.

What questions on the medical history are important to explore in this patient?

What manifestations of systemic diseases might be present? How should this patient be evaluated?

Review Questions

1. **The anterior pituitary gland secretes two main types of hormones. Which one of the following is NOT secreted by the anterior pituitary gland?**
   A. Antidiuretic hormone (ADH)
   B. Adrenocorticotropic hormone (ACTH)
   C. Growth hormone (GH)
   D. Follicle stimulating hormone (FSH)

2. **Elevation of growth hormone after the closure of bone growth plates results in which one of the following diseases?**
   A. Gigantism
   B. Acromegaly
   C. Dwarfism
   D. Cushing's disease

3. **Thyrotoxicosis is defined as elevated serum levels of free T3 and T4 and presents with many signs. Which of the following is NOT a sign of thyrotoxicosis?**
   A. Tremor and emotional instability
   B. Heat intolerance
   C. Decreased appetite with weight gain
   D. Elevated blood pressure with palpitations

4. **Diagnosis of hyperparathyroidism is based on blood serum assay. Which of the following results of a blood serum assay is positive in hyperparathyroidism?**
   A. Decreased PTH, elevated serum calcium levels
   B. Decreased PTH, decreased serum calcium levels
   C. Elevated PTH, elevated serum calcium levels
   D. Elevated PTH, decreased serum calcium levels

5. **Signs and symptoms of hyperparathyroidism include all of the following EXCEPT**
   A. loss of lamina dura.
   B. renal stones.
   C. supernumerary teeth.
   D. gastric ulcers.

6. **Which of the following statements about the adrenal gland and its disorders is false?**

    A. The adrenal glands are located on the superior poles of the kidneys.
    B. In Cushing's syndrome, the adrenals produce too much cortisol.
    C. In Addison's disease, the adrenals produce too little cortisol.
    D. The adrenal glands produce too much ACTH in CREST syndrome.

7. **Which of the following is NOT a clinical feature of Addison's disease?**

    A. Hyperpigmentation of the skin
    B. Hypocortisolism
    C. Adrenal insufficiency
    D. Bruises and purplish striae

8. **You notice your patient has been sweating excessively while you are treating her. She also appears to have a wide staring gaze, exophthalmos, and sagging eyelids. She mentions that her recent physical examination showed a decrease in TSH levels and increased free T3 and T4 levels. What condition does she most likely have?**

    A. Addison's disease
    B. Cushing's disease
    C. Graves' disease
    D. Ehlers-Danlos syndrome

9. **Uncontrolled diabetes mellitus may cause all of the following EXCEPT**

    A. immune suppression.
    B. ketoacidosis.
    C. elevated insulin levels.
    D. elevated blood glucose levels.

10. **Common oral manifestations of diabetes mellitus include all of the following EXCEPT**

    A. oral candidiasis.
    B. xerostomia.
    C. erythema migrans.
    D. burning tongue.

11. **Which of the following statements about diabetes mellitus is incorrect?**

    A. Type 2 diabetes is more common than type 1 diabetes.
    B. Patients with diabetes mellitus have a higher incidence of gingivitis and periodontitis.
    C. If a hypoglycemic episode occurs, it is usually not an emergency and discontinuation of dental treatment is not necessary.
    D. Type 1 diabetes is an idiopathic autoimmune disorder of the pancreas, whereas type 2 diabetes is due to insulin resistance and insufficient secretion of insulin by the pancreas.

12. **Which test is used to confirm the diagnosis of Cushing's syndrome?**

    A. Fasting blood cortisol level
    B. 24-hour free cortisol level
    C. Random cortisol level
    D. Random ACTH levels

13. **Which of the following are common clinical features seen in a patient with thalassemia?**

    A. Enlarged maxilla and mandible
    B. Altered trabecular pattern
    C. "Hair-on-end" appearance on skull radiograph
    D. All of the above

14. **Which of the following is NOT a common etiologic factor of iron deficiency anemia?**

    A. Lack of dietary iron intake
    B. Excessive acute or chronic blood loss
    C. Frequent blood transfusion
    D. Impaired absorption of iron by the body

15. **Which of the following is NOT a common oral manifestation of iron deficiency anemia?**

    A. Bleeding gums
    B. Atrophic glossitis
    C. Angular cheilitis
    D. Burning sensation of the tongue

16. Pyostomatitis vegetans is an inflammatory condition characterized by yellow pustules in the oral mucosal surfaces. It is associated with which one of the following conditions?

    A. Vitamin A deficiency
    B. Crohn's disease
    C. Hepatitis A infection
    D. Addison's disease

17. Jaundice is a clinical presentation that indicates an underlying liver disease. Which of the following is NOT a cause of jaundice?

    A. Increased production of bilirubin
    B. Decreased uptake of bilirubin into the liver
    C. Increased excretion of bilirubin
    D. Decreased excretion of bilirubin

18. Radiographic examination of a 42-year-old woman reveals bilateral, generalized, diffuse decrease in bone density and apparent loss of lamina dura and cortical plates. Serum calcium levels are elevated. Based on this information, which of the following is the most likely diagnosis?

    A. Hyperparathyroidism
    B. Cushing's syndrome
    C. Graves' disease
    D. Addison's disease

19. A 19-year-old male has multiple red papules on the tongue and vermilion zone of the lips. The papules are 1 to 2 mm in size and blanch upon pressure. The patient has a history of multiple episodes of epistaxis. Based on this information, which of the following is the most likely diagnosis?

    A. Hereditary hemorrhagic telangiectasia
    B. Pyostomatitis vegetans
    C. Peutz-Jeghers syndrome
    D. Vitamin D deficiency

20. A 48-year-old female with anemia complains of a burning tongue and tingling and numbness of the fingers and toes. Laboratory studies reveal decreased levels of intrinsic factor and vitamin B12. Based on this information, what specific type of anemia does this patient most likely have?

    A. Iron deficiency anemia
    B. Pernicious anemia
    C. Plummer-Vinson syndrome
    D. Folic acid deficiency

REFERENCES
Books

Tamparo, L: Diseases of the Human Body, ed. 5. F.A. Davis, Philadelphia, 2011.

Underwood, J, Simon, S: General and Systematic Pathology, ed. 5. Churchill-Livingston, Elsevier, London, 2009.

Wardlaw GM, Smith AM: Contemporary Nutrition, A Functional Approach, ed. 3. McGraw-Hill Higher Education, New York, 2013.

Zelman M, Tompary, R, Holdaway, M: Human Diseases: A Systemic Approach, ed. 7. Prentiss Hall, Upper Saddle River, NJ, 2010.

Journals

Chrysomali, E, Piperi, E, Sklavounou-Andrikopoulou, A: Oral acanthosis nigricans in chronic hepatitis B with a 21 year follow up. Journal of Dermatology 38(12):1172–1176, December 2011.

Clayton, B: Stroke, dysphagia and oral care: What is best practice? Alta RN 68(1):26–27, Spring 2012.

Genco, RJ: Periodontal disease and association with diabetes mellitus and diabetes: Clinical implications. Journal of Dental Hygiene 83(4):186–187, Fall 2009.

Jen, M, Yan, AC: Syndromes associated with nutritional deficiency and excess. Clinical Dermatology 28(6):669–685, November-December 2010.

Khocht, A, Schleifer, SJ, Janal, MN, Keller, S: Dental care and oral disease in alcohol-dependent persons. Journal of Substance Abuse Treatment 37(2):214–218, September 2009.

Wilkins, T, Jarvis, K, Patel J: Diagnosis and management of Crohn's disease. American Family Physician 84(12):1365–1375, December 15, 2011.

Answers to Review Questions

Chapter 1

1. D
2. B
3. D
4. C
5. A
6. D
7. B
8. D
9. B
10. C
11. C
12. A
13. C
14. B
15. A
16. D
17. A
18. D
19. B
20. B

Chapter 2

1. D
2. A
3. A
4. C
5. C
6. C
7. D
8. D
9. A
10. A

11. B
12. D
13. A
14. B
15. C
16. B
17. B
18. C
19. A
20. D
21. A
22. C
23. A
24. C
25. B

Chapter 3

1. C
2. B
3. D
4. C
5. C
6. B
7. B
8. D
9. C
10. A
11. B
12. C
13. B
14. A
15. D
16. A
17. B

18. A
19. D
20. C

Chapter 4

1. A
2. B
3. A
4. B
5. D
6. B
7. C
8. D
9. B
10. C
11. B
12. D
13. A
14. B
15. C
16. B
17. D
18. A
19. B
20. D
21. D
22. A
23. B
24. C
25. C
26. B
27. D
28. D

Chapter 5

1. C
2. A
3. D
4. A
5. C
6. B
7. A
8. C
9. A
10. D
11. C
12. B
13. D
14. A
15. B
16. C
17. A
18. D
19. C
20. C

Chapter 6

1. A
2. C
3. C
4. A
5. D
6. A
7. D
8. B
9. A
10. C

11. A
12. D
13. D
14. A
15. A
16. A
17. B
18. D
19. A
20. C
21. B
22. A
23. D
24. C
25. C
26. B
27. B
28. D

Chapter 7

1. D
2. A
3. C
4. D
5. B
6. D
7. C
8. A
9. D
10. C
11. B
12. D
13. B
14. B

15. B

16. A

17. B

18. A

19. B

20. D

Chapter 8

1. B

2. D

3. A

4. C

5. A

6. B

7. A

8. B

9. D

10. B

11. C

12. A

13. B

14. A

15. D

Chapter 9

1. A

2. B

3. C

4. C

5. C

6. D

7. D

8. C

9. C

10. C

11. C

12. B

13. D

14. C

15. A

16. B

17. C

18. A

19. A

20. B

Glossary

A

Abfraction: Loss of cervical tooth structure due to flexing pressures on the tooth

Abrasion: Loss of tooth structure from mechanical forces; example: toothbrush abrasion

Abscess: A collection of pus within an enclosed body space

Actinic: Relating to or caused by sunlight or ultraviolet light

Actinic damage: Damage to the skin caused by exposure to sunlight or ultraviolet light

Active immunity: Type of immunity that happens naturally when the body fights an infection, antibodies are produced in response to an antigen; also occurs artificially through vaccination

Acute: A disease condition of abrupt onset; disease of short duration that is rapidly progressive; example: the common cold

Acute inflammation: Type of inflammation characterized by exudative process in which fluid, plasma proteins, and cells leave the bloodstream and enter the tissues: polymorphonuclear neutrophils (PMNs) predominate

Acute phase response: Rapid systemic reaction of the body to deal with tissue damage caused by the inflammatory response; includes fever, elevated cortisol levels, leukocytosis and lymphadenopathy

Adenocarcinoma: A malignant neoplasm that originates within glandular tissue; example: breast adenocarcinoma

Adenoma: A benign neoplasm that originates within glandular tissue; example: pleomorphic adenoma

Aglossia: Congenital absence of the tongue

Allele: DNA coding on genes responsible for hereditary variation; example: 2 alleles are inherited for eye color, one from each parent, the dominant allele is expressed and determines eye color

Allergen: A substance that causes an allergic or hypersensitivity reaction

Allergy: Abnormal reaction of the immune system to an otherwise harmless substance (allergen) previously encountered

Alopecia: Partial or complete absence of hair from defined areas of the body where it normally grows; example: baldness

Anaphylactic reactions: Acute multisystem severe type I hypersensitivity reactions associated with hypotension, urticaria, or difficulty breathing, caused by exposure to an allergen; example: reaction to a bee sting

Anaplasia: Loss of differentiation of cells with reversion to a more primitive state; a characteristic of malignant cells; anaplastic cells

Anemia: A deficiency of red blood cells or hemoglobin resulting in decreased oxygen-carrying capacity of the blood

Anodontia: Congenital absence of teeth; may be partial (oligodontia) or complete; seen in ectodermal dysplasia

Anorexia: A lack or loss of appetite for food, or a refusal to eat

Antibiotic resistance: The ability of bacteria to resist the effects of an antibiotic to which they once were sensitive

Antibody: A specific protein produced by plasma cells in response to exposure to a specific antigen, which it can neutralize

Antigen: A foreign substance that induces an immune response and production of antibodies

Antioxidant: A chemical compound or substance that removes potentially damaging free radicals from the body; molecules that inhibit or counteract oxidation

Apoptosis: The process of programmed or planned cell death; may be physiologic in embryonic development or pathologic in disease states

Atopy: An allergic reaction that occurs within a few minutes when a sensitized individual comes into contact with a particular antigen

Atrophy: Decrease in the size of an organ or tissue due to disease, injury, or lack of use; typically due to degeneration of cells; example: atrophy of muscles occurs over time when an arm or leg is immobilized in a cast

Attrition: Loss of tooth tissue due to tooth-to-tooth contact; example: chronic tooth grinding, bruxism

Auscultation: Listening to body sounds to evaluate if a structure is normal or abnormal. Example: using a stethoscope to hear sounds made by internal organs such as the heart and lungs

Autoantibodies: Antibodies inappropriately produced by an individual in response to a component of one's own tissue

Autoimmune disease: A disease in which the immune system mistakenly attacks one's own body cells and tissues; example: rheumatoid arthritis

Autoimmunity: The inappropriate production of antibodies against one's own tissues

Autoinoculation: Spreading an infection from a part of one's body to another by transferring the microorganism, usually with contaminated hands

Autosomal recessive disorder: A genetic disease that appears only in individuals who receive two copies of a particular disease allele, one from each parent

Autosome: A chromosome that is not a sex chromosome

B

Bacterium: (Pl. Bacteria) A unicellular microorganism, some are capable of causing disease

Benign: A tumor that does not threaten life by invading and destroying tissue, or metastasizing; example: lipoma

Betel quid: A concoction composed of areca nut and other herbal drugs wrapped in the leaf of a betel palm and chewed for its intoxicant properties; a habit seen in Asian countries

Bifid: Divided into two parts; example: bifid tongue

Biopsy: The surgical removal of tissue or cells for microscopic examination; may be incisional or excisional

Bone marrow transplant: Replacement of diseased or damaged bone marrow with healthy bone marrow; the replacement bone marrow may be the patient's own (autologous) or it may come from a donor (allogeneic)

Bradycardia: A heart rate slower than normal heart rate (usually less than 60 bpm)

Bruxism: Wear of teeth due to clenching or grinding; a form of attrition

C

Capsule: A membranous structure made of fibrous connective tissue that envelops an organ or tumor

Carcinoma: A malignancy arising from structures of epithelial origin; example: squamous cell carcinoma

Carrier: A person who harbors an infectious microorganism without clinical evidence of the disease; may transmit the infection to others. In genetics, an individual who inherits a trait or mutation, but does not show signs of the disorder

Cell aging: Over time, the decrease in ability of the cell to divide or proliferate

Cellular response: Immune process characterized by direct attack on foreign antigens by sensitized T cells, and secretion of lymphokines that activate the humoral response

Central: Developing within bone

Chancre: A painless ulcer, the primary lesion of syphilis; occurs at a microorganism's site of entry

Chemotherapy: Treatment of disease by use of chemical substances; typically using drugs to destroy cancer cells, but can refer to other drug therapies

Chromosome: A structure composed of nucleic acids and proteins located within the nucleus of living cells that carries genetic information in the form of DNA; humans have 23 pairs of chromosomes (22 pairs of autosomes and 1 pair of sex chromosomes)

Chronic: Persisting for a long period of time; gradual onset over time and of longer duration

Cicatricial: Pertaining to a scar; cicatrix is synonymous with scar

Cleft: An opening or cleavage resulting from failure of parts to fuse during embryonic development; example: cleft lip

Clinical trial: Research based upon the scientific method in which a control group and a test group are compared over a period of time in order to study a single, differing factor; a highly reliable form of research

Coloboma: A congenital malformation of the eye, often seen as a defect or failure of a part of the eye to form

Congenital: A condition, defect, or lesion that is present at birth

Conjunctivitis: Inflammation of the conjunctiva of the eye

Constitutional symptoms: A group of symptoms that may affect many different systems in the body simultaneously; affecting the whole body; examples are fever, fatigue, weight loss

Craniosynostosis: Premature fusion of the sutures between the growth plates in the skull that prevents normal skull expansion and growth

Culture: Microorganisms grown in a special medium; often used to isolate and identify infectious organisms and test for antibiotic resistance

Cyst: An epithelial-lined cavity filled with fluid or semi-solid material

Cytokine: Protein released by cells of the immune system that acts as an intercellular mediator in generating the immune response; examples: interleukins and lymphokines

Cytology: Study of the anatomy, chemistry, pathology, and physiology of individual cells; use of cells for diagnosis; example: Pap smear

D

Debulking: Partial removal of a large tumor that cannot be completely resected

Deletion: Occurs when a segment of DNA on a chromosome goes missing during cell division

De novo: From the beginning; anew

Dental fluorosis: Abnormal discoloration and hypoplasia of teeth caused by excessive intake of fluoride during tooth development

Deoxyribonucleic acid (DNA): A nucleic acid that carries genetic information and is capable of self-replication

Dermatitis: Inflammation of the skin caused by any irritating or allergenic substance

Desquamative gingivitis: A clinical term used to describe diffuse gingival erythema and mucosal sloughing as a result of atrophy of the epithelial cells; has many different causes

Developmental disorder: A condition or disease caused by interruption of a particular stage in development often causing developmental delay

Diabetic ketoacidosis: A complication of diabetes that occurs when blood sugar levels are extremely high, fat breakdown produces increased ketones in blood, generalized decrease in pH results; a hallmark of uncontrolled diabetes

Diagnosis: The precise identification or naming of a disease based on its signs and symptoms.

Differential diagnosis: The identification of a condition through a process of comparing all pathologic processes that share similar signs and symptoms

Differentiation: The process by which an embryonic cell becomes specialized to perform a particular function; example: cells of the inner enamel epithelium differentiate into ameloblasts; in the study of tumors, refers to the degree to which diseased cells resemble their normal counterparts

Disease: Variation from a normal state, may be caused by developmental disturbances; genetic or metabolic factors; microorganisms; physical, chemical, or radiant energy; or other unknown causes

Disseminated: Widespread; remote from site of origin

Dominant: In genetics, when one of many genes is expressed over others

Dysesthesia: Distortion of any sense especially touch; unpleasant abnormal sensation

Dysphagia: Difficulty swallowing

Dysplasia: Lack of proper maturation of a tissue; examples: cleidocranial dysplasia with lack of proper maturation of the clavicles and skull, and premalignant epithelial dysplasia with lack of proper maturation of epithelial cells in the oral mucosa

Dyspnea: Shortness of breath

Dystrophic calcifications: Deposition of calcium into diseased or degenerating tissues

E

Ecchymosis: Escape of blood from ruptured vessels under skin or mucous membranes causing purple discoloration of skin, larger than petechiae; a bruise

Ectopic: Developing in an abnormal location or position; example: ectopic sebaceous glands in the buccal mucosa

Embolus: (Pl. Emboli) A foreign object or detached blood clot carried through a blood vessel that blocks blood flow

Embryology: The study of embryos and their development

Enamel hypoplasia: Underdevelopment of the enamel matrix resulting in defective enamel formation that appears abnormal

Encephalitis: Inflammation of the brain, most often due to infection

Endemic: A disease or condition regularly present in a specific region or within a specific group of people

Endocrine: Related to secretion of hormones directly into the bloodstream rather than through a duct system

Endogenous: Caused by factors within the body or arising from internal causes; example: endogenous bilirubin stain of teeth in a child with liver disease

Endophytic: Extends down and below the level of the surrounding normal tissue

Enucleation: Complete surgical removal of a cyst or tumor without cutting it into fragments

Epidemiology: Branch of medicine that studies disease within a population rather than in an individual

Eponymous: Named after a person; example is Gorlin syndrome, named after Dr. Robert Gorlin

Epistaxis: Nosebleed

Epulis: Any raised mass of the gingiva

Erosion: Loss of tooth hard tissue due to exposure to chemicals with a low pH or stomach acid; example vomiting in bulimia

Erythroleukoplakia: A clinical descriptive term meaning red and white epithelial or mucosal color change to the mucosa or skin

Erythroplakia: A clinical descriptive term meaning red epithelial or mucosal patch

Etiologic agent: A microorganism or substance, such as a toxin, that causes a disease; example: mycobacterium tuberculosis is the etiologic agent of tuberculosis

Etiologic factor: An agent or condition that contributes to the production of a disease; example: smoking as an etiologic factor for lung disease

Etiology: The cause of a disease

Exacerbation: Worsening; increase in severity of the disease

Excisional biopsy: The removal of an entire lesion including a significant margin of normal tissue for microscopic examination and diagnosis

Exfoliative cytology: Removal of surface epithelial or mucosal cells for microscopic examination of individual cells to determine a diagnosis; example: cytologic smear to diagnose candidiasis

Exogenous stain: An external agent/substance that imparts color or discoloration to a tissue or cells (extrinsic); example: tobacco stain

Exophthalmos: Abnormal protrusion of the eyes from the orbit caused by disease; seen in hyperthyroidism

Exophytic: Protrudes from the surface

Exostosis: Exophytic growth of normal bone; tori are an example

Expression: Process by which information from a gene is used in the synthesis of a functioning gene product

Extraglandular: Associated with a gland but occurring outside the glandular tissues

Extraosseous: Occurring within soft tissues that surround bone, but not within the bone itself

Extrapulmonary: Outside of or unrelated to the lungs

Extrinsic stain: A substance that imparts color to a tissue or cells or a discoloration caused by external agents (exogenous); example: tobacco stain

F

Factitial: Self-induced injury either intentionally or unintentionally; example: a pizza burn is a factitial injury

Fibromatosis: Formation of multiple fibrous, tumor-like nodules

Field cancerization: Generalized carcinogen-induced changes within a tissue from which multiple independent lesions may occur; example: skin cancers arising in sun-damaged skin

Five-year survival rate: The percentage of patients who are living 5 years after being diagnosed with a life-threatening condition

Foramen caecum: A shallow depression in the posterior dorsal tongue that is a remnant of the embryonic thyroglossal duct

Foreign body reaction: An immunologic reaction to substances not recognized by the immune system as "self"; capable of inducing an inflammatory response

Forensic medicine: The branch of medicine that uses anatomic structures and physical characteristics for legal purposes

Forensic odontology: Branch of forensic medicine that uses dental characteristics for legal purposes

Formalin: A colorless solution of formaldehyde in water; a 10 percent solution is used to fix and preserve tissues for study under the microscope

Free radicals: A highly unstable and reactive group of atoms that have at least one unpaired electron in their outer shell, responsible for aging, tissue damage, and some diseases

Friable: Easily crumbled

Frictional keratosis: Benign reactive phenomenon in which excess keratin builds up to protect the underlying tissues from persistent irritation; a form of hyperkeratosis

Fulminant: Occurring suddenly and with great severity

Fungi: A group of single-celled or complex multicellular organisms, includes yeasts and molds

Fusion: The process of merging and making one unit; example: fusion of two tooth germs to form one large tooth

G

Gastritis: Inflammation of the mucosal lining of the stomach

General pathology: The branch of pathology that studies disease processes occurring in any organ system such as inflammation, infection, genetic disorders, and neoplasia

Genetics: The study of inheritance, a branch of biology that deals with heritable factors that influence development and maintenance of an organism

Genotype: The genetic makeup of an individual; type of genes expressed; genotype predicts phenotype or appearance, the way a person looks

Globulomaxillary: An anatomic location that describes any lesion located between the maxillary canine and lateral incisor

Glossitis: Inflammation of the tongue, often but not always producing pain

Glucometer: A medical device for determining the approximate concentration of glucose in the blood; used as a monitor in diabetes

Granulation tissue: Nonspecific vascular fibrous connective tissue that replaces a fibrin clot in wound healing, as the body repairs injury

Granuloma: A specific form of chronic inflammation that attempts to wall off substances perceived as foreign but impossible or difficult to eliminate

Gummas: Soft, rubbery tissue masses associated with tertiary syphilis

H

Hamartoma: A benign tumor-like malformation composed of an overgrowth of tissue elements normally found at the anatomic site where it develops

Hemarthosis: Bleeding into a joint space

Hematocrit: A blood test that measures the percentage of whole blood made up of red blood cells

Hematoma: A localized collection of blood that accumulates outside blood vessels causing a bluish discoloration and enlargement of the surrounding tissues, most often due to local trauma and rupture of blood vessels

Hematuria: Blood in the urine

Hemoglobin: Oxygen-carrying pigment in red blood cells

Hemolysis: Breakdown or destruction of red blood cells with the resulting release of hemoglobin

Hemoptysis: Coughing up blood due to bleeding in any portion of the respiratory tract

Hemostasis: The stoppage of blood loss from a damaged blood vessel

Histamine: A neurotransmitter released by cells (often mast cells) in response to injury and during an allergic reaction, triggers the inflammatory response

Hormone: A chemical released by a cell with the ability to affect or regulate cells in other parts of the body

Humoral response: The portion of the immune system that is mediated by transformation of B cells into plasma cells producing antibodies; humoral refers to the non-cellular components of blood

Hutchinson's Triad: Three common clinical features of congenital syphilis: 1) Hutchinson's teeth with notched incisors and mulberry molars, 2) ocular keratitis, and 3) eighth cranial nerve deafness

Hypercalcemia: Abnormally high levels of calcium in the blood

Hyperchromatism: Intense deep blue coloration to cell nucleus

Hyperglycemia: Abnormally high levels of glucose in the blood

Hyperkeratosis: Thickening of the stratum corneum of the skin or superficial keratin layer of the mucous membranes, most commonly caused by chronic irritation

Hypermelanosis: Abnormal darkening of the skin or mucous membrane resulting from increased melanin production by normal melanocytes without an increase in the number of melanocytes

Hyperplasia: Increase in the size of an organ or tissue due to an increase in the number of cells

Hypersensitivity reaction: Excessive or inappropriate reaction to an allergen; an allergic reaction

Hypertelorism: Abnormal increase in distance between two organs or parts; example: ocular hypertelorism indicates wide spacing of the eyes

Hypertrophy: Increase in the size of an organ or tissue due to increase in the size of individual cells

Hypodontia: Partial congenital absence of teeth

Hypohidrotic: Decreased ability to sweat

Hypoxia: Decreased concentration or lack of oxygen within body tissues

I

Iatrogenic: Clinician-induced injury, occurs as a result of treatment; example: accidental trauma or laceration from a dental instrument

Icteric/Icterus: Jaundiced, yellowing of the skin and sclera of the eyes, etc.

Idiopathic: Term used when the cause of a disease is unknown

Immune system: A complex of organs involving the thymus, bone marrow, and lymphoid tissues that protects the body from foreign substances and pathogenic microorganisms

Immunodeficiency: Inability to produce a normal immune or inflammatory response

Immunoglobulins: Large glycoproteins secreted by plasma cells; function as antibodies

Immunomodulary: Refers to a class of drugs capable of modifying or regulating the immune response

Immunosuppressive: A substance that has the ability to lower the body's normal immune response; example: corticosteroid medications that suppress the inflammatory response

In situ: In its original place or position; example: squamous cell carcinoma-in-situ that remains within the surface epithelium and has not infiltrated or metastasized

Incidence: In epidemiology, the number of new cases of the disease during a designated period of time; example: the incidence of hepatitis B in the United States was 8,064 cases in 2002

Incisional biopsy: Surgical removal of part of a lesion to be used in establishing the diagnosis, most often used when the lesion is large and will require a more extensive procedure to totally remove it

Indigenous microflora: Microorganisms regularly found at any anatomical site; also known as the normal flora

Indolent: Slow-growing; causing few symptoms; example: prostate cancer tends to be an indolent disease in many cases and not discovered until autopsy

Indurated: Soft tissue that is abnormally firm due to influx of fibrous or cellular tissue elements or exudate; example: oral cancer tends to be indurated

Infarction: Obstruction of the blood supply to an organ or tissue typically by a thrombus or embolus resulting in local death of the tissue; example: myocardial infarction or heart attack

Infectious agent: An agent (microorganism) capable of producing infection

Infectious disease: A disease caused by microorganisms; may or may not be contagious

Infiltration: Permeation into adjacent normal structures or tissues

Injury: Damage, harm, or wounding

Inspection: The process of critically appraising a lesion or condition: involves examination, measurement, and comparing the findings with normal.

Insulin: A hormone produced in the pancreas by the islets of Langerhans that regulates glucose levels in the blood

Intermaxillary segment: Wedge of tissue formed by growth of the medial nasal processes, participates in formation of the primary palate

Intraosseous: Located within bone

Intrinsic: Caused by factors within the body or arising from internal causes; example: intrinsic (endogenous) bilirubin stain of teeth in a child with liver disease

Inversion: Occurs when a chromosome breaks and the part is reinserted in the wrong location

Ischemia: Temporary deficiency of blood in a body part due to obstruction or constriction of local blood vessels; example: angina pectoris is caused by ischemia of the heart muscle

K

Keloid: Exuberant proliferation of scar tissue resulting from excess collagen production during healing

Keratinaceous: Composed of, containing, or characterized by keratin

Keratin: An insoluble protein that makes up the uppermost layer of surface skin and some mucous membranes

Keratosis: Refers to rough raised areas of epithelium with extra keratin build-up

Ketoacidosis: A change in the pH of blood due to increased accumulation of ketone bodies in the blood from excess fat breakdown; seen in diabetes

Koplik's spots: Highly characteristic sign of early measles, small red spots with white centers on mucous membranes of cheeks and lips

L

Latent: Lying dormant or hidden; example: herpes simplex can lie dormant in nerve ganglia. Also a symptom-and lesion-free stage in syphilis

Lesion: Any pathologic change in an organ or tissue that alters normal form or function

Leukocytosis: Increase in circulating white blood cells (leukocytes) in the blood, due to additional release of these cells from the bone marrow

Leukopenia: Abnormal decrease in the number of circulating white blood cells

Leukoplakia: A white plaque that cannot be wiped off or attributed to a specific cause

Local recurrence: Reappearance of a tumor in a localized area close to the original or primary site

Lymphadenitis: Painful inflammation and swelling of the lymph nodes; commonly referred to as "swollen glands"; however, lymph nodes are not glands

Lymphadenopathy: Enlargement of the lymph nodes, usually as a result of disease; may or may not be painful

Lymphocytes: Small mononuclear, nongranular white blood cells that play a role in the body's immune response; B and T cells are two types

Lymphokines: Substances produced by T lymphocytes that have been activated by antigens; act upon other cells of the immune system, such as macrophages

Lysis: The disintegration or dissolution of cells

M

Macule: A flat, discolored, usually red or brown lesion that is not elevated above the normal adjacent surface

Maculopapular skin rash: A skin rash containing both macules and papules, characterized clinically by flat red discolored areas (macules) covered with small raised bumps (papules)

Malar: Pertaining to the malar, or cheek, bone

Malignant: A process that potentially threatens life by invading and destroying tissue, cancer; example: squamous cell carcinoma

Melanin: Protective brown pigment produced by melanocytes in epithelium

Metachronous: Identical tumors appearing at different times, multiple separate occurrences

Metaplasia: Reversible change from one mature cell type to another mature cell type

Metastasis: Spread of cancerous cells from site of origin to distant sites in the body

Microorganism: An organism that is microscopic in size such as a bacterium, virus, or protozoan

Microscope: An instrument containing a powerful lens that magnifies objects for viewing

Morbidity: The incidence or prevalence of disease in a population

Mortality: Fatal outcome, death

MSM: Men having sex with men

Mucositis: Inflammation of the mucous membranes; typically painful

Mucous patch: Elevated membrane-covered lesion found on mucosal surfaces, usually a feature of secondary syphilis

Mutation: Permanent damage to the DNA sequence that makes up a gene; damaged trait may be transmitted to subsequent generations

Myelogenous: Related to, produced by, or originating in the bone marrow; example: myelogenous leukemia

N

Nasopalatine duct: A canal between the oral and nasal cavities in the embryo

Necrosis: Death of cells and tissues, often the result of cells failing to adapt to changes in their environment

Neoplasm: Any swelling or collection of cells appearing as a mass or lump

Neoplasia: The formation of a new abnormal growth of tissue

Neoplastic: Relating to a neoplasm

Neural crest cells: Specialized cells from neuroectoderm in the embryo that migrate to distant sites to form portions of the endocrine system, connective tissues, and pigment cells

Neuralgia: Pain or burning along the course of a nerve or group of nerves caused by nerve irritation or damage

Neuritis: Inflammation of the peripheral nerve causing pain and loss of function

Neuropathy: A dysfunction or disturbance in the peripheral nervous system

Neurotropic: Tending to affect the nervous system preferentially; example: herpes simplex is a neurotropic virus

Neurotropism: Having an affinity for neural tissue

Neutropenia: A decrease in the number of circulating neutrophils

Nikolsky's sign: Phenomenon where gentle rubbing results in sloughing of surface epithelium; seen in vesiculobullous disorders of the skin and mucous membranes

Nodule: A solid mass that is greater than 5 mm in diameter

Nonodontogenic: Arising from cells or tissue unrelated to tooth development

Nosocomial infection: A disease originating in a health-care setting; an infection acquired in a hospital, nursing home, or other health-care facility

O

Obturator: A prosthetic device used to close an opening, often due to a developmental defect or disease process

Odontogenic: Arising from cells or tissues related to tooth development

Odontogenic cysts: Cysts arising from remnants of epithelium associated with tooth development

Oncogene: Altered gene capable of causing a neoplasm

Oncogenic: Agent with potential to cause development of a cancer or neoplasm

Operculum: Flap or hood of fibrotic tissue around or over an erupting tooth, most often third molars

Opportunistic infection: An infection by a microorganism that normally does not cause disease; however, due to an impaired immune system infection occurs

Oral pathologist: One who studies the characteristics, causes, and effects of diseases of the mouth, oral cavity, and associated structures

Oropharyngeal: Relating to the mouth and pharynx

Osteoradionecrosis: Death of bone following irradiation; radiation exposure may be therapeutic or accidental; bone death results from destruction of the blood supply within bone

P

Palliative: Treatment provided to relieve the symptoms of the disease rather than cure it

Palpation: A procedure in which the sense of touch is used to gather data for diagnosis

Palsy: An involuntary uncontrollable tremor or paralysis

Papillary: Having a finger-like protuberances or projections

Papule: A circumscribed, solid, elevated lesion; less than 5 mm

Parulis: Mass of granulation tissue on the alveolar ridge or gingiva, contains the opening through which an abscess drains

Passive immunity: Short-term immunity resulting from administration of antibodies produced by another person or animal

Pathogenic: Capable of causing or producing disease

Pathogenicity: The ability of microorganisms to produce pathological changes or disease

Pathognomonic: Relating to a sign or symptom unique to a particular disease, which distinguishes it from other diseases; example: blistering skin lesions following a dermatome are pathognomonic of herpes zoster (shingles)

Pathologic atrophy: Atrophy due to a physical process, such as disuse of muscles, reversible

Pathologic calcification: Abnormal deposition of calcium in tissues other than bones and teeth

Pathologic hyperplasia: Increase in the size of an organ or tissue due to an increase in the number of cells due to underlying disease

Pathologic hypertrophy: Increase in the size of an organ or tissue due to an increase in the size of individual cells, due to underlying disease

Pathophysiology: The study of physiologic processes that are altered in the presence of disease or injury

Pedunculated: A raised mass with a stalk

Penetrance: The proportion of individuals who carry a particular variant of a gene for a trait; complete penetrance refers to the trait being present in all individuals who carry the allele; incomplete penetrance refers to the trait being expressed in only a portion of the individuals carrying the allele

Percussion: The act of tapping on a surface to determine the condition of the underlying structure; example: percussion is used on teeth to help identify which tooth is most sensitive and has associated inflammation of the periodontium

Peripheral: Developing outside the bone within the overlying soft tissues

Petechiae: Small red or purple pinpoint spots, due to hemorrhage of capillaries

Pharyngotonsillitis: Concurrent inflammation of the pharynx and tonsils

Phenotype: Observable physical characteristics of an individual that are determined by the individual's genetic makeup (genotype) and effects of environmental factors

Physiologic atrophy: Irreversible atrophy, often due to aging of an organ or body part

Physiologic hyperplasia: An increase in the size of an organ or tissue due to an increase in the number of cells in response to normal metabolic function

Physiologic hypertrophy: An increase in the size of an organ or tissue due to an increase in the size of individual cells in response to normal metabolic function

Plasma cells: Antibody-producing cells found in lymphoid tissue derived from B lymphocytes

Pleomorphism: Wide range in cell size and shape (cells are dissimilar to the size and shape of normal cells; *pleo* = many; *morphism* = shape)

Polydipsia: Excessive thirst

Polyphagia: Excessive hunger

Polyuria: Excessive urination

Prevalence: The total number of cases of a disease within a population; example: the prevalence of hepatitis B in the United States is approximately 730,000 people

Primary tumor: The original neoplasm from which metastatic disease originated

Protozoa: Single-celled microscopic microorganisms, many of which are motile; example: amoebas

Pruritic: Severe itching

Pseudocyst: A cavity that is not lined by epithelium; example: traumatic bone cavity, formerly called traumatic bone cyst

Purpura: Discoloration of the skin comprised of purple spots caused by hemorrhage into surface skin or mucosa; generally greater than 3 mm in diameter

Pus: A thick creamy yellow-or green-colored fluid produced by infected tissue, composed of dead white blood cells (primarily neutrophils), bacteria, and tissue debris

R

Radiation therapy: Treatment of disease using ionizing x-rays or other forms of radiation to destroy or shrink a lesion

Radiosensitive: Vulnerable to the effects of ionizing radiation; example: white blood cells are radiosensitive

RBCs: Abbreviation for red blood cells, also known as erythrocytes

Recessive: A gene that produces its characteristics when the two inherited alleles are identical, in the homozygous state

Remission: A period of time during which symptoms of disease disappear or are greatly reduced

Resectable: Capable of being excised

Resection: Surgical excision

Resorption: Loss or reduction of volume of a tissue by physiologic or pathologic means; example: root resorption occurs prior to exfoliation of the primary teeth

Rests of Malassez: Epithelial remnants of Hertwig's root sheath that remain within the periodontal ligament space

Rests of Serres: Epithelial remnants of the dental lamina

Reticular: Resembling a network; a net-like form; intricate

Risk factor: A characteristic statistically associated with, but not causally related to, increase of disease; example: smoking is a risk factor for heart disease

S

Saliva substitutes: Sprays and rinses that temporarily replace lost saliva and provide relief from the physical discomfort of dry mouth

Sarcoma: A cancer arising from nonepithelial or connective tissues, such as muscle or bone

Sclera: The white external covering of the eyeball; known as "the white of the eye"

Sclerotic: Becoming rigid; losing the ability to adapt; hardening; example: atherosclerosis

Self-limiting: A disease that runs a limited or defined course; self-limiting diseases tend to end without treatment; example: the common cold

Septicemia: Presence of microorganisms or toxins within the blood; blood poisoning

Serologic: Pertaining to the study of blood serum

Sessile: Exophytic lesion in which the base is broader than the mass; example: the common wart

Sex chromosomes: Chromosomes that carry the genes that transmit sex-linked traits and conditions; can be X or Y

Sialadenosis: Enlargement of the salivary glands often seen in alcoholism and malnutrition

Sialogogue: A drug that increases the flow of saliva

Sign: Any objective evidence of a disease; example: radiolucency is a sign of apical tooth pathology in the jaws

Sinus tract: Communication between a pathologic space and an anatomic body cavity or the skin

Sinusitis: Inflammation of the nasal and/or paranasal sinuses

Sporadic: A disease that occurs as single and scattered cases, which are usually self-limiting and acute

Sputum: A mixture of mucous and saliva expelled by coughing or clearing the throat

Staging: Describes the extent to which cancer has spread in a patient's body

Stasis: Stoppage of the flow of a body fluid

Stem cell transplant: A cancer treatment that involves removal of stem cells from a donor for placement into a new patient; the stem cells migrate to the bone marrow of the recipient where they replace the diseased marrow; stem cells are "blank" cells capable of developing (differentiating) into many different types of cells

Stomatitis: Inflammation occurring in the mouth (stoma)

Symptom: Any evidence of disease such as altered function or sensation; experienced by the patient (subjective); examples are the sensations of itching, burning, numbness, or dizziness

Synchronous: Two or more diseases or lesions occurring at the same time

Syndactyly: Completely or partially fused fingers or toes, as in web-footed animals

Syndrome: A group of symptoms or signs linked by a common pathologic history; example: Down syndrome

Systemic pathology: The branch of pathology that studies disease by organ system

T

Tachycardia: Abnormally rapid heartbeat, generally exceeding 100 beats per minute

Telangiectasias: Permanent dilation of pre-existing small blood vessels creating focal red lesions

Teratogen: An agent or factor that adversely affects the normal development of the embryo or fetus; examples: chemicals, drugs, radiation, microorganisms

Teratology: The study of abnormalities of physiologic development, both before and after birth

Thrombocytopenia: Abnormally decreased number of platelets in circulating blood

Thrombus: A blood clot formed along the wall of a blood vessel that may be of sufficient size to obstruct blood flow

Thyroglossal duct: Embryologic structure forming the connection between the foramen cecum in the tongue to the thyroid gland in the neck; marks the path of descent for the thyroid gland

Tonsils: Generally refers to organized lymphoid tissue located in the back of the throat on either side of the oropharynx: palatine tonsils

Torus: (Pl. Tori) Convex semicircular structure composed of an excessive growth of normal bone

Translocation: A chromosome abnormality caused by two different chromosomes exchanging portions of genetic material

Trismus: An inability to open the mouth completely due to spasm or weakness of the muscles of mastication

Tumor: Literally a swelling; an abnormal growth of tissue, malignant or benign

U

Ubiquitous: Present or appearing everywhere; example: flu viruses are ubiquitous

Ulcer: The loss of surface epithelium from skin or mucous membranes, with exposure of the underlying connective tissue; usually covered by a fibrinopurulent membrane

V

Vaccine: An agent that produces active immunity to induce antibody formation and kill microbes; example: human papilloma virus (HPV) vaccine to prevent cervical cancer

Variable expressivity: Variations of phenotype among individuals carrying a particular genotype: varying range of signs and symptoms in different people with the same genetic condition

Vector: A carrier (person, animal, or insect) that transmits an infective agent from one animal to another; example: the mosquito is a vector for West Nile virus infection and malaria

Venereal: Transmitted by sexual intercourse; example: syphilis

Verrucous: Thick and wart-like; on the skin it can mean scaly; example: verruca vulgaris

Virulence: The power of a microorganism to produce disease versus the capacity of the individual to overcome the resistance of the microorganism

Virus: A noncellular infective agent too small to be seen by light microscopy, composed of a nucleic acid molecule with a protein coat; can only replicate within living cells

Viscosity: Thickened, condition or property of resistance to flow of a fluid, semifluid

W

WBCs: Abbreviation for white blood cells, also known as leukocytes

X

Xerophthalmia: Dry eyes caused by diminished or absent tear production

Xerostomia: Dry mouth caused by diminished or absent salivary flow

X-linked recessive disorders: Genetic diseases caused by a mutation on the X chromosome; males are more frequently affected than females

Z

Zoonotic infection: A disease that normally occurs in animals, but can infect humans; example: rabies

Index